Williams Obstetrics

22nd Edition Study Guide

Susan M. Cox, MD

Associate Dean for Professional Education
Gillette Professor of Obstetrics and Gynecology
Director of Maternal-Fetal Medicine Fellowship Program
The University of Texas Southwestern Medical Center
Dallas, Texas

Claudia L. Werner, MD

Associate Professor
Department of Obstetrics and Gynecology
The University of Texas Southwestern Medical Center
Dallas, Texas

Barbara L. Hoffman

Assistant Professor
Department of Obstetrics and Gynecology
The University of Texas Southwestern Medical Center
Dallas, Texas

F. Gary Cunningham, MD

Professor and Chairman
Department of Obstetrics and Gynecology
Beatrice & Miguel Elias Distinguished Chair in Obstetrics &
* Gynecology*
The University of Texas Southwestern Medical Center at Dallas
Chief of Obstetrics and Gynecology
Parkland Memorial Hospital
Dallas, Texas

D1440271

McGRAW-HILL
Medical Publishing Division

New York   Chicago   San Francisco   Lisbon   London   Madrid   Mexico City
Milan   New Delhi   San Juan   Seoul   Singapore   Sydney   Toronto

Williams Obstetrics, Twenty Second Edition Study Guide

1234567890 QPD/QPD 098765

ISBN: 0-07-142782-1

This book was set in Garamond by TechBooks.
The editors were Andrea Seils, Karen G. Edmonson, and Patrick Carr.
The production supervisor was Richard Ruzycka.
The indexer was Victoria Boyle.
Quebecor World Dubuque was printer and binder.

This book is printed on acid-free paper.

We lovingly dedicate this study guide to our mothers:

Joyce L. Cox
Joan Marie Hoffman
Margot R. Werner
Frances May Outland

Thank you for giving us the guidance and freedom to find our own answers
to life's many multiple choice questions.

Contents

Preface

This *Williams Obstetrics 22nd Edition Study Guide* is designed to assess comprehension and retention of materials covered in the 22nd edition of *Williams Obstetrics*.

The questions for each section are based on the key points from each chapter and are in the same order as the text. There are a total of 2674 questions from the 59 chapters. The questions are in multiple choice format with one single best answer. It is suggested that the user first read the question and think of the answer prior to choosing the correct answer from the four choices given. The questions are followed by a section that contains the answers and the page numbers in the textbook where answers can be found.

We hope that the simplified format used in this study guide will make the task of assimilating the information from the 22nd edition of *Williams Obstetrics* less formidable.

Susan M. Cox, MD
Claudia L. Werner, MD
Barbara L. Hoffman, MD
F. Gary Cunningham, MD

Williams
Obstetrics

Study Guide

1

Obstetrics in Broad Perspective

1–1. What year was the Bureau of the Census established?

    a. 1858
    b. 1902
    c. 1928
    d. 1952

1–2. At present, what agency coordinates the 57 registration centers that collect vital statistics in the United States?

    a. Bureau of the Census
    b. National Center for Health Statistics (part of the CDC)
    c. National Institutes of Health
    d. Vital Statistics Bureau

1–3. Which of the following time periods corresponds to the perinatal period?

    a. 20 weeks gestation to 4 weeks postpartum
    b. 22 weeks gestation to 2 weeks postpartum
    c. 34 weeks gestation to 3 months postpartum
    d. 38 weeks gestation to 1 year postpartum

1–4. The term "birth" usually refers to fetuses born weighing at least what amount?

    a. 250 g
    b. 500 g
    c. 1000 g
    d. 1500 g

1–5. Which of the following is defined as the number of livebirths per 1000 population?

    a. fertility rate
    b. birth rate
    c. perinatal birth rate
    d. delivery rate

1–6. Of the following, what is the number of deaths per 1000 births occurring during the first 28 days of life?

    a. stillbirth rate
    b. fetal death rate
    c. perinatal mortality rate
    d. neonatal mortality rate

1–7. The perinatal mortality rate (per 1000 total births) is calculated by adding the number of neonatal deaths to which of the following?

    a. number of stillbirths
    b. number of infant deaths
    c. spontaneous abortions
    d. all of the above

1–8. An infant death is one that takes place at a time between birth and what age?

    a. 3 months
    b. 6 months
    c. 12 months
    d. 24 months

1–9. How is low birthweight defined for the purpose of vital statistics?

    a. <1000 g
    b. <1500 g
    c. <2000 g
    d. <2500 g

1–10. A birth is defined as *preterm* when it is below which gestational age?

    a. 29 weeks
    b. 33 weeks
    c. 35 weeks
    d. 37 weeks

1–11. How is a neonate classified that is born between 260 and 294 days of gestation?

    a. preterm
    b. term
    c. postterm
    d. postmature

1–12. How would a maternal death secondary to mitral stenosis be classified?

    a. direct maternal death
    b. indirect maternal death
    c. nonmaternal death
    d. nonobstetrical death

1–13. Currently, American women on average are pregnant how many times over their lifetimes?

    a. 1.6
    b. 2.5
    c. 3.2
    d. 4.8

1–14. Approximately what percentage of pregnancies in the United States are wanted or planned?

    a. 25
    b. 50
    c. 75
    d. 95

1–15. What is the average number of livebirths per woman in the United States?

    a. 1
    b. 2
    c. 3
    d. 4

1–16. Approximately what percentage of pregnancies in the United States result in livebirths?

    a. 50
    b. 60
    c. 70
    d. 90

1–17. Approximately what percentage of pregnancies in the United States end by induced termination?

    a. 5
    b. 10
    c. 15
    d. 20

1–18. Approximately what percentage of pregnancies in the United States end as spontaneous abortions?

    a. 5
    b. 10
    c. 15
    d. 20

1–19. What is the most common cause of nondelivery-related hospitalization during pregnancy?

    a. preterm labor
    b. preeclampsia
    c. gestational diabetes
    d. pyelonephritis

1–20. What percentage of infant deaths involve low birthweight neonates?

    a. 25
    b. 33
    c. 50
    d. 66

1–21. Although thought to be an underestimation, approximately how many maternal deaths in the United States in 2002 were identified by vital statistics?

    a. 336
    b. 3360
    c. 33,600
    d. 336,000

1–22. Between 1900 and the 1980s, the maternal mortality rate decreased by what percentage?

    a. 65
    b. 75
    c. 85
    d. 99

1–23. Which of the following is NOT among the top three causes of pregnancy-related death?

    a. cardiomyopathy
    b. embolism
    c. hemorrhage
    d. hypertensive disorders

1–24. At the beginning of the 1900s, what proportion of women giving birth died of pregnancy-related complications?

    a. 1 in 10
    b. 1 in 50
    c. 1 in 100
    d. 1 in 1000

1–25. What is the maternal mortality rate per 100,000 livebirths in the United States as of 1982?

    a. 2
    b. 8
    c. 12
    d. 28

1–26. In 2002, what percentage of births in the United States were by cesarean delivery?

    a. 6
    b. 10
    c. 26
    d. 36

1–27. The rise in the cesarean delivery rate is related to which of the following?

    a. breech presentation management
    b. dystocia increasing
    c. vaginal birth after cesarean delivery attempted less often
    d. all of the above

1–28. At present, what percentage of U.S. resident physicians training in obstetrics and gynecology are women?

    a. 30
    b. 50

    c. 70
    d. 90

1–29. On average, how many times is an obstetrician sued for malpractice?

    a. <1
    b. 1
    c. 1.5
    d. 2.5

1–30. What percentage of medically uninsured in the United States belong to working families?

    a. 20
    b. 40
    c. 60
    d. 80

1–31. Despite a 23 to 4 vote by a committee of experts to make *Plan B* emergency contraception available without a prescription, application for this status was denied primarily because of

    a. political opposition.
    b. religious group opposition.
    c. widespread public opposition.
    d. pharmacist opposition.

2

Maternal Anatomy

2–1. The labia majora are homologous with which of the following male structures?

    a. glans penis

    b. scrotum

    c. gubernaculum testis

    d. corpora cavernosa

2–2. The clitoris is homologous with which of the following male structures?

    a. penis

    b. scrotum

    c. gubernaculum testis

    d. corpora cavernosa

2–3. What is the principal erogenous organ or area in women?

    a. vagina

    b. clitoris

    c. labia minora

    d. G-spot

2–4. The prepuce of the clitoris is formed from tissues of which of the following?

    a. urethra

    b. mons pubis

    c. labia minora

    d. labia majora

2–5. The entire clitoral length rarely exceeds which of the following?

    a. 0.5 cm

    b. 1 cm

    c. 2 cm

    d. 3 cm

2–6. From which embryonic structure does the vestibule arise?

    a. genital ridge

    b. urogenital sinus

    c. müllerian ducts

    d. mesonephric ducts

2–7. All of the following typically open onto the vestibule EXCEPT

    a. urethra

    b. Skene ducts

    c. Bartholin ducts

    d. müllerian ducts

2–8. Which of the following are characteristics of the hymen?

    a. richly innervated

    b. contains sebaceous glands

    c. contains muscular elements

    d. covered by stratified squamous epithelial

2–9. Your patient brings her 14-year-old daughter for examination with concerns that her daughter is sexually active. The hymen easily admits an examining finger and has a tear inferiorly. Based on your physical findings, you advise your patient which of the following?

    a. her daughter has been sexually active

    b. her daughter has been sexually assaulted

    c. these same findings may be seen with tampon use

    d. a virginal hymenal opening should be 0.5 cm in diameter or less

2–10. From which embryonic structure does the upper vagina arise?

a. genital ridge
b. urogenital sinus
c. müllerian ducts
d. mesonephric ducts

2–11. From which embryonic structure does the lower vagina arise?

a. genital ridge
b. urogenital sinus
c. müllerian ducts
d. mesonephric ducts

2–12. A victim of sexual assault presents to your emergency room. A 3-cm, deep, penetrating laceration is found in the upper posterior one fourth of her vagina. Anatomically, the most likely structure injured includes which of the following?

a. bladder
b. rectum
c. anus
d. any structure in the cul-de-sac of Douglas

2–13. The vagina is lined most with what type of epithelium?

a. cuboidal epithelium
b. glandular epithelium
c. cornified squamous epithelium
d. noncornified squamous epithelium

2–14. Which of the following is the predominant type of bacteria in the vagina during pregnancy?

a. *Lactobacillus* sp.
b. *Peptostreptococcus* sp.
c. *Listeria monocytogenes*
d. *Streptococcus agalactiae*

2–15. You find a locally invasive vaginal cancer in the lower third of your patient's vagina. Based on anatomical lymphatic drainage patterns, which of the following lymph nodes would be primarily involved?

a. aortic
b. inguinal
c. hypogastric
d. internal iliac

2–16. Significant physical support of the perineum comes from diaphragms which include all of the following muscles EXCEPT

a. coccygeus
b. iliococcygeus
c. ischiocavernosus
d. deep transverse perineal

2–17. Which part of the uterus becomes the lower uterine segment during pregnancy?

a. cervix
b. cornua
c. corpus
d. isthmus

2–18. During postpartum surgery for sterilization, you grasp a tubular structure for ligation through a small infraumbilical incision. Correct anatomical information regarding the round ligaments that may assist you include which of the following?

a. extend to the pelvic sidewalls
b. are not covered by peritoneum
c. lie superior to the fallopian tubes
d. originate from the posterior uterine surface

2–19. Your patient presents for physical examination. Findings that indicate she may have previously given birth vaginally include which of the following?

a. closely apposed labia majora
b. cervix length equaling corporal length
c. labia minora projecting past the labia majora
d. small, smooth-bordered oval-shaped external cervical os

2–20. Approximately what percentage of the normal cervix is composed of muscle?

a. <1
b. 10
c. 25
d. 50

2–21. Uterine enlargement in pregnancy is due to which myometrial process?

a. hypertrophy
b. hyperplasia
c. decidualization
d. collagen dissociation

2–22. The infundibulopelvic ligament is contiguous with which of the following structures?

a. broad ligament
b. lateral uterine wall
c. uterosacral ligament
d. supravaginal portion of the cervix

2–23. Ovarian vessels are found in which of the following ligaments?

a. broad
b. round
c. uterosacral
d. infundibulopelvic

2–24. The thick medial portion on the broad ligament which is firmly connected to the supravaginal portion of the cervix is given what name?

a. round ligament
b. uterosacral ligament
c. Mackenrodt ligament
d. infundibulopelvic ligament

2–25. The uterine artery is a main branch of which of the following arteries?

a. aorta
b. internal iliac artery
c. external iliac artery
d. common iliac artery

2–26. At which of the following locations does the uterine artery most commonly cross over the ureter?

a. 1 cm lateral to the cervix
b. 2 cm lateral to the cervix
c. 3.5 cm lateral to the cervix
d. 4.5 cm lateral to the cervix

2–27. The ovarian artery is a main branch of which of the following arteries?

a. aorta
b. internal iliac artery
c. external iliac artery
d. common iliac artery

2–28. The right ovarian vein empties into which of the following veins?

a. vena cava
b. renal vein
c. internal iliac vein
d. external iliac vein

2–29. Lymphatic drainage from the cervix empties mainly into which group of nodes?

a. iliac
b. inguinal
c. hypogastric
d. internal iliac

2–30. Which of the following nerve roots provide sensory fibers from the uterus that are associated with the painful stimuli of uterine contractions?

a. T-9 and T-10
b. T-11 and T-12
c. L-1 and L-2
d. S-2, S-3, and S-4

2–31. Which of the following correctly describes the anatomical portions of the fallopian tube from most lateral to most medial?

a. interstitial, isthmus, ampulla, infundibulum
b. infundibulum, ampulla, interstitial, isthmus
c. interstitial, ampulla, infundibulum, isthmus
d. infundibulum, ampulla, isthmus, interstitial

2–32. The uterus and fallopian tubes arise embryologically from which of the following?

a. müllerian ducts
b. wolffian ducts
c. urogenital sinus
d. mesonephric ducts

2–33. Anatomical changes associated with physiological aging of the ovaries include all of the following EXCEPT

a. increased volume
b. diminution of oocyte number
c. corrugation of the tunica albuginea
d. marked atrophy of the cortical layer

2–34. What is the estimated number of oocytes present at puberty?

a. 50,000 to 100,000
b. 200,000 to 400,000
c. 750,000 to 1 million
d. 3 to 5 million

2–35. What is the mean number of oocytes in women over age 36?

a. 3400
b. 34,000
c. 340,000
d. 3,400,000

2–36. During an ultrasonographic examination of your patient for menstrual irregularity, you identify a unilocular, smooth-bordered, thin-walled, anechoic structure within the plane of the broad ligament. It is adjacent yet distinct from the right ovary. The most likely diagnosis is which of the following?

a. parovarian cyst
b. fallopian tube diverticula
c. tuboovarian abscess
d. pedunculated uterine myoma

2–37. Gartner duct cysts are remnants of which of the following?

a. mesonephric ducts
b. paramesonephric ducts
c. metanephric ducts
d. parametanephric ducts

2–38. Which of the following is NOT a part of the innominate bone?

   a. ilium
   b. ischium
   c. pubis
   d. sacrum

2–39. Shoulder dystocia occurs during the delivery of your patient. The McRoberts position takes advantage of laxity in which of the following?

   a. vaginal wall
   b. sacroiliac joint
   c. symphysis pubis
   d. perineal body

2–40. Which of the following serve as landmarks when assessing descent of the fetal head?

   a. ischial spines
   b. symphysis pubis
   c. ischial tuberosities
   d. sacral promontory

2–41. Which is the narrowest diameter of the pelvic inlet through which the fetal head must pass?

   a. true conjugate
   b. diagonal conjugate
   c. transverse diameter
   d. obstetrical conjugate

2–42. What does the obstetrical conjugate normally measure (at minimum)?

   a. 9 cm
   b. 10 cm
   c. 11 cm
   d. 12 cm

2–43. How is the obstetrical conjugate computed?

   a. add 1.5 cm to the diagonal conjugate
   b. subtract 1.5 cm from the diagonal conjugate
   c. average the diagonal and true conjugate
   d. add 1.5 cm to the true conjugate

2–44. What is the narrowest pelvic dimension that must be navigated by the fetal head?

   a. inferior strait
   b. obstetrical conjugate
   c. interspinous diameter
   d. transverse diameter of the pelvic inlet

2–45. Which of the following terms best describes the pelvis type with a small posterior sagittal diameter, convergent sidewalls, prominent ischial spines, and narrow pubic arch?

   a. android
   b. gynecoid

   c. anthropoid
   d. platypelloid

2–46. Which of the following terms best describes the pelvis type with a round inlet, straight sidewalls, nonprominent spines, and a wide pubic arch?

   a. android
   b. gynecoid
   c. anthropoid
   d. platypelloid

2–47. Which of the following terms best describes the pelvis type with convergent sidewalls and anteroposterior diameter greater than the transverse?

   a. android
   b. gynecoid
   c. anthropoid
   d. platypelloid

2–48. The type of pelvis within the Caldwell-Moloy classification is determined by which of the following?

   a. the posterior component of the pelvic inlet
   b. the anterior component of the pelvic inlet
   c. the posterior component of the midpelvis
   d. the anterior component of the midpelvis

2–49. The diagonal conjugate is calculated by measuring the distance between which of the following anatomical structures?

   a. coccyx and inner margin of symphysis pubis
   b. tip of sacrum and inner margin of symphysis pubis
   c. ischial spine and external margin of symphysis pubis
   d. sacral promontory and inferior point of symphysis pubis

2–50. Engagement occurs when the biparietal diameter of the fetal head descends below the level of which of the following?

   a. midpelvis
   b. pelvic inlet
   c. pelvic floor
   d. ischial tuberosities

2–51. During pelvic assessment, when physicians place a closed fist against their obstetrical patient's perineum, they are measuring all of the following EXCEPT

   a. the intertuberous diameter
   b. the transverse diameter of the pelvic outlet
   c. a clinically insignificant diameter of the pelvic outlet
   d. a diameter that should be greater than 8 cm in an adequate pelvis

3

Implantation, Embryogenesis, and Placental Development

3–1. For women below the age of 35, an average of how many ovarian follicles are depleted each month?

- **a.** 1
- **b.** 10
- **c.** 1000
- **d.** 100,000

3–2. Recruitment of resting follicles and the initial stages of their growth are orchestrated by which of the following?

- **a.** pituitary hormones
- **b.** hypothalamic gonadotropins
- **c.** locally produced growth factors
- **d.** unknown

3–3. Which of the following ovarian components exclusively express FSH receptors?

- **a.** endothelium
- **b.** stromal tissue
- **c.** granulosa cells
- **d.** theca lutein cells

3–4. The granulosa cell aromatase enzyme allows conversion of androstenedione to which of the following?

- **a.** estradiol
- **b.** progesterone
- **c.** 17-hydroxyprogesterone
- **d.** dehydroepiandrosterone

3–5. Granulosa cell aromatase activity is induced by which of the following?

- **a.** LH
- **b.** FSH

- **c.** inhibin B
- **d.** growth differentiation factor-10

3–6. Changing levels of which of the following affect selection of the dominant follicle during the late follicular phase?

- **a.** FSH levels
- **b.** estradiol levels
- **c.** inhibin B levels
- **d.** all of the above

3–7. LH levels typically peak approximately how many hours prior to ovulation?

- **a.** 12
- **b.** 24
- **c.** 48
- **d.** 72

3–8. Which of the following changes will maintain the corpus luteum?

- **a.** decreased LH
- **b.** increased FSH
- **c.** increased hCG
- **d.** decreased inhibin B

3–9. Which of the following is the most potent of the naturally occurring estrogens?

- **a.** estriol
- **b.** estrone
- **c.** estradiol
- **d.** ethinyl estradiol

3–10. Selective estrogen receptor modulators (SERMS) exploit which of the following qualities of the estrogen receptors ERα and ERβ?

  a. Estradiol binding differs greatly.
  b. ERβ levels are greatest during the secretory phase of the menstrual cycle.
  c. Each binds estrogens, other than estradiol, to a greater or lesser degree.
  d. ERα is a nuclear hormone receptor, whereas ERβ is cell-membrane bound.

3–11. Progesterone receptors exist in how many biologically distinct isoforms?

  a. 2
  b. 3
  c. 4
  d. 5

3–12. By which day of the endometrial cycle is restoration of the epithelial surface of the endometrium complete?

  a. 2
  b. 5
  c. 8
  d. 12

3–13. Using histological criteria to date endometrial development, which of the following is the earliest sign of ovulation?

  a. gland coiling
  b. stromal edema
  c. neovascularization
  d. glycogen accumulation

3–14. Sloughing of the endometrium during menstruation is thought to be triggered by which of the following?

  a. pressure necrosis from stromal edema
  b. vascular stasis from spiral artery coiling
  c. atrophy from cessation of stromal cell mitosis
  d. pressure necrosis from inspissated gland glycoproteins

3–15. Which of the following is thought to be a mediator of dysmenorrhea?

  a. interleukin-8
  b. enkephlinase
  c. prostaglandin $F_{2\alpha}$
  d. monocyte chemotactic factor-1

3–16. The decidua found directly beneath the site of blastocyst invasion is termed which of the following?

  a. vera
  b. basalis
  c. parietalis
  d. capsularis

3–17. The zone of fibrinoid degeneration known as the Nitabuch layer is found at the junction of which of the following?

  a. decidua parietalis and decidua vera
  b. decidua basalis and trophoblastic layer
  c. decidua capsularis and decidua parietalis
  d. decidua capsularis and trophoblastic layer

3–18. The prolactin found in amnionic fluid is produced by which of the following?

  a. decidua
  b. chorion
  c. amnion
  d. anterior pituitary of the fetus

3–19. The physiological role of the prolactin found in amnionic fluid is theorized to be which of the following?

  a. implantation angiogenesis
  b. amnionic fluid volume balance
  c. modulation of local immune function
  d. all of the above

3–20. The time window surrounding ovulation that allows for fertilization of an oocyte in humans is which of the following?

  a. 3 days
  b. 5 days
  c. 7 days
  d. 9 days

3–21. What is the solid ball of cells formed by 16 or more blastomeres?

  a. zygote
  b. morula
  c. embryo
  d. blastocyst

3–22. The morula leaves the fallopian tube and enters the uterine cavity after approximately what period of time postfertilization?

  a. 1 day
  b. 3 days
  c. 5 days
  d. 7 days

3–23. Which of the following is the stage at which cells destined to be either trophoblast or fetus first differentiate?

  a. zygote
  b. morula
  c. embryo
  d. blastocyst

3–24. The blastocyst typically implants into the endometrium how many days postfertilization?

    a. 4 to 5
    b. 6 to 7
    c. 8 to 9
    d. 10 to 11

3–25. The most common site for blastocyst implantation in humans involves which of the following uterine walls?

    a. upper anterior
    b. lower anterior
    c. upper posterior
    d. lower posterior

3–26. The process early in implantation that involves loose adherence of the blastocyst to the endometrium is called which of the following?

    a. apposition
    b. margination
    c. juxtaposition
    d. approximation

3–27. Characteristics of cytotrophoblasts include which of the following?

    a. active mitosis
    b. single nucleus
    c. distinct cell borders
    d. all of the above

3–28. True placental circulation is established approximately how many days postfertilization?

    a. 9
    b. 13
    c. 17
    d. 28

3–29. Villi in contact with the decidua basalis proliferate to form which of the following?

    a. chorion leave
    b. chorion basalis
    c. chorion capsularis
    d. chorion frondosum

3–30. At the end of which week of gestation are the amnion and chorion in intimate contact and no longer separated by the extracoelomic cavity?

    a. 6
    b. 9
    c. 12
    d. 15

3–31. Fetal fibronectin is a protein that can be measured to help determine risk for preterm labor. What is its role in placental physiology?

    a. activates matrix metalloproteinases
    b. digests endometrial extracellular matrix
    c. connects trophoblastic and decidual cells
    d. stimulates trophoblastic invasion of spiral - arteries

3–32. The average placental diameter at term approximates which of the following?

    a. 10 cm
    b. 20 cm
    c. 30 cm
    d. 40 cm

3–33. What is the average weight of a term placenta?

    a. 100 g
    b. 500 g
    c. 1000 g
    d. 1500 g

3–34. Which eponym is used for fetal macrophages found in the villous stroma?

    a. Kupffer
    b. Werner
    c. Hofbauer
    d. Langerhans

3–35. End-diastolic flow, which can be measured with Doppler velocimetry as an assessment tool of fetal well-being, develops within the umbilical arteries at what approximate week of gestation?

    a. 10
    b. 16
    c. 20
    d. 24

3–36. Blood flow into the intervillous space is regulated by which of the following?

    a. uterine contractions
    b. intrauterine pressure
    c. maternal arterial blood pressure
    d. all of the above

3–37. Passage of fetal cells into maternal circulation may be responsible for which of the following?

    a. scleroderma
    b. maternal thyroiditis
    c. D-antigen isoimmunization
    d. all of the above

3–38. What is the dominant type of leukocyte present at implantation and thought responsible in large part for the immunotolerance seen during pregnancy?

    a. elliptical macrophages
    b. round clear eosinophils
    c. small cystic monocytes
    d. large granular lymphocytes

3–39. Highly localized cytotrophoblastic expression of which of the following is likely to be a key immunological component of maternal–fetal immunotolerance?

    a. cytokines
    b. interleukins
    c. HLA-G
    d. rhesus antigen

3–40. Presence of which of the following is found in the amnion?

    a. neurons
    b. macrophages
    c. endothelial cells
    d. smooth muscle cells

3–41. Chemical contributions of the amnion include which of the following?

    a. fetal fibronectin
    b. prostaglandin E2
    c. corticotrophin-releasing hormone
    d. all of the above

3–42. Amnionic fluid reaches maximum volume at which of the following gestational weeks?

    a. 26
    b. 30
    c. 34
    d. 38

3–43. The most common vascular anomaly involving the umbilical cord is which of the following?

    a. arterial aneurysm
    b. single umbilical artery
    c. arteriovenous malformation
    d. persistent right umbilical vein

3–44. What is the average umbilical cord length in centimeters?

    a. 25
    b. 55
    c. 95
    d. 125

3–45. Which of the following umbilical cord characteristics is NOT designed to help prevent blood flow obstruction?

    a. false knots
    b. Wharton jelly
    c. cord vessel dextral spiraling
    d. cord vessel sinistral spiraling

3–46. HCG is structurally LEAST similar to which of the following hormones?

    a. LH
    b. TSH
    c. FSH
    d. ACTH

3–47. In comparing structurally related glycoproteins, the biologically distinct portion of the hCG molecule consists of which of the following?

    a. α-subunit
    b. β-subunit
    c. both subunits
    d. carbohydrate moieties

3–48. All of the genes coding for the hCG molecule are located on which of the following chromosomes?

    a. 1
    b. 9
    c. 19
    d. X

3–49. The maximum levels of hCG in maternal serum occur at approximately which week of pregnancy?

    a. 4
    b. 10
    c. 16
    d. 20

3–50. The hCG molecule is first detectable in maternal serum approximately how many days after the midcycle LH surge?

    a. 3
    b. 8
    c. 13
    d. 18

3–51. Which of the following abnormalities is associated with lower hCG levels compared with that of a normal singleton gestation at an equivalent gestational age?

    a. Down syndrome
    b. ectopic pregnancy
    c. complete hydatidiform mole
    d. D-antigen erythroblastosis fetalis

3–52. Functions of hCG include all EXCEPT which of the following?

    a. maintenance of corpus luteum function
    b. stimulation of the maternal thyroid gland
    c. promotion of sexual differentiation in the male fetus
    d. stimulation of estrogen production in female fetal ovaries

3–53. The hCG receptor is also the receptor for what other hormone?

　　a. LH
　　b. FSH
　　c. estriol
　　d. progesterone

3–54. Human placental lactogen (hPL) is structurally MOST similar to which of the following hormones?

　　a. LH
　　b. FSH
　　c. insulin
　　d. prolactin

3–55. The genes coding for hPL are located on which of the following chromosomes?

　　a. 1
　　b. 7
　　c. 17
　　d. X

3–56. Highest levels of hPL can be found in which of the following?

　　a. fetal urine
　　b. fetal serum
　　c. amnionic fluid
　　d. maternal serum

3–57. Actions of hPL are believed to include which of the following?

　　a. lipolysis
　　b. angiogenesis
　　c. insulin antagonism
　　d. all of the above

3–58. Which of the following placental hormones does NOT appear to have effects on myometrial contractility?

　　a. relaxin
　　b. progesterone
　　c. growth hormone-variant
　　d. parathyroid hormone-related protein

3–59. Which of the following placental hormones is a likely contributor to the insulin resistance of pregnancy?

　　a. relaxin
　　b. progesterone
　　c. growth hormone-variant
　　d. parathyroid hormone-related protein

3–60. Placental-derived GnRH has which of the following functions?

　　a. relaxes the myometrium
　　b. regulates trophoblastic hCG production

　　c. increases trophoblastic ACTH secretion
　　d. no known function

3–61. The probable role of placental inhibin involves suppression of which of the following?

　　a. FSH
　　b. TRH
　　c. CRH
　　d. GnRH

3–62. After which week of gestation (approximately) is the ovary no longer producing appreciable amounts of progesterone?

　　a. 3
　　b. 7
　　c. 11
　　d. 15

3–63. During early pregnancy, which of the following replaces the ovary as the main source of progesterone production?

　　a. amnion
　　b. chorion
　　c. trophoblast
　　d. myometrium

3–64. Which of the following is the main precursor of progesterone production in the placenta?

　　a. IDL
　　b. HDL
　　c. LDL
　　d. VLDL

3–65. What is the immediate precursor for estrogen biosynthesis in the human placenta?

　　a. acetate
　　b. cholesterol
　　c. progesterone
　　d. dehydroepiandrosterone sulfate

3–66. Placental conversion of dehydroepiandrosterone sulfate (DHEAS) to estrogen takes place in which of the following?

　　a. amnion
　　b. chorion
　　c. cytotrophoblast
　　d. syncytiotrophoblast

3–67. Quantitatively, what is the most important source of placental estrogen precursors in humans?

　　a. cytotrophoblast
　　b. fetal adrenal gland
　　c. syncytiotrophoblast
　　d. maternal adrenal gland

3–68. At term, which of the following fetal endocrine glands equals its eventual size in the adult human?

    a. testis
    b. ovary
    c. adrenal
    d. pituitary

3–69. The fetal zone component of the fetal adrenal gland undergoes which of the following developmental changes?

    a. involutes postnatally
    b. gives rise to the zona fasciculata
    c. becomes incorporated into its juxtaposed kidney
    d. none of the above

3–70. What is the major source of fetal plasma low-density lipoprotein (LDL)?

    a. fetal liver
    b. maternal transfer
    c. placental synthesis
    d. fetal adrenal gland

3–71. Which of the following fetal conditions is NOT associated with low maternal serum plasma levels of estrogen?

    a. anencephaly
    b. Down syndrome
    c. oligohydramnios
    d. congenital adrenal hypoplasia

3–72. Which of the following maternal situations is associated with low maternal serum plasma levels of estrogen?

    a. Addison disease
    b. glucocorticoid treatment
    c. beta-lipoprotein deficiency
    d. all of the above

3–73. What type of disorder is placental sulfatase deficiency?

    a. multifactorial
    b. X-linked recessive
    c. autosomal recessive
    d. autosomal dominant

4

Fetal Growth and Development

4–1. How many days does human pregnancy last, on average, counting from the first day of the last menstrual period?

    a. 260
    b. 270
    c. 280
    d. 290

4–2. Pregnancy is said to consist of 10 lunar months. How long is a real lunar month?

    a. 25 days
    b. 26 1/2 days

    c. 28 days
    d. 29 1/2 days

4–3. Given the date of a pregnant woman's last menstrual period (LMP), what method is used to quickly estimate the due date?

    a. subtract 7 days, subtract 3 months
    b. add 7 days, subtract 3 months
    c. add 7 days, add 3 months
    d. subtract 7 days, add 3 months

4–4. What are the products of conception called prior to implantation?

   a. embryo
   b. fetus
   c. ovum
   d. zygote

4–5. Which of the following best represents the embryonic period?

   a. fertilization to 6 weeks
   b. implantation to 6 weeks
   c. 3rd to 8th week after fertilization
   d. first 11 to 12 weeks of pregnancy

4–6. During which embryonic week is the chorionic sac 1 cm in diameter?

   a. 3
   b. 4
   c. 5
   d. 6

4–7. The embryonic heart is completely formed by how many weeks after fertilization?

   a. 4
   b. 6
   c. 10
   d. 12

4–8. What is the approximate crown-rump length of the fetus by the end of the 12th week of pregnancy?

   a. 1 to 2 cm
   b. 3 to 5 cm
   c. 6 to 7 cm
   d. 8 to 9 cm

4–9. In general, spontaneous fetal movements begin at what gestational age (weeks)?

   a. 6
   b. 12
   c. 16
   d. 20

4–10. Gender of the fetus is first evident by what gestational age (weeks)?

   a. 6
   b. 8
   c. 12
   d. 16

4–11. What is the approximate weight of the fetus at 24 gestational weeks?

   a. 210 g
   b. 420 g

   c. 630 g
   d. 840 g

4–12. At what gestational age (weeks) is the canalicular phase of lung development nearly complete, but terminal air sacs have not yet formed?

   a. 18
   b. 24
   c. 28
   d. 32

4–13. What is the approximate weight of the fetus at 28 gestational weeks?

   a. 750 g
   b. 890 g
   c. 1100 g
   d. 1500 g

4–14. By what gestational age (weeks) has the pupillary membrane disappeared?

   a. 10
   b. 20
   c. 24
   d. 28

4–15. What is the intact survival rate of an otherwise normal infant born at 28 weeks gestation?

   a. 25%
   b. 50%
   c. 75%
   d. 90%

4–16. What is the average weight of the fetus at 32 gestational weeks?

   a. 1200 g
   b. 1500 g
   c. 1800 g
   d. 2000 g

4–17. What is the average weight of the fetus at 36 gestational weeks?

   a. 2000 g
   b. 2500 g
   c. 3000 g
   d. 3500 g

4–18. What is the average crown-rump length and weight of a term fetus?

   a. 28 cm, 3000 g
   b. 32 cm, 3200 g
   c. 36 cm, 3400 g
   d. 40 cm, 3600 g

4-19. In the fetus or neonate, what are the two sutures between the posterior margin of the parietal bones and the upper margin of the occipital bone called?

    a. occipitalis
    b. sagittal
    c. lambdoid
    d. coronal

4-20. In the fetus or neonate, what are the two sutures between the frontal and parietal bones called?

    a. frontal
    b. sagittal
    c. lambdoid
    d. coronal

4-21. Which of the following diameters has the greatest transverse diameter?

    a. occipitofrontal
    b. biparietal
    c. occipitomental
    d. suboccipitobregmatic

4-22. The plane of which of the following diameters represents the greatest circumference of the head?

    a. occipitofrontal
    b. suboccipitobregmatic
    c. bitemporal
    d. biparietal

4-23. The plane of which of the following diameters represents the smallest circumference of the head?

    a. occipitofrontal
    b. suboccipitobregmatic
    c. bitemporal
    d. biparietal

4-24. What is the name of the process by which fetal skull bones shift during labor to accommodate the maternal bony pelvis?

    a. accommodation
    b. conformation
    c. craniosyntosis
    d. molding

4-25. What is the approximate uteroplacental blood flow near term?

    a. 100 to 200 mL/min
    b. 300 to 450 mL/min
    c. 700 to 900 mL/min
    d. 1200 to 1400 mL/min

4-26. What is the residual volume of the intervillous space at term?

    a. 140 mL
    b. 210 mL
    c. 280 mL
    d. 350 mL

4-27. Direct transfer of nutrients and oxygen from mother to fetus occurs primarily across which of the following interfaces?

    a. decidua capsularis
    b. fetal membranes
    c. syncytiotrophoblast
    d. yolk sac

4-28. What is the mechanism of transfer of anesthetic gases across the placenta?

    a. simple diffusion
    b. facilitated diffusion
    c. active transport
    d. pinocytosis

4-29. Which of the following is an example of a large high-molecular-weight substance that readily crosses the placenta?

    a. IgG
    b. thyrotropin
    c. insulin
    d. IgM

4-30. What is the mechanism by which IgG crosses the placenta?

    a. simple diffusion
    b. active diffusion
    c. specific trophoblast receptor-mediated
    d. blood flow limited

4-31. What is the PO_2 (mm Hg) of intervillous space blood?

    a. 10 to 20 mm Hg
    b. 30 to 35 mm Hg
    c. 65 to 75 mm Hg
    d. 90 to 95 mm Hg

4-32. What is the average oxygen saturation of intervillous space blood?

    a. 10 to 15%
    b. 25 to 35%
    c. 65 to 75%
    d. 90 to 95%

4-33. How is glucose transferred across the placenta?

    a. active transport
    b. simple diffusion
    c. facilitated diffusion (carrier-mediated)
    d. endocytosis

4–34. Of the following proteins involved in glucose transport, which are located in the syncytiotrophoblast plasma membrane?

    a. Glut-3
    b. HPL
    c. FGF-2
    d. IGF-1

4–35. After being concentrated in the syncytiotrophoblasts, how are amino acids transferred across the placenta?

    a. active transport
    b. diffusion
    c. phagocytosis
    d. endocytosis

4–36. How does IgG cross the placenta?

    a. active transport
    b. simple diffusion
    c. facilitated diffusion
    d. endocytosis

4–37. Which of the following proteins accounts for the low level of Cu^{2+} in cord blood?

    a. metallothionein-1
    b. insulin
    c. Glut-3
    d. parathyroid hormone-related protein (PTH-rP)

4–38. How do calcium and phosphorus cross the placenta?

    a. active transport
    b. simple diffusion
    c. facilitated diffusion
    d. endocytosis

4–39. At what gestational age (weeks) does the fetal kidney begin producing urine?

    a. 8
    b. 12
    c. 16
    d. 20

4–40. Which of the following factors found in amnionic fluid may play a significant role in fetal lung development?

    a. vitamin A
    b. cholecalciferol
    c. prolactin
    d. epidermal growth factors

4–41. Which of the following fetal vessels empties directly into the inferior vena cava?

    a. umbilical vein
    b. portal vein
    c. ductus venosus
    d. hepatic vein

4–42. Which of the following contains the most oxygenated blood in the fetus?

    a. superior vena cava
    b. blood deflected by the crista dividens into the left heart
    c. ductus arteriosus
    d. right ventricle

4–43. Which of the following structures represents the intra-abdominal remnants of the umbilical vein?

    a. umbilical ligaments
    b. ligamentum teres
    c. ligamentum venosus
    d. ligamentum portalis

4–44. Which of the following fetal structures is NOT a site of early hematopoiesis?

    a. yolk sac
    b. liver
    c. bone marrow
    d. kidney

4–45. What is the average fetal hemoglobin concentration at term?

    a. 10 g/dL
    b. 13 g/dL
    c. 15 g/dL
    d. 18 g/dL

4–46. Fetal erythropoiesis is primarily controlled by which hormone?

    a. fetal erythropoietin
    b. maternal erythropoietin
    c. fetal thyroxine
    d. maternal thyroxine

4–47. What is the approximate fetoplacental blood volume at term?

    a. 50 mL/kg
    b. 75 mL/kg
    c. 100 mL/kg
    d. 125 mL/kg

4–48. Which of the following hemoglobins contain a pair of alpha chains and a pair of beta chains?

    a. Gower-1
    b. hemoglobin F
    c. hemoglobin A
    d. hemoglobin A_2

4-49. What percentage of total hemoglobin at birth is hemoglobin F?

a. 50
b. 67
c. 75
d. 100

4-50. Which of the following vitamins is given prophylactically to infants soon after birth (especially in the breast-feeding newborn)?

a. vitamin K
b. vitamin A
c. vitamin C
d. vitamin D

4-51. Which of the following mutations is associated with thrombosis and infarctions in the fetus?

a. protein C deficiency
b. antithrombin III deficiency
c. factor V Leiden mutation
d. all of the above

4-52. The bulk of IgG acquired by the fetus from its mother occurs during which of the following time periods?

a. 10 to 14 weeks
b. 16 to 20 weeks
c. 24 to 28 weeks
d. last 4 weeks of pregnancy

4-53. Which of the following immunological factors ingested in colostrum provides protection against enteric infections?

a. IgG
b. IgM
c. IgA
d. IgE

4-54. At the time of birth, the spinal cord extends to which vertebra?

a. L_1
b. L_3
c. S_1
d. S_3

4-55. At what gestational age (weeks) are fetal respiratory movements first evident?

a. 8 to 10
b. 14 to 16
c. 18 to 20
d. 22 to 24

4-56. At what gestational age might the fetus hear sound in utero?

a. 12 weeks
b. 18 weeks
c. 24 weeks
d. 30 weeks

4-57. Which of the following can lead to intrauterine passage of meconium?

a. cord compression
b. hypoxia
c. normal bowel peristalsis
d. all of the above

4-58. What is the fate of most of the unconjugated bilirubin produced in the fetus?

a. transferred across the placenta to maternal circulation
b. excreted into and stored in fetal gut
c. conjugated by fetal liver
d. not well understood

4-59. At what gestational age (weeks) is insulin first detectable in fetal plasma?

a. 6
b. 12
c. 16
d. 20

4-60. From what fetal anlage does the bladder arise?

a. intermediate mesoderm
b. mesonephros
c. pronephros
d. urogenital sinus

4-61. What is the approximate daily urine output of a term fetus?

a. 100 mL
b. 350 mL
c. 650 mL
d. 1000 mL

4-62. Where is surfactant primarily produced in the fetal lung?

a. type II pneumocytes
b. alveoli macrophages
c. alveoli basement membrane cells
d. interstitial cells

4-63. Which of the following glycerophospholipids is the principal active component of surfactant?

a. phosphatidylinositol
b. phosphatidylethanolamine
c. phosphatidylglycerol
d. phosphatidylcholine

4–64. What is the major surfactant-associated protein (apoprotein)?

   a. SP-A
   b. SP-B
   c. SP-C
   d. SP-D

4–65. SP-A genes are located on chromosome 10 and are differentially regulated. Which of the following decreases SP-A$_2$ expression?

   a. TRH
   b. beta-mimetics
   c. dexamethasone
   d. antimicrobials

4–66. When can movements of the fetal chest wall first be detected by ultrasound?

   a. 11 weeks
   b. 18 weeks
   c. 24 weeks
   d. 26 weeks

4–67. Which of the following adenohypophysis cells produces growth hormone?

   a. corticotropes
   b. gonadotropes
   c. lactotropes
   d. somatotropes

4–68. At what gestational age (weeks) does the fetus begin to produce thyroxine?

   a. 7 to 8
   b. 10 to 12
   c. 14 to 16
   d. 22 to 24

4–69. When can corticotropin first be detected in the fetal pituitary?

   a. 7 weeks
   b. 11 weeks
   c. 15 weeks
   d. 19 weeks

4–70. The gene for testes development (TDF) or sex-determining region (SR4) is located on which chromosome?

   a. 4
   b. 11
   c. X
   d. Y

4–71. What is the most likely explanation for the 46,XX phenotypical male?

   a. production of müllerian-inhibiting substance by the ovary
   b. Y chromosome was lost from a 47,XXY fetus
   c. translocation of portions of the Y chromosome containing TDF to the X chromosome
   d. error in karyotyping

4–72. Which of the following statements is correct regarding müllerian-inhibiting substance?

   a. It is an endocrine hormone.
   b. It is produced by the Leydig cells.
   c. It acts locally near its site of formation.
   d. It appears after testosterone.

4–73. The virilizing effect of testosterone on the external genitalia in the male fetus is amplified by its local conversion to which of the following androgens?

   a. 7,21α-epiandrosterone
   b. androstenedione
   c. 5α-dihydrotestosterone
   d. DHEA

4–74. In newborns with either male external genitalia and bilateral cryptorchidism or completely ambiguous external genitalia, what diagnosis should be immediately ruled out?

   a. congenital adrenal hyperplasia
   b. 5α-reductase deficiency
   c. gonadal dysgenesis
   d. maternal androgen-secreting tumor

4–75. Which of the following is NOT characteristic of female pseudohermaphroditism?

   a. Müllerian-inhibiting substance is not produced.
   b. The fetus is exposed to excess androgen.
   c. The karyotype is 46,XX.
   d. A testis is present on one side.

4–76. Which of the following is NOT characteristic of male pseudohermaphroditism?

   a. Müllerian-inhibiting substance is produced.
   b. Androgenic representation is variable.
   c. Karyotype is 47,XXY.
   d. Testes or no gonads are present.

4–77. Which of the following is NOT characteristic of androgen insensitivity syndrome?

   a. female phenotype
   b. short, blind-ending vagina
   c. no uterus or fallopian tubes
   d. ovarian remnants on one side

4–78. Androgen insensitivity syndrome is characterized by increased testicular secretion of which hormone as compared with a normal male?

    a. androstenedione
    b. estradiol-17β
    c. müllerian-inhibiting factor
    d. testosterone

4–79. The gene encoding for androgen receptor has had over 100 mutations identified and is located on which chromosome?

    a. 6
    b. 16
    c. X
    d. Y

4–80. Which of the following is a feature of dysgenetic gonads?

    a. karyotype is variable, often abnormal
    b. müllerian-inhibiting substance is produced
    c. normal ovaries or testes may be present
    d. uterus is usually absent

5

Maternal Physiology

5–1. What is the average uterine weight at term?

    a. 200 g
    b. 450 g
    c. 780 g
    d. 1100 g

5–2. Uterine enlargement in pregnancy is primarily due to what process involving myocytes?

    a. hyperplasia (new myocyte production)
    b. hypertrophy and stretching
    c. atrophy with replacement by collagen
    d. hyperplasia and hypertrophy play equal roles

5–3. At what gestational age does the uterus become too large to lie totally within the pelvis?

    a. 10 weeks
    b. 12 weeks
    c. 14 weeks
    d. 16 weeks

5–4. For whom are the painless, irregular uterine contractions that begin early in gestation named?

    a. Braxton Hicks
    b. Casey Alexander

    c. Sheffield Yost
    d. Wendel Smith

5–5. What is the approximate uteroplacental blood flow at term?

    a. 100 mL/min
    b. 250 mL/min
    c. 550 mL/min
    d. 800 mL/min

5–6. Uteroplacental blood flow is apparently sensitive to the regulatory effects of which of the following?

    a. catecholamines
    b. estrogens
    c. nitric oxide
    d. all of the above

5–7. Which of the following is a factor responsible for the softening and cyanosis of the cervix in early pregnancy?

    a. increased vascularity
    b. decreased stromal edema
    c. decreased venous oxygen concentration
    d. atrophy of cervical glands

5–8. Surgical removal of the corpus luteum of pregnancy consistently results in spontaneous abortion if performed prior to what gestational age?

  a. 7 weeks
  b. 9 weeks
  c. 11 weeks
  d. 13 weeks

5–9. What is the major biological target of relaxin in assisting accommodation to pregnancy?

  a. cardiovascular system
  b. musculoskeletal system
  c. nervous system
  d. reproductive tract

5–10. What is the most likely complication resulting from a large pregnancy luteoma?

  a. ambiguous genitalia in a male fetus
  b. virilization of a pregnant woman
  c. virilization of a female fetus
  d. no fetal or maternal effects result

5–11. Which of the following conditions predisposes to the development of theca-lutein cysts?

  a. diabetes
  b. gestational trophoblastic disease
  c. multiple gestation
  d. all of the above

5–12. How does hyperreactio luteinalis differ from a pregnancy luteoma?

  a. cystic, not solid
  b. may cause maternal virilization
  c. has a different cellular pattern
  d. associated with low serum chorionic gonadotropin levels

5–13. In pregnancy, what is the Chadwick sign?

  a. bluish discoloration of the hyperemic vaginal mucosa
  b. lower uterine segment softening
  c. tenderness of breasts with enlargement
  d. uterus palpable above the pubic symphysis

5–14. What is pigmentation of the midline, anterior abdominal skin during pregnancy called?

  a. striae gravidarum
  b. linea nigra
  c. chloasma
  d. melasma

5–15. Which of the following skin conditions, common in pregnancy, is likely related to hyperestrogenemia?

  a. angiomas
  b. melasma gravidarum

  c. palmar erythema
  d. all of the above

5–16. What are hypertrophic sebaceous glands visible on the breast areolae in pregnancy called?

  a. Gatcliffe nodules
  b. glands of Montgomery
  c. mammary vesicles
  d. papillae of Li

5–17. What is the average weight gain during pregnancy?

  a. 5.5 kg
  b. 9.5 kg
  c. 12.5 kg
  d. 15.5 kg

5–18. What is the minimum amount of extra water that the average woman accrues during normal pregnancy?

  a. 1.0 L
  b. 3.5 L
  c. 6.5 L
  d. 8.0 L

5–19. Of the total 1000 g net gain of protein in normal pregnancy, how much is used by the fetus and placenta?

  a. 100 g
  b. 300 g
  c. 500 g
  d. 750 g

5–20. Which of the following characterizes carbohydrate metabolism in pregnancy relative to the nonpregnant state?

  a. hypoinsulinemia
  b. mild fasting hypoglycemia
  c. postprandial hypoglycemia
  d. fasting hyperglycemia

5–21. Plasma levels of which of the following continuously increases into the late third trimester of pregnancy?

  a. high-density lipoprotein (HDL) cholesterol
  b. low-density lipoprotein (LDL) cholesterol
  c. lipostatin
  d. none of the above

5–22. What happens to total maternal serum levels of calcium and magnesium in pregnancy?

  a. decrease
  b. increase throughout pregnancy
  c. increase during the third trimester
  d. remain unchanged

5–23. What is the average increase in maternal blood volume during pregnancy?

   a. 10%
   b. 25%
   c. 40%
   d. 75%

5–24. What is the average increase in the volume of circulating erythrocytes during pregnancy?

   a. 150 mL
   b. 250 mL
   c. 450 mL
   d. 850 mL

5–25. Despite increased red cell volume, hemoglobin and hematocrit decrease slightly during normal pregnancy. Below what hemoglobin concentration is a pregnant woman considered anemic?

   a. 9 g/dL
   b. 10 g/dL
   c. 11 g/dL
   d. 12 g/dL

5–26. Total body iron of an adult woman is 2.0 to 2.6 mg. What is the average iron store of a healthy young woman?

   a. 300 mg
   b. 500 mg
   c. 1000 mg
   d. 1500 mg

5–27. What are the iron requirements of normal pregnancy?

   a. 300 mg
   b. 500 mg
   c. 1 g
   d. 4 g

5–28. Approximately how much iron is required by the fetus and placenta during pregnancy?

   a. 150 mg
   b. 300 mg
   c. 500 mg
   d. 1 g

5–29. What is the average daily iron requirement during the second half of pregnancy?

   a. 1 to 2 mg/day
   b. 3 to 4 mg/day
   c. 6 to 7 mg/day
   d. 15 to 20 mg/day

5–30. What volume of blood is lost on average with a singleton vaginal delivery?

   a. 250 mL
   b. 500 mL
   c. 750 mL
   d. 1000 mL

5–31. What is the average blood loss with cesarean delivery of a singleton fetus?

   a. 500 mL
   b. 750 mL
   c. 1000 mL
   d. 1500 mL

5–32. Which of the following is NOT increased in pregnancy?

   a. cervical mucous IgA and IgG
   b. C-reactive protein
   c. leukocyte alkaline phosphate activity
   d. interferon

5–33. What is the average increase in fibrinogen concentration during pregnancy?

   a. 10%
   b. 25%
   c. 50%
   d. 75%

5–34. Which of the following coagulation factors is NOT increased during pregnancy?

   a. factor VII
   b. factor VIII
   c. factor IX
   d. factor XI

5–35. Which of the following inhibits coagulation?

   a. antithrombin
   b. protein C
   c. protein S
   d. all of the above

5–36. Factor V Leiden mutation causes resistance to which of the following?

   a. activated protein C
   b. free protein S
   c. antithrombin III
   d. none of the above

5–37. Increased maternal cardiac output is detectable as early as what gestational age?

   a. 5 weeks
   b. 10 weeks
   c. 20 weeks
   d. 15 weeks

5–38. What is the average increase in the resting pulse during pregnancy?

    a. 0 bpm
    b. 5 bpm
    c. 10 bpm
    d. 20 bpm

5–39. Which of the following does NOT contribute to enlargement of the cardiac silhouette noted in radiographs in normal pregnant women?

    a. displacement of the heart to the left and upward
    b. right atrial and ventricular dilatation
    c. increase in uterine size
    d. benign pericardial effusion of pregnancy

5–40. What is the only characteristic ECG finding in normal pregnancy?

    a. shortening of the QRS complex
    b. shortening of the ST segment
    c. slight depression of the ST segment
    d. slight left axis deviation

5–41. Which of the following changes in cardiac sounds is commonly found during pregnancy?

    a. muffling of the first heart sound
    b. wide splitting of the second heart sound
    c. systolic murmur
    d. diastolic murmur

5–42. In which of the following positions is cardiac output most increased in the pregnant patient?

    a. left lateral recumbent
    b. right lateral recumbent
    c. standing
    d. supine

5–43. Which of the following hemodynamic values remains unchanged in pregnancy?

    a. systemic vascular resistance
    b. pulmonary vascular resistance
    c. colloid osmotic pressure
    d. pulmonary capillary wedge pressure

5–44. Which of the following characterizes arterial blood pressure in normal pregnancy?

    a. nadir in midpregnancy, rising thereafter
    b. nadir in the first trimester, rising thereafter
    c. peaks in the first trimester, falling thereafter
    d. peaks in the second trimester, falling thereafter

5–45. Which of the following is decreased in normotensive pregnant women?

    a. renin activity and concentration
    b. angiotensinogen

    c. sensitivity to pressor effects of angiotensin II
    d. aldosterone

5–46. Alteration of the ratio of which of the following is thought to be important in the etiology of preeclampsia?

    a. atrial natriuretic peptide:B-type natriuretic peptides
    b. angiotensin:angiotensinogen
    c. progesterone:dihydroprogesterone
    d. prostacyclin:thromboxane

5–47. What is the average change in elevation of the diaphragm during normal pregnancy?

    a. 0 to 1 cm
    b. 2 cm
    c. 4 cm
    d. 6 cm

5–48. Which of the following is decreased in normal pregnancy?

    a. tidal volume
    b. minute ventilatory volume
    c. minute oxygen uptake
    d. functional residual capacity

5–49. What compensated acid–base state exists during normal pregnancy?

    a. metabolic acidosis
    b. metabolic alkalosis
    c. respiratory acidosis
    d. respiratory alkalosis

5–50. Which of the following is decreased during normal pregnancy?

    a. glomerular filtration rate
    b. renal plasma flow
    c. creatinine clearance
    d. serum concentration of urea nitrogen

5–51. Which of the following is commonly excreted in large amounts in the urine of a normal pregnant woman?

    a. amino acids
    b. glucose
    c. hemoglobin
    d. protein

5–52. At what level does compression of the ureters by the gravid uterus occur?

    a. bladder trigone
    b. pelvic brim
    c. sacrospinous ligaments
    d. ureterovesical junction

5–53. What alterations in bladder function characterize term pregnancy?

    a. increased bladder pressure
    b. reduced bladder capacity
    c. increased in functional urethral length
    d. all of the above

5–54. Approximately what percentage of women report new onset stress urinary incontinence during pregnancy?

    a. 10
    b. 20
    c. 50
    d. 80

5–55. Which of the following shows an increased incidence during pregnancy?

    a. epulis
    b. hemorrhoids
    c. pyrosis
    d. all of the above

5–56. With regard to liver function in pregnancy, which of the following shows the largest decrease compared with nonpregnant values?

    a. total serum alkaline phosphatase activity
    b. bilirubin levels
    c. plasma albumin concentration
    d. plasma globulin levels

5–57. Pruritus gravidarum is caused by elevated tissue levels of which of the following?

    a. bile salts
    b. bile acids
    c. bilirubin, direct
    d. bilirubin, indirect

5–58. Which of the following is NOT true of the maternal pituitary gland during pregnancy?

    a. Function is essential for the maintenance of pregnancy.
    b. Prolactin-secreting macroadenomas tend to enlarge.
    c. The pituitary gland enlarges by approximately 135%.
    d. Pituitary enlargement does not cause significant visual changes.

5–59. Although of uncertain significance, onset of labor coincides with peak concentrations of which of the following?

    a. cortisol
    b. placental growth hormone
    c. prolactin
    d. thyroxine

5–60. Which of the following has a positive effect on prolactin secretion?

    a. estrogen
    b. serotonin
    c. thyroid releasing hormone
    d. all of the above

5–61. Prolactin is essential to which of the following?

    a. initiation of labor
    b. lactation
    c. myometrial quiescence
    d. placental growth

5–62. Which of the following has a pronounced stimulatory effect on maternal thyroid function?

    a. chorionic gonadotropin
    b. placental growth hormone
    c. prolactin
    d. vasopressin

5–63. Which of the following does NOT increase as a result of maternal physiological hyperparathyroidism?

    a. bone resorption
    b. kidney reabsorption of calcium
    c. intestinal absorption of calcium
    d. serum phosphate levels

5–64. Which hormone opposes the action of parathyroid hormone, protecting skeletal calcium content?

    a. calcitonin
    b. gastrin
    c. thyroxine
    d. vasopressin

5–65. Which of the following is NOT known to increase the conversion of 25-hydrovitamin D_3 to 1,25-dihydrovitamin D_3?

    a. calcitonin
    b. low plasma calcium levels
    c. low plasma phosphate levels
    d. parathyroid hormone

5–66. Which of the following is increased during pregnancy?

    a. adrenal cortisol secretion
    b. cortisol half-life
    c. cortisol clearance rate
    d. none of the above

5–67. Which of the following shows decreased plasma levels during pregnancy?

    a. aldosterone
    b. dehydroepiandrostenedione sulfate
    c. deoxycorticosterone
    d. androstenedione

5–68. What is the level of testosterone in umbilical venous plasma likely to be in a pregnant woman with an androgen-secreting tumor?

  a. undetectable
  b. slightly lower than maternal serum levels
  c. equal to maternal serum levels
  d. higher than maternal serum levels

5–69. The increased joint mobility seen in pregnancy correlates with increased levels of which hormone?

  a. estradiol
  b. progesterone
  c. relaxin
  d. none of the above

5–70. Which of the following central nervous system and cognitive changes has been observed in late pregnancy?

  a. concentration deficit
  b. increased irritability
  c. memory decline
  d. sleep quality improvement

6

Parturition

6–1. What phase of parturition corresponds with the clinical stages of labor?

  a. phase 0
  b. phase 1
  c. phase 2
  d. phase 4

6–2. Myometrial contractions that do not result in labor are characterized by which of the following?

  a. low intensity
  b. brief duration
  c. unpredictable
  d. all of the above

6–3. Phase 1 of parturition begins how many weeks before labor?

  a. 1 to 2
  b. 2 to 4
  c. 6 to 8
  d. 8 to 10

6–4. Which of the following characterizes phase 1 of parturition?

  a. ↓ myometrial oxytocin receptors plus ↑ connexin-43
  b. ↓ myometrial oxytocin receptors plus ↓ connexin-43
  c. ↑ myometrial oxytocin receptors plus ↑ connexin-43
  d. ↑ myometrial oxytocin receptors plus ↓ connexin-43

6–5. What is the most plausible hypothesis for the cause of labor pain?

  a. myometrial hypoxia
  b. cervical stretching
  c. peritoneum stretching
  d. compression of nerve ganglia in the cervix

6–6. What is the average amnionic fluid pressure generated by uterine contractions?

  a. 1 mm Hg
  b. 10 mm Hg
  c. 40 mm Hg
  d. 100 mm Hg

6–7. What causes the pathological Bandl ring?

    a. thinning of the lower uterine segment
    b. thinning of the upper uterine segment
    c. thickening of the lower uterine segment
    d. a band of fibromuscular tissue at the level of the internal os

6–8. After complete cervical dilatation, what is the most important force in the expulsion of the fetus?

    a. amnionic fluid hydrostatic pressure
    b. uterine contractions
    c. maternal intra-abdominal pressure
    d. levator ani tensile strength

6–9. Which of the following is NOT a factor contributing to the progress of labor?

    a. intra-abdominal pressure
    b. cervical position
    c. resistance of maternal tissues
    d. uterine contractions

6–10. Which of the following is NOT considered a structural component of the cervix?

    a. smooth muscle
    b. collagen
    c. ground substance
    d. oncofibronectin

6–11. What is the direction of cervical effacement?

    a. above downward
    b. below upward
    c. lateral inward
    d. lateral outward

6–12. Which of the following is NOT a part of the urogenital diaphragm?

    a. deep transverse perineal muscle
    b. levator ani muscle
    c. coccygeus muscle
    d. ischiorectal fascia

6–13. What is the most important muscle of the pelvic floor?

    a. bulbocavernosus
    b. ischiocavernosus
    c. levator ani
    d. superficial transverse perineal muscle

6–14. What mechanism refers to peripheral separation of the placenta so that blood collects between the membranes and uterine wall and then escapes causing the maternal surface of the placenta to present upon delivery?

    a. Schultze
    b. Duncan
    c. Cunningham
    d. Pritchard

6–15. Which of the following is NOT associated with normal phase 3 of parturition?

    a. uterine contractions
    b. milk ejection
    c. restoration of fertility
    d. uterine eversion

6–16. What is an agent that helps bring about the "awakening" of the uterus in terms of its ability to contract?

    a. contracting agent
    b. uterotropin
    c. uterotonin
    d. growth factor

6–17. Which of the following are essential for myometrial contractions?

    a. tubulin–actin
    b. actin–myosin
    c. myosin–tubulin
    d. all of the above

6–18. Which of the following is essential for the generation of smooth muscle contractions?

    a. prostaglandins
    b. intracellular free calcium
    c. extracellular free calcium
    d. oxytocin

6–19. Which of the following activates the phosphorylation reaction responsible for myometrial contractions?

    a. free intracellular calcium
    b. adenosine triphosphatase
    c. adenosine triphosphatase hydrolysis
    d. myosin light chain kinase

6–20. What is the gap junction protein?

    a. actin
    b. myosin
    c. connexin
    d. laminin

6–21. Which of the following characterizes phase 0 of parturition?

    a. myometrial tranquility
    b. uterine awakening
    c. cervical effacement
    d. cervical dilatation

6–22. In most mammals, the implementation of phase 1 of parturition is due to which of the following?

   a. cortisol withdrawal
   b. progesterone withdrawal
   c. increase in oxytocin receptors
   d. inflammatory responses

6–23. Which of the following can block progesterone action?

   a. steroids
   b. RU-486
   c. aspirin
   d. β-blockers (i.e., propranolol)

6–24. During what weeks of gestation are plasma relaxin levels the highest?

   a. 4 to 6
   b. 8 to 12
   c. 16 to 20
   d. 24 to 28

6–25. Plasma levels of relaxin peak at which concentration?

   a. 0.1 ng/mL
   b. 1.0 ng/mL
   c. 10 ng/mL
   d. 100 ng/mL

6–26. Which of the following agents may be a uterorelaxant as well as a uterotonin?

   a. relaxin
   b. corticotropin-releasing hormone
   c. parathyroid hormone-related protein
   d. thromboxane

6–27. What is the possible action of parathyroid hormone-related protein (PTH-rP)?

   a. maintains uterine tranquility
   b. vasoconstricts
   c. increases oxytocin receptors
   d. stimulates cervical ripening

6–28. What is the initial and rate-limiting enzyme in prostaglandin inactivation?

   a. cyclooxygenase
   b. prostaglandin dehydrogenase
   c. enkephalinase
   d. oxytocinase

6–29. Which of the following enzymes catalyzes the degradation of endothelin-1?

   a. endothelinase
   b. oxytocinase

   c. placental sulfatase
   d. enkephalinase

6–30. Receptors for which of the following have decreased activity late in pregnancy?

   a. oxytocin
   b. progesterone
   c. glucocorticoid
   d. prostaglandin

6–31. Which of the following is NOT a primary regulator of oxytocin receptor expression?

   a. estradiol
   b. progesterone
   c. pitocin
   d. all of the above

6–32. Which of the following is NOT a uterotonin?

   a. endothelin-1
   b. prostaglandins
   c. oxytocin
   d. calcium

6–33. Where is oxytocin primarily synthesized?

   a. adrenal gland
   b. placenta
   c. posterior pituitary
   d. ovary

6–34. What is the carrier protein for oxytocin transport to the posterior pituitary?

   a. neurophysin
   b. relaxin
   c. binding globulin
   d. actin

6–35. Platelet-activating factor (PAF) has which of the following actions on myometrial cells?

   a. no effects
   b. decreases myosin light chain kinase levels
   c. decreases intracellular Ca^{2+}
   d. increases intracellular Ca^{2+}

6–36. What is the action of endothelin-1 on myometrial cells?

   a. decreases intracellular K^+
   b. decreases intracellular Ca^{2+}
   c. increases intracellular K^+
   d. increases intracellular Ca^{2+}

6–37. Which of the following tissues is avascular?

   a. amnion
   b. syncytium
   c. decidua
   d. placenta

6–38. What are the likely sources of the bioactive agent set in the amnionic fluid?

    a. chorion laeve; mononuclear cells
    b. chorion laeve; amnion
    c. decidual cells; mononuclear cells
    d. decidual cells; amnion

6–39. Which of the following matrix metalloproteinases (MMP) are found in higher concentrations in the amnionic fluid from pregnancies with preterm premature rupture of the membranes (PPROM)?

    a. MMP 2
    b. MMP 3
    c. MMP 9
    d. all of the above

6–40. What percentage of pregnancies delivered preterm are likely caused by intrauterine infection?

    a. 10
    b. 20
    c. 40
    d. 60

6–41. Which of the following bioactive agents is NOT a normal constituent of amnionic fluid?

    a. IL-1β
    b. IL-6
    c. macrophage colony stimulating factor (MCSF)
    d. prostaglandins

6–42. What is the cell source of interleukin-1β in amnionic fluid?

    a. amnion
    b. chorion laeve
    c. cytotrophoblast
    d. mononuclear phagocytes

6–43. Which receptor is activated by bacterial toxins to cause the inflammatory response?

    a. LPS receptor
    b. oxytocin receptor
    c. toll-like receptor
    d. IL-6 receptor

7

Preconceptional Counseling

7–1. Which of the following is an important goal of preconceptional counseling?

    a. prevent unintended pregnancy
    b. initiate preventive care measures
    c. identify genetic and obstetrical risk factors
    d. all of the above

7–2. What hypothesis states that the intrauterine fetal environment greatly impacts the health of an individual into adulthood?

    a. Amsterdam consensus
    b. Barker hypothesis
    c. Parkland proclamation
    d. Richmond statement

7–3. Approximately what percentage of pregnancies in the United States are unplanned and, therefore, at greater risk of preventable complications?

    a. 10
    b. 20
    c. 30
    d. 50

7–4. Preconceptional counseling of diabetics has been shown to have what effect on subsequent pregnancy?

    a. decreased fetal malformations
    b. lower maternal hemoglobin A_{1c} levels
    c. less fetal growth restriction and macrosomia
    d. all of the above

7–5. A 34-year-old insulin-dependent diabetic woman presents for prenatal care 8 weeks past missed menses. Her glycosylated hemoglobin level is 11%. What is the likelihood her fetus has a major anomaly?

    a. 1 in 100
    b. 1 in 50
    c. 1 in 10
    d. 1 in 4

7–6. Above what glycosylated hemoglobin level is there a marked rise in fetal anomalies?

    a. 4%
    b. 9%
    c. 14%
    d. 19%

7–7. What is the increased risk of fetal anomalies if the mother is epileptic, particularly if she takes anticonvulsants?

    a. 2×
    b. 5×
    c. 10×
    d. 20×

7–8. Which preconceptional intervention is recommended for epileptic women using antiseizure medications?

    a. control seizures with smaller doses of multiple medications
    b. discontinue antiseizure medications in all cases and treat periodically
    c. switch to the least teratogenic monotherapy at the lowest needed dose
    d. prescribe thiamine supplementation prior to conception

7–9. What periconceptional vitamin supplementation is very effective at reducing birth defects in the offspring of epileptic women who are using anticoagulants?

a. B_6
b. C
c. folic acid
d. thiamine

7–10. What is the leading cause of infant death?

a. birth defects
b. infections
c. preterm birth
d. sudden infant death syndrome

7–11. What is the incidence of neural-tube defects?

a. 1 to 2 per 10,000 live births
b. 8 per 10,000 live births
c. 1 to 2 per 1000 live births
d. 8 per 1000 live births

7–12. Some neural-tube defects are associated with a mutation in the gene for what enzyme?

a. acid phosphatase
b. folate decarboxylase
c. methylene tetrahydrofolate reductase
d. 5-alpha reductase

7–13. A woman who has a child with a neural-tube defect can reduce the rate of recurrence in subsequent pregnancy by taking preconceptional folic acid supplementation. What is the magnitude of this reduction?

a. 10%
b. 30%
c. 50%
d. 70%

7–14. Which of the following is true regarding preconceptional counseling of women with phenylketonuria (PKU)?

a. Only a fetus homozygous for PKU is at risk for birth defects.
b. The heterozygous fetus is at no increased risk.
c. Strict preconceptional dietary control decreases fetal risk.
d. Women with PKU should not reproduce under any circumstances.

7–15. The incidence of which genetic disorder has plummeted as a result of preconceptional screening and counseling?

a. phenylketonuria
b. polycystic kidney disease
c. sickle-cell anemia
d. Tay-Sachs disease

7–16. What is the most common single-gene disorder worldwide?

a. cystic fibrosis
b. fragile X
c. phenylketonuria (PKU)
d. thalassemia

7–17. Which group has been successfully targeted for preconceptional counseling regarding the risk of β-thalassemia?

a. African descent
b. Asian descent
c. Jewish descent
d. Mediterranean descent

7–18. Teenagers are NOT at higher risk for which of the following pregnancy complications?

a. anemia
b. fetal growth restriction
c. gestational diabetes
d. sexually transmitted infections

7–19. Increased risks of pregnancy over maternal age 35 are decreased by which of the following?

a. preconceptional counseling
b. lack of significant medical problems
c. socioeconomic advantage
d. all of the above

7–20. What is the predominant genetic abnormality in the fetus seen with advanced maternal age?

a. aneuploidy
b. fragile X
c. single gene mutation
d. translocation

7–21. What is the relationship between advanced paternal age and genetic birth defects?

a. decreased
b. increased slightly
c. increased markedly
d. no relationship

7–22. Currently, what is the most important cause of dyzygotic twinning?

a. advanced maternal age
b. assisted reproductive technology
c. high parity
d. racial predisposition

7–23. Which of the following is NOT increased by smoking during pregnancy?

   a. attention deficit hyperactivity disorder in child
   b. birth defects
   c. fetal growth restriction
   d. preterm labor

7–24. Pregnant women should limit their weekly dietary intake of fish to 12 ounces and should eliminate consumption of certain kinds of fish in order to minimize exposure to which neurotoxin?

   a. algae-related toxin
   b. cadmium
   c. mercury
   d. organic phosphate

7–25. A 19-year-old G3P2002 at 28 weeks gestation is embarrassed to admit she has been craving and eating ice and clay dirt. She thinks she must be "going crazy." What test is most likely to be abnormal?

   a. drug-alcohol screen
   b. electroencephalogram
   c. hemoglobin
   d. liver function tests

7–26. Maternal obesity is related to an increase in which of the following maternal complications?

   a. hypertension
   b. gestational diabetes
   c. preeclampsia
   d. all of the above

7–27. What adverse fetal outcomes are associated with maternal obesity?

   a. late fetal death
   b. spina bifida
   c. ventral wall defects
   d. all of the above

7–28. Risk from domestic abuse shows what general pattern during pregnancy as compared with before pregnancy?

   a. decreases
   b. approximately the same
   c. increases
   d. difficult to draw conclusions from available studies

7–29. How should a woman be counseled if she inadvertently becomes pregnant within 3 months of receiving a live-virus vaccine?

   a. no fetal risk
   b. theoretical, but no definite risks
   c. serious fetal risks, but are uncommon
   d. significant risk and pregnancy termination is recommended

Prenatal Care

8–1. In 2001, what was the median number of prenatal visits per pregnancy?

   a. 6
   b. 8
   c. 10
   d. 12

8–2. In 1998, approximately what percentage of pregnant women in the United States received no prenatal care?

   a. 1
   b. 5
   c. 10
   d. 20

8–3. The Kessner Index for measuring adequacy prenatal care incorporates all of the following information recorded on birth certificates EXCEPT:

   a. birthweight
   b. length of gestation
   c. number of prenatal visits
   d. timing of first prenatal visit

8–4. According to the Kessner Index, what percentage of women delivering in 2000 received inadequate prenatal care?

   a. 2
   b. 12
   c. 22
   d. 32

8–5. According to the Centers for Disease Control and Prevention (CDC), which of the following is NOT among the top three reasons for no or delayed prenatal care?

   a. appointment difficult to obtain
   b. financial obstacles
   c. indifference or lack of education
   d. not aware early of pregnancy diagnosis

8–6. Prenatal care has contributed to the dramatic decline in maternal mortality from 690 per 100,000 births in 1920, to what U.S. maternal mortality rate today?

   a. 1 per 100,000
   b. 8 per 100,000
   c. 80 per 100,000
   d. 180 per 100,000

8–7. In a population-based study from North Carolina (Harper and colleagues, 2003), how much was the risk of maternal death decreased among recipients of prenatal care?

   a. twofold
   b. fivefold
   c. tenfold
   d. twentyfold

8–8. A comprehensive program of prenatal care includes which of the following?

   a. preconceptual care
   b. prompt pregnancy diagnosis
   c. prenatal care visits
   d. all of the above

8–9. During pregnancy, the loss of cervical mucus ferning when air dried on a slide and examined microscopically is due to which of the following?

   a. high estrogen, high sodium chloride concentration

   b. high progesterone, low sodium chloride concentration
   c. low estrogen, high phosphate concentration
   d. low progesterone, low phosphate concentration

8–10. On examination of a 22-year-old whose last menses began 12 weeks ago, you notice the vaginal mucosa has a bluish hue. What is this physical sign suggestive of pregnancy called?

   a. Berry sign
   b. Chadwick sign
   c. Hoffman sign
   d. McDonnell sign

8–11. What is the Hegar sign in pregnancy?

   a. breast tenderness on exam
   b. cervical mucus ferning
   c. isthmus of uterus softens
   d. perception of fetal movement by examiner

8–12. What is the mean gestational age at which the fetal heartbeat can be detected by auscultation with a stethoscope?

   a. 17 weeks
   b. 19 weeks
   c. 21 weeks
   d. 23 weeks

8–13. The auscultated sound of blood rushing through the umbilical or uterine vessels is referred to by what term?

   a. murmur
   b. pate
   c. souffle
   d. thrill

8–14. At what gestational age can an examiner typically first detect fetal movements?

   a. 14 weeks
   b. 16 weeks
   c. 20 weeks
   d. 24 weeks

8–15. In early pregnancy, what is the approximate doubling time of maternal plasma hCG concentration?

   a. 12 to 18 hours
   b. 36 to 48 hours
   c. 48 to 72 hours
   d. 72 to 96 hours

8–16. Maternal hCG levels peak at how many days following implantation?

   a. 30 to 40
   b. 60 to 70
   c. 90 to 100
   d. 120 to 130

8–17. Pregnancy testing targets which subunit of hCG to optimize specificity?

    a. α (alpha)
    b. β (beta)
    c. Δ (delta)
    d. γ (gamma)

8–18. What are the most common serum factors causing some women to test falsely positive for hCG?

    a. antinuclear antibodies
    b. heterophilic antibodies
    c. illicit drugs
    d. lupus anticoagulant

8–19. What is the approximate sensitivity of home pregnancy tests performed by patients?

    a. 65%
    b. 75%
    c. 85%
    d. 95%

8–20. A pregnant patient presents to you at 6.5 weeks gestation calculated by date of last menses. She has had some vaginal bleeding on and off. A transvaginal sonogram fails to reveal a gestational sac in the uterus. By how many days (menstrual age) should all normal gestational sacs be visualized?

    a. 25
    b. 30
    c. 35
    d. 40

8–21. An early crown-rump length is predictive of gestational age within how many days?

    a. 4
    b. 7
    c. 14
    d. 17

8–22. A woman is classified as a nulligravida if she has

    a. never delivered a live-born baby
    b. had one miscarriage
    c. never been pregnant
    d. had only one pregnancy

8–23. A woman has had two pregnancies, both ending in spontaneous abortion. What is her obstetrical designation?

    a. multipara
    b. nulligravida
    c. nullipara
    d. none of the above

8–24. What is a primiparous woman?

    a. pregnant once, regardless of outcome
    b. delivered once of a fetus of at least 20 weeks' gestation
    c. delivered once of a fetus weighing at least 550 g
    d. has had one pregnancy lasting at least 12 weeks

8–25. A woman's parity is determined by the number of which of the following?

    a. total number of pregnancies
    b. live fetuses delivered
    c. fetuses reaching viability
    d. pregnancies reaching 20 weeks' gestation

8–26. An obstetrical notation showing a woman to be a gravida 4 para 3-1-0-2 indicates a history of which of the following?

    a. 2 abortions
    b. 3 living children
    c. 3 term deliveries
    d. 0 preterm deliveries

8–27. What is the mean duration of pregnancy from the first day of the last menstrual period (LMP)?

    a. 250 days
    b. 260 days
    c. 270 days
    d. 280 days

8–28. The Naegele rule estimates gestational age based on which of the following formulas?

    a. add 7 days to LMP and count back 3 months
    b. subtract 7 days from LMP and count back 3 months
    c. add 21 days to LMP and count back 3 months
    d. subtract 21 days from LMP and count back 3 months

8–29. By convention, pregnancy trimesters divide which of the following gestational time periods (weeks) into three equal parts?

    a. 36
    b. 39
    c. 40
    d. 42

8–30. Duration of pregnancy is most correctly measured clinically by which of the following units?

    a. completed weeks since first day of LMP
    b. number of weeks, rounded to the nearest whole week, since the first day of LMP
    c. completed weeks since estimated date of conception
    d. number of weeks, rounded to the nearest whole week, since the estimated date of conception

8–31. In 2001, what percentage of women reported smoking during their pregnancy?

   a. 8
   b. 12
   c. 18
   d. 22

8–32. Cigarette smoking has been linked to increases in which of the following?

   a. fetal growth restriction
   b. preterm birth
   c. spontaneous abortion
   d. all of the above

8–33. Which of the following is NOT a characteristic of fetal alcohol syndrome?

   a. central nervous system dysfunction
   b. facial abnormalities
   c. growth restriction
   d. limb deformities

8–34. What proportion of pregnant women are exposed to domestic violence?

   a. 1 in 10
   b. 1 in 100
   c. 1 in 1000
   d. 1 in 10,000

8–35. According to the American College of Obstetricians and Gynecologists (ACOG, 1999), when should prenatal screening for domestic violence be carried out?

   a. first prenatal visit
   b. each trimester
   c. postpartum
   d. all of the above

8–36. A primigravida presents at 20 weeks' gestation. Which of the following laboratory tests is NOT obtained during the first prenatal visit?

   a. antibody screen
   b. Group B streptococcus culture
   c. HIV screen
   d. Pap smear

8–37. At which of these gestational ages is maternal serum alpha-fetoprotein screening best carried out?

   a. 7 weeks
   b. 12 weeks
   c. 17 weeks
   d. 22 weeks

8–38. There is close correlation of fundal height in centimeters with gestational age during which weeks of gestation?

   a. 14 to 35
   b. 17 to 34
   c. 20 to 31
   d. 25 to 38

8–39. At what gestational age are audible fetal heart sounds heard with a fetal stethoscope in 100% of live pregnancies?

   a. 16 weeks
   b. 18 weeks
   c. 20 weeks
   d. 22 weeks

8–40. At what gestational age should laboratory testing for gestational diabetes be performed?

   a. 10 to 16 weeks
   b. 20 to 24 weeks
   c. 24 to 28 weeks
   d. 32 to 36 weeks

8–41. For which of the following is universal prenatal screening currently recommended?

   a. chlamydia
   b. cystic fibrosis carrier status
   c. fetal fibronectin
   d. HIV

8–42. What approach does ACOG and the CDC currently recommend for universal Group B streptococcus screening during pregnancy?

   a. vaginal culture at 30 to 32 weeks
   b. rectal and urine cultures at 30 to 32 weeks
   c. vaginal swab for rapid test in labor
   d. rectal and vaginal cultures at 35 to 37 weeks

8–43. A couple of Indian or Pakistani descent is at greatest risk for which of the following genetic diseases?

   a. α-thalassemia
   b. β-thalassemia
   c. cystic fibrosis
   d. Tay-Sachs disease

8–44. A total maternal weight gain of less than 16 lb is associated with which of the following?

   a. fetal malformations
   b. impaired mental development of the infant or child
   c. low birthweight
   d. pregnancy-induced hypertension

8–45. Which is considered to be a normal weight gain during pregnancy for a woman with a normal body mass index (BMI)?

    a. 10 lb
    b. 15 lb
    c. 20 lb
    d. 30 lb

8–46. Excessive maternal weight gain is most strongly associated with which of the following?

    a. fetal macrosomia
    b. preterm delivery
    c. placental abruption
    d. oligohydramnios

8–47. Which nutrients can exert toxic effects if taken in excessive amounts during pregnancy?

    a. vitamins A and B_6
    b. vitamins C and D
    c. iron, zinc, and selenium
    d. all of the above

8–48. During pregnancy, a daily caloric increase of how much is recommended?

    a. 50 to 100 kcal
    b. 100 to 300 kcal
    c. 300 to 500 kcal
    d. 500 to 700 kcal

8–49. Which nutrient during pregnancy is NOT adequately provided in diet alone?

    a. calcium
    b. magnesium
    c. iron
    d. folate

8–50. What is the average daily iron requirement during the latter half of pregnancy?

    a. 1 mg/d
    b. 3 mg/d
    c. 5 mg/d
    d. 7 mg/d

8–51. To minimize the gastrointestinal side effects of iron, when is it recommended that patients take their iron?

    a. at bedtime
    b. with breakfast
    c. during the first trimester
    d. only if the hemoglobin is less than 10 mg/dL

8–52. During pregnancy, how much calcium is retained?

    a. 30 g
    b. 60 g
    c. 90 g
    d. 120 g

8–53. What characterizes intestinal calcium absorption during pregnancy?

    a. It decreases.
    b. It remains the same.
    c. It increases.
    d. It increases with vitamin E supplementation.

8–54. Which of the following is NOT associated with severe zinc deficiency?

    a. impaired wound healing
    b. poor appetite
    c. dwarfism in the fetus
    d. seizures

8–55. What are the current recommendations for daily zinc intake during pregnancy?

    a. 6 mg
    b. 12 mg
    c. 60 mg
    d. 120 mg

8–56. Severe maternal hypothyroidism has been linked to which of the following in offspring?

    a. cretinism
    b. dwarfism
    c. hypogonadism in children
    d. limb reduction deformities

8–57. In general, dietary iodine intake has shown what trend over the past 15 years?

    a. stable
    b. increasing
    c. decreasing
    d. unknown

8–58. Supplementation of which of the following minerals has been shown to improve pregnancy outcome?

    a. chromium
    b. copper
    c. manganese
    d. none of the above

8–59. In the People's Republic of China, selenium deficiency is associated with which of the following in children?

    a. cardiomyopathy
    b. renal failure
    c. seizures
    d. short stature

8–60. What percentage of neural-tube defects are related to folic acid metabolism and therefore, preventable by folic acid supplementation?

a. 5
b. 15
c. 25
d. 50

8–61. What amount of daily folic acid intake is currently recommended during the preconceptual period and early pregnancy?

a. 40 μg
b. 100 μg
c. 400 μg
d. 1000 μg

8–62. What is the recurrence risk of neural-tube defect for a woman with a prior affected fetus?

a. 3%
b. 13%
c. 23%
d. 33%

8–63. Your patient, a Para 1, is considering a second pregnancy. Her first child was anencephalic and died soon after birth. You recommend what daily dose of folic acid periconceptually to reduce the risk of recurrence?

a. 0.4 mg
b. 4 mg
c. 40 mg
d. 400 mg

8–64. Excessive intake of vitamin A in pregnancy is suspected of causing which of the following in the fetus?

a. blindness
b. congenital heart block
c. limb malformations
d. seizures

8–65. Strict vegetarianism may cause maternal and fetal deficiency of which vitamin due to its availability exclusively from animal sources?

a. A
b. B_{12}
c. C
d. K

8–66. Excessive ingestion of which vitamin can lead to a functional vitamin B_{12} deficiency?

a. A
b. B_6
c. C
d. D

8–67. What is the recommended daily dietary allowance for vitamin C during pregnancy (usually provided by an adequate diet)?

a. 10 mg
b. 30 mg
c. 50 mg
d. 80 mg

8–68. Which of the following activities poses the MOST risk to the mother and fetus during pregnancy and should be avoided?

a. cycling
b. running
c. scuba diving
d. swimming

8–69. Approximately what proportion of pregnant employed women are advised to stop working at some point due to medical indications?

a. 1 in 10
b. 1 in 4
c. 1 in 3
d. 1 in 2

8–70. What are the hazards for pregnant women who work at jobs that require prolonged standing or are physically demanding?

a. fetal growth retardation
b. preeclampsia
c. preterm delivery
d. all of the above

8–71. In general, what risk does travel pose to the healthy pregnant woman?

a. decreased birthweight with frequent travel
b. increased pulmonary embolus
c. increased hypertensive complications
d. no increased risks identified

8–72. ACOG has concluded that pregnant women can safely engage in air travel until what gestational age?

a. 30 weeks
b. 32 weeks
c. 34 weeks
d. 36 weeks

8–73. Which of the following is true regarding safe automobile use during pregnancy?

a. Air bags should be disabled.
b. Three-point belt restraints should be used.
c. Lap belts should not be used.
d. Shoulder belts should not be used.

8–74. Which is a risk of coitus during pregnancy?

 a. unknown
 b. increased preterm delivery
 c. increased chorioamnionitis
 d. increased maternal musculoskeletal complaints

8–75. What is the recommendation for the administration of hepatitis A and B vaccines to pregnant women?

 a. contraindicated throughout pregnancy
 b. given pre- and postexposure to women at risk
 c. given postexposure only
 d. restricted to second or third trimester

8–76. What is the recommendation for the administration of tetanus toxoid to pregnant women?

 a. contraindicated
 b. for postexposure prophylaxis
 c. only if traveling to endemic area
 d. only if immunocompromised

8–77. What is the recommendation for the administration of measles vaccine to pregnant women?

 a. contraindicated
 b. same as for nonpregnant women
 c. for postexposure only
 d. only if risk factors are present

8–78. What is the recommendation for the administration of pneumococcus vaccine to pregnant women?

 a. contraindicated
 b. same as for nonpregnant women
 c. for postexposure only
 d. only if asplenic

8–79. What is the recommendation for the administration of varicella vaccine to pregnant women?

 a. contraindicated
 b. same as for nonpregnant women
 c. for postexposure only
 d. only if risk factors are present

8–80. Which is true for the administration of influenza vaccine during pregnancy?

 a. given IM, one dose, annually
 b. given after the first trimester during the flu season in average-risk women
 c. given any trimester in women at high risk of pulmonary complications
 d. all of the above

8–81. In which group should anthrax vaccination be most strongly considered?

 a. airline attendants
 b. medical students
 c. schoolteachers
 d. veterinarians

8–82. Which of the following statements regarding caffeine consumption during pregnancy is most strongly supported by research?

 a. Teratogenic in lab animals.
 b. Increases the risk of pregnancy-induced hypertension.
 c. Increases the risk of preterm birth.
 d. Increases the risk of spontaneous abortion at extremely high levels.

8–83. What percentage of women take one or more prescribed medications during pregnancy?

 a. 15
 b. 35
 c. 75
 d. 95

8–84. Ninety percent of women with nausea and vomiting of pregnancy have resolution of this problem by what gestational age (weeks)?

 a. 10
 b. 14
 c. 18
 d. 22

8–85. Although high levels of human chorionic gonadotropin have been implicated in the past as the etiology of nausea during pregnancy, which hormone is currently suspected to be the real culprit?

 a. estrogen
 b. human placental lactogen
 c. progesterone
 d. prolactin

8–86. Appearance or exacerbation of which of the following conditions commonly occurs during pregnancy?

 a. backache
 b. heartburn
 c. varicosities in lower extremities
 d. all of the above

8–87. Which of the following is most strongly associated with pica during pregnancy?

 a. domestic abuse
 b. intestinal parasites
 c. iron deficiency anemia
 d. schizophrenia

8–88. Excessive fatigue typical of early pregnancy is thought to be due to which hormone?

a. estrogen
b. human placental lactogen
c. progesterone
d. prolactin

8–89. Treatment of which of the following vaginal infections improves pregnancy outcome?

a. bacterial vaginosis
b. candidiasis
c. trichomoniasis
d. none of the above

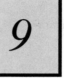

9

Abortion

9–1. By convention, abortion would include which of the following?

a. pregnancy intentionally ended prior to 20 weeks
b. pregnancy spontaneously ended prior to 20 weeks
c. pregnancy intentionally ended with a fetus weighing <500 g
d. all of the above

9–2. What is the term for no visible fetus in the gestational sac?

a. blighted ovum
b. miscarriage
c. septic abortion
d. polar body

9–3. Which of the following is most commonly associated with spontaneous abortion?

a. aneuploidy
b. listeriosis
c. antiphospholipid syndrome
d. anti-Kell antibodies

9–4. Which of the following is NOT associated with an increased abortion rate?

a. advanced maternal age
b. advanced paternal age

c. pregnancy within 3 months of a live birth
d. class A_1 diabetes mellitus

9–5. A correct statement regarding aneuploid spontaneous abortions includes which of the following?

a. They compose a small fraction of all spontaneous abortions.
b. Triploidy is most frequently identified.
c. Advanced maternal age does not affect the incidence of triploidy.
d. They typically occur after 12 weeks gestation.

9–6. A correct statement regarding euploid spontaneous abortions includes which of the following?

a. They tend to abort earlier than aneuploid pregnancies.
b. Their incidence is unaffected by maternal age.
c. The majority occur before 8 weeks gestation.
d. None of the above are correct.

9–7. Maternal factors associated with an increased risk of spontaneous abortion include all of the following EXCEPT

a. advanced maternal age
b. herpes simplex infection
c. antiphospholipid antibodies
d. uncontrolled insulin-dependent diabetes

9–8. Which of the following nutritional factors have been linked with an increased risk of spontaneous abortion?

    a. drinking >5 cups of coffee per day
    b. maternal hyperemesis
    c. folic acid deficiency
    d. iron-deficiency anemia

9–9. Occupational exposure to which of the following environmental agents has been linked with an increased risk of spontaneous abortion?

    a. anesthetic gases
    b. ultrasound
    c. *Chlamydia trachomatis*
    d. electromagnetic radiation from computer display screens

9–10. Which of the following is associated with an increased risk of spontaneous abortion?

    a. uncomplicated laparotomy
    b. maternal tuberculosis
    c. uterine fibroids
    d. Asherman syndrome

9–11. Your patient presents for evaluation following her third spontaneous abortion. Which of the following might be a logical next step for this patient?

    a. herpes simplex antibody assay
    b. lupus anticoagulant assay
    c. protein C assay
    d. antinuclear antibody assay

9–12. Your patient has had two first-trimester and one second-trimester spontaneous abortions. Her screen for anticardiolipin antibodies is positive. The most appropriate treatment option for this patient during her next pregnancy includes which of the following?

    a. low-dose aspirin plus heparin
    b. low-dose aspirin plus plaquenil sulfate
    c. low-dose aspirin plus steroids
    d. reassurance

9–13. What causes pregnancy loss in women with antiphospholipid antibodies?

    a. placental thrombosis and infarction
    b. increased vascularization of decidua basalis
    c. increased prostacyclin release
    d. protein C activation

9–14. Your 26-year-old patient, G5 P2 A3, presents with a history of two spontaneous vaginal deliveries followed by three first-trimester spontaneous abortions. Her second delivery was complicated by a postpartum hemorrhage with dilatation and curettage to remove placental fragments. The most likely cause of this patient's abortions is which of the following?

    a. large uterine fibroids
    b. antiphospholipid syndrome
    c. Asherman syndrome
    d. systemic lupus erythematosus

9–15. Which of the following is the most appropriate and accurate test to confirm the diagnosis of Asherman syndrome?

    a. ultrasonography
    b. antinuclear antibody assay
    c. hysteroscopy
    d. lupus anticoagulant assay

9–16. Treatment options for the patient in Question 14 include which of the following?

    a. uterine myomectomy
    b. low-dose aspirin therapy
    c. oral corticosteroids
    d. adhesiolysis and intrauterine device placement

9–17. Your patient describes events relating to her first pregnancy, which spontaneously aborted at 18 weeks. She tells of arriving in labor and delivery with complaints of pelvic pressure but without contractions. Examination showed bulging membranes and a dilated cervix. Her membranes ruptured shortly thereafter with spontaneous expulsion of the abortus. You explain to her that in some cases one of the underlying causes for this type of abortion may include which of the following?

    a. prior cervical conization
    b. prior syphilitic infection
    c. maternal toxoplasmosis infection during pregnancy
    d. colposcopic examination during pregnancy

9–18. You explain to your patient in Question 17 that the most valuable information for establishing this diagnosis is which of the following?

    a. "funneling" found on ultrasonographic examination during pregnancy
    b. detailed obstetrical history
    c. cervical shortening found on physical examination during pregnancy
    d. cervical shortening found on hysterography prior to pregnancy

9–19. You explain to the patient in Question 17 that the most effective treatment option during her next pregnancy for this problem is which of the following?

   a. oral tocolytics
   b. oral indomethacin
   c. strict bed rest
   d. cerclage procedure

9–20. In women with a classical history of cervical incompetence, which of the following is true of cerclage procedures?

   a. The modified Shirodkar type is preferred as a first-line treatment.
   b. The transabdominal approach carries an equal complication rate as the transvaginal approach.
   c. Success rates to prevent preterm delivery are 40 to 50%.
   d. The transabdominal approach is used for patients with prior McDonald cerclage failures.

9–21. Optimally, when should prophylactic cerclage procedures be performed?

   a. preconceptionally
   b. between 6 to 12 weeks' gestation
   c. between 12 to 16 weeks' gestation
   d. at first sign of cervical dilatation

9–22. Management options for patients with a McDonald cerclage who present with clinical infection include which of the following?

   a. intravenous antimicrobials and bed rest
   b. cerclage removal and labor induction
   c. intravenous antimicrobials and tocolytic administration
   d. oral indomethacin and serial ultrasonographic examinations

9–23. At 8 weeks' gestation, if vaginal bleeding develops, what is the risk of spontaneous abortion?

   a. 10%
   b. 30%
   c. 50%
   d. 70%

9–24. Which of the following is NOT an associated sequela of bleeding at 8 weeks' gestation?

   a. preterm labor
   b. low birthweight
   c. neonatal mortality
   d. fetal malformations

9–25. At 8 weeks' gestation a woman has vaginal bleeding of supracervical origin. Which of the following is most helpful with regard to prognosis?

   a. serum β-HCG level
   b. plasma estriol level
   c. serum progesterone level
   d. ultrasonographic examination of fetus for fetal heart motion

9–26. Your patient presents with bleeding at 8 weeks' gestation. She is afebrile and isovolemic. Physical examination reveals tissue protruding through her cervical os. Which of the following is the next best management step for this patient?

   a. suction curettage
   b. observation and bed rest
   c. serial ultrasonographic examinations
   d. intramuscular progesterone

9–27. Your patient with a pregnancy at 8 weeks' gestation by last menstrual period presents with vaginal bleeding and complaints of lower abdominal pain. She is afebrile and isovolemic. Physical examination reveals a closed cervical os and 6-week size, soft, nontender uterus. An appropriate next management step includes which of the following?

   a. reassurance and bed rest
   b. ultrasonographic examination
   c. Doppler auscultation of fetal heart tones
   d. measurement of serum progesterone level

9–28. Your patient with a pregnancy at 14 weeks' gestation presents with fever (38.5°C) and lower abdominal pain, but without bleeding. She describes a small leakage of vaginal fluid that occurred the previous day. The next management step of this patient should include which of the following?

   a. urinalysis
   b. dilatation and curettage
   c. bed rest and observation
   d. antimicrobials and observation

9–29. Appropriate management of first-trimester missed abortion includes which of the following?

   a. intravaginal misoprostol
   b. dilatation and curettage
   c. expectantly await spontaneous abortion
   d. all of the above

9–30. Early first-trimester induced abortion techniques include all of the following EXCEPT

   a. sharp curettage
   b. manual vacuum curettage
   c. oral misoprostol plus intravenous oxytocin
   d. intramuscular methotrexate plus oral misoprostol

9–31. Complications of vacuum aspiration first-trimester abortion include all of the following EXCEPT

    a. uterine synechiae
    b. cervical laceration
    c. retained products of conception
    d. preterm delivery in future pregnancies

9–32. Which of these complications following surgical abortion occurs LEAST commonly?

    a. infertility
    b. endometritis
    c. cervical laceration
    d. retained products of conception

9–33. The dilatation and evacuation method of surgical abortion should be used beginning at which of the following gestational ages?

    a. 12 weeks
    b. 16 weeks
    c. 18 weeks
    d. 20 weeks

9–34. You place laminaria in your patient in preparation for termination of her 16-week pregnancy. The next day your patient asks about NOT proceeding with the abortion. You remove the laminaria and counsel her which of the following?

    a. Abortion will spontaneously occur in most of these cases.
    b. Cerclage placement is required to sustain the pregnancy.
    c. Observation is recommended.
    d. Oral antimicrobials are required to prevent infection.

9–35. Prior to surgical abortion, the cervix may commonly be dilated using all of the following EXCEPT

    a. Pratt dilators
    b. oral mifepristone
    c. *Laminaria japonica*
    d. vaginal misoprostol

9–36. Common complications of surgical abortion can be minimized by which of the following?

    a. adequate cervical dilatation
    b. preoperative enema
    c. postsurgical D-immunoglobulin administration for all patients
    d. curette grasped firmly by the entire hand during curettage

9–37. The American College of Obstetricians and Gynecologists supports outpatient medical abortion as an acceptable alternative to surgical abortion for pregnancies less than how many weeks?

    a. 5
    b. 7
    c. 9
    d. 11

9–38. Contraindications to medical abortion include which of the following maternal conditions?

    a. severe anemia
    b. hypothyroidism
    c. cervical dysplasia
    d. systemic lupus erythematosus

9–39. Safe, effective second-trimester abortifacients include all of the following EXCEPT

    a. oxytocin
    b. indomethacin
    c. prostaglandin E_1
    d. prostaglandin E_2

9–40. Common side effects of prostaglandin E_2 include which of the following?

    a. fever
    b. dysuria
    c. seizure
    d. arthralgia

9–41. How many weeks after an abortion does ovulation usually occur?

    a. 2 to 3
    b. 4 to 5
    c. 5 to 6
    d. 6 to 7

10

Ectopic Pregnancy

10–1. What is the approximate incidence of ectopic versus normal pregnancy in the United States?

    a. 1 in 50
    b. 1 in 500
    c. 1 in 1000
    d. 1 in 1500

10–2. Which poses the greatest risk of maternal death in the first trimester?

    a. ectopic pregnancy
    b. elective abortion
    c. term pregnancy
    d. all pose equal risk

10–3. With which of the following are tubal pregnancies NOT increased?

    a. assisted reproduction
    b. history of pelvic infection
    c. previous tubal surgery
    d. abnormal embryos

10–4. What is the approximate rate of recurrent ectopic pregnancy after one previous ectopic?

    a. 1%
    b. 10%
    c. 50%
    d. 90%

10–5. Which method of contraceptive failure has an increased *relative* risk of ectopic pregnancy?

    a. intrauterine device
    b. progestin-only minipills
    c. tubal sterilization
    d. all of the above

10–6. Ectopic pregnancies account for what percentage of pregnancy-related deaths?

    a. 5
    b. 10
    c. 20
    d. 25

10–7. What is the most common ectopic tubal implantation site?

    a. fimbria
    b. ampulla
    c. isthmus
    d. cornua

10–8. Which of the following is true about interstitial pregnancy?

    a. represents 3% of tubal pregnancies
    b. frequently ruptures later (8 to 16 weeks)
    c. is usually associated with massive hemorrhage if ruptured
    d. all of the above

10–9. Which has caused an increase in the incidence of heterotypic pregnancy?

    a. assisted reproduction
    b. dietary factors
    c. obesity
    d. progestin-only contraceptives

10–10. Which of the following signs or symptoms most strongly indicates a ruptured ectopic pregnancy with sizable intraperitoneal hemorrhage?

    a. heavy vaginal bleeding
    b. lower abdominal pain, unilateral
    c. nausea and vomiting
    d. shoulder pain on inspiration

10–11. What is the most common symptom of ectopic pregnancy?

    a. gastrointestinal symptoms
    b. heavy vaginal bleeding
    c. pain
    d. syncope

10–12. Results of enzyme-linked immunosorbent assays (ELISA) for chorionic gonadotropin are positive in what percentage of ectopic pregnancies?

    a. 50
    b. 70
    c. 80
    d. >99

10–13. A patient with a positive pregnancy test result and a serum progesterone level of less than 5 ng/mL strongly suggests which of the following?

    a. corpus luteum decline (physiological)
    b. inconclusive level
    c. a nonviable pregnancy
    d. a viable intrauterine pregnancy

10–14. Sonographic evidence of an ectopic pregnancy includes which of the following?

    a. adnexal mass
    b. fluid in the cul de sac
    c. lack of intrauterine gestational sac
    d. all of the above

10–15. At what level of serum hCG can intrauterine gestations be detected with 50% sensitivity using vaginal sonography?

    a. 100 mIU/mL
    b. 500 mIU/mL
    c. 1000 mIU/mL
    d. 5000 mIU/mL

10–16. Approximately what percentage of ectopic pregnancies are diagnosed prior to rupture?

    a. 60
    b. 70
    c. 80
    d. 90

10–17. What is the mean doubling time for β-hCG levels in early pregnancy?

    a. 24 hr
    b. 48 hr
    c. 72 hr
    d. 96 hr

10–18. What is the lowest normal increase for β-hCG levels in early normal pregnancies during a 48-hour interval?

    a. 33%
    b. 44%
    c. 55%
    d. 66%

10–19. A gravida with a history of tubal reanastomosis presents with vaginal spotting several days after missed menses. Physical exam is nonspecific. The patient is stable. Serum hCG is 1012 mIU/mL. Vaginal sonography is negative for intrauterine pregnancy, adnexal mass, or free fluid. What would a reasonable next step be?

    a. laparoscopy
    b. repeat serum hCG in 48 hr
    c. serum progesterone
    d. all are reasonable approaches

10–20. In which surgical approach to ectopic pregnancy is the tube opened to remove the gestational products, then left unsutured?

    a. salpingectomy
    b. salpingotomy
    c. salpingorrhaphy
    d. salpingostomy

10–21. Compared with laparotomy, laparoscopic surgery for ectopic pregnancy offers what advantage?

    a. lower risk of subsequent ectopic pregnancy
    b. higher rate of subsequent intrauterine pregnancy
    c. lower risk of tubal rupture
    d. lower cost and recovery time

10–22. By how many days following resection of an ectopic pregnancy does serum chorionic gonadotropin decrease to 10% of preoperative levels?

    a. 2
    b. 4
    c. 8
    d. 12

10–23. Persistent trophoblast following salpingostomy is rarely a problem if the serum hCG level falls by what amount on postoperative day 1?

    a. 5%
    b. 10%
    c. 25%
    d. 50%

10–24. Which of the following would make methotrexate therapy for ectopic pregnancy less likely to succeed?

    a. pregnancy of 5 weeks duration
    b. tubal mass 3.5 cm
    c. fetal heart motion
    d. a primigravid patient

10–25. What is the ultimate success rate of methotrexate therapy for ectopic pregnancy (cases needing multiple doses included)?

    a. 60%
    b. 70%
    c. 80%
    d. 90%

10–26. In what percentage of cases does tubal rupture occur after methotrexate therapy for ectopic pregnancy?

    a. <1
    b. 5 to 10
    c. 25 to 30
    d. >50

10–27. Patients undergoing methotrexate therapy for ectopic pregnancy should be counseled to avoid which of the following?

    a. alcohol
    b. folic acid supplements and multivitamins
    c. sexual intercourse
    d. all of the above

10–28. What is the usual dose of methotrexate given for medical treatment of ectopic pregnancy (single-dose regimen)?

    a. 1 mg/m^2
    b. 5 mg/m^2
    c. 50 mg/m^2
    d. 500 mg/m^2

10–29. Which is NOT an expected possible complication of methotrexate therapy for ectopic pregnancy?

    a. cardiac arrhythmia
    b. gastroenteritis
    c. liver toxicity
    d. stomatitis

10–30. Following successful single-dose methotrexate therapy for ectopic pregnancy, serum levels of β-hCG should decrease by how much between days 4 and 7?

    a. 15%
    b. 25%

    c. 33%
    d. 50%

10–31. Abdominal pregnancy most commonly results from reimplantation after which of the following?

    a. dehiscence of uterine scar
    b. physical trauma
    c. rupture of tubal pregnancy
    d. induced abortion

10–32. Which of the following maternal serum laboratory values may be elevated due to the presence of abdominal pregnancy?

    a. alpha-fetoprotein
    b. creatinine
    c. glucose
    d. hematocrit

10–33. The diagnosis of abdominal pregnancy is missed by sonography in what percentage of cases?

    a. 10
    b. 25
    c. 50
    d. 75

10–34. What is the common approach to an abdominal pregnancy of 16 weeks' gestation?

    a. expectant management
    b. laparotomy with delivery of fetus
    c. methotrexate
    d. uterine artery embolization, then await fetal resorption

10–35. Which of the following has caused an increase in the incidence of cervical pregnancies?

    a. high cesarean delivery rates
    b. in vitro fertilization
    c. advancing maternal age
    d. increased incidence of cervical neoplasia

10–36. What is the preferred therapy for a cervical pregnancy in a stable patient?

    a. hysterectomy
    b. cerclage
    c. embolization
    d. methotrexate

11

Gestational Trophoblastic Disease

11–1. Complete molar pregnancies most commonly have which of the following genetic compositions?

a. 45,XO
b. 46,XY
c. 46,XX
d. 47,XXY

11–2. Partial molar pregnancies most commonly have which of the following genetic compositions?

a. 45,XO
b. 46,XY
c. 46,XX
d. 69,XXY

11–3. You performed a dilatation and curettage for your patient with a missed abortion. Pathologic evaluation of the specimen revealed swelling within the stroma and avascularity of the chorionic villi. Chromosomal analysis of the tissue revealed a composition of 69,XXX. You counsel that her risk of persistent trophoblastic disease is which of the following?

a. 1%
b. 10%
c. 20%
d. 30%

11–4. The incidence of persistent trophoblastic disease following a complete mole is closest to which of the following?

a. 1%
b. 10%
c. 20%
d. 30%

11–5. What is the etiology of theca-lutein cysts?

a. abnormal karyotype
b. increased prolactin receptors

c. increased chorionic gonadotropin
d. increased follicle-stimulating hormone

11–6. Bilateral ovarian theca-lutein cysts in association with molar pregnancies may portend a greater risk of which of the following?

a. gestational hypertension
b. maternal thyrotoxicosis
c. trophoblastic tissue embolization
d. gestational trophoblastic neoplasia

11–7. Risk factors for molar pregnancy include which of the following?

a. age younger than 15 years
b. >2 prior pregnancies
c. type I diabetes mellitus
d. prior cesarean delivery

11–8. What causes the increase in plasma thyroxine in women with partial molar pregnancy?

a. increased fetal thyroxine production
b. estrogen-induced increased total thyroxine
c. increased levels of human chorionic gonadotropin
d. unknown

11–9. Symptoms commonly associated with molar pregnancy include which of the following?

a. nausea
b. diarrhea
c. dyspnea
d. loss of lateral visual fields

11–10. Clinical findings commonly associated with molar pregnancy include all of the following EXCEPT

a. absent fetal heart sounds
b. iron-deficiency anemia
c. uterine size > gestational age
d. harsh maternal systolic cardiac murmur

11–11. What imaging technique is most useful in diagnosing molar pregnancy?

    a. radiography
    b. ultrasonography
    c. magnetic resonance imaging
    d. computed tomographic imaging

11–12. Primary treatment of molar pregnancy is which of the following?

    a. hysterotomy
    b. suction curettage
    c. oxytocin induction
    d. misoprostol induction

11–13. Routine postevacuation treatment of molar pregnancy typically includes which of the following?

    a. oral contraceptive pills
    b. methotrexate chemotherapy
    c. methotrexate plus actinomycin D chemotherapy
    d. methotrexate plus cisplatin chemotherapy

11–14. Gestational trophoblastic neoplasia may develop after which of the following?

    a. evacuation of a partial mole
    b. delivery of a normal term pregnancy
    c. abortion of a genetically normal abortus
    d. all of the above

11–15. The diagnosis of gestational trophoblastic neoplasia typically is determined by which of the following?

    a. CT imaging
    b. serum hCG levels
    c. tissue pathology
    d. physical examination findings

11–16. A common site of gestational trophoblastic disease metastasis includes which of the following?

    a. vagina
    b. bone
    c. spleen
    d. breast

11–17. Choriocarcinoma is spread metastatically by which of the following methods?

    a. lymphatic
    b. hematogenous
    c. contiguous invasion
    d. disseminated via peritoneal fluid

11–18. Gestational trophoblastic neoplasia includes all of the following EXCEPT

    a. invasive mole
    b. choriocarcinoma
    c. hydatidiform mole
    d. placenta site trophoblastic tumor

11–19. The hallmark sign of gestational trophoblastic neoplasia is which of the following?

    a. fever
    b. seizures
    c. uterine bleeding
    d. pelvic vein thrombosis

11–20. Your patient presents with complaints of persistent, heavy, dark brown vaginal bleeding 8 weeks after delivery of a term neonate. Initial testing in her evaluation, in addition to a serum hCG level, should include which of the following?

    a. uterine curettage
    b. chest radiography
    c. CT imaging of the head
    d. MR imaging of the abdomen

11–21. According to the International Federation of Gynecology and Obstetrics (FIGO), when staging gestational trophoblastic neoplasia, which of the following is assessed and assigned a rating score?

    a. parity
    b. patient age
    c. presence of thyrotoxicosis
    d. presence and size of theca-lutein cysts

11–22. Your patient is assigned a FIGO score of 4 for choriocarcinoma. She may be treated effectively with methotrexate OR with which of the following?

    a. radical hysterectomy
    b. external beam pelvic radiation
    c. EMA-CO combination chemotherapy
    d. actinomycin D single-agent chemotherapy

11–23. High-risk choriocarcinoma is most effectively treated by which of the following?

    a. radical hysterectomy
    b. EMA-CO combination chemotherapy
    c. methotrexate plus external beam pelvic radiation
    d. methotrexate single-agent therapy plus radical hysterectomy

11–24. Your patient has been assigned a FIGO score of 5 for choriocarcinoma and has received standard treatment. You counsel her that her chances for cure are closest to which of the following?

    a. 40%
    b. 50%
    c. 80%
    d. 95%

11–25. Concerns regarding future pregnancy plans following treatment of gestational trophoblastic disease include which of the following?

    a. decrease fertility
    b. increased risk of fetal trisomy
    c. increased risk of a second molar pregnancy
    d. increased risk of first-trimester pregnancy loss

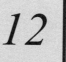

12

Genetics

12–1. What percentage of newborns have a structural anomaly?

    a. <1
    b. 2 to 3
    c. 7 to 8
    d. 10

12–2. Approximately how many genes comprise the haploid human genome?

    a. 20,000
    b. 40,000
    c. 80,000
    d. 120,000

12–3. Which of the following is NOT a cause of birth defects?

    a. malformation
    b. deformation
    c. interruption
    d. disruption

12–4. Which of the following is NOT an associated defect in CHARGE?

    a. heart defects
    b. growth deficiency
    c. coloboma
    d. gonad anomalies

12–5. What is the approximate percentage of chromosomal abnormalities in live-born infants?

    a. 0.009
    b. 0.09
    c. 0.9
    d. 9.0

12–6. What is the frequency of chromosomal abnormalities among stillbirths and neonatal deaths?

    a. <1%
    b. 1 to 3%
    c. 6 to 11%
    d. 15 to 20%

12–7. What is the most common chromosomal abnormality in early spontaneous abortions?

    a. 45,X
    b. 47,XXY
    c. 47,XXX
    d. trisomy 16

12–8. In the majority of cases, triploidy results from fertilization of which of the following?

    a. one egg by two sperm
    b. two eggs with one sperm
    c. one egg joined to polar body
    d. polar body with three sperm

12–9. Which of the following types of genetic disease is related to paternal age?

    a. trisomy
    b. multifactorial disease
    c. translocation
    d. autosomal dominant disease

12–10. What is the frequency of new, dominant mutations in newborns whose fathers are older than 40?

    a. 0.3%
    b. 1.0%
    c. 3.0%
    d. 10.0%

12–11. In conceptions induced by intracytoplasmic sperm injection (ICSI), the fetuses are at risk for which of the following?

    a. monosomy X
    b. trisomy 16
    c. trisomy 21
    d. Y chromosome deletion

12–12. Which of the following is NOT a characteristic finding in newborns with Down syndrome?

    a. large head
    b. flattened occiput
    c. up-slanting palpebral fissures
    d. clinodactyly

12–13. What is the recurrence risk of trisomy 21 in the subsequent children of young mothers?

    a. 1%
    b. 5%
    c. 12%
    d. 25%

12–14. What is the approximate risk of trisomy 21 in a 33-year-old woman?

    a. 1 in 70
    b. 1 in 150
    c. 1 in 500
    d. 1 in 1400

12–15. What is the approximate risk of trisomy 21 in a 40-year-old woman?

    a. 1 in 70
    b. 1 in 150
    c. 1 in 500
    d. 1 in 1200

12–16. Approximately what percentage of Down syndrome pregnancies in women 35 years and older will be lost by 16 weeks (time of amniocentesis)?

    a. <5
    b. 10
    c. 30
    d. 50

12–17. Trisomy 18 (Edwards syndrome) occurs in how many newborns?

    a. 1 in 1000
    b. 1 in 8000
    c. 1 in 16,000
    d. 1 in 24,000

12–18. Which of the following is NOT a facial feature of trisomy 18?

    a. prominent occiput
    b. malformed auricles
    c. short palpebral fissures
    d. large mouth

12–19. Which of the following is NOT an anomaly of trisomy 13 or Patau syndrome?

    a. cleft lip/palate
    b. omphalocele
    c. macrocephaly
    d. radial aplasia

12–20. Which of the following is usually NOT found in offspring with 47,XXY (Klinefelter syndrome)?

    a. small testicles
    b. gynecomastia
    c. short stature
    d. azoospermia

12–21. Which of the following traits is NOT characteristic of offspring with an extra Y chromosome (47,XYY)?

    a. tall
    b. normal intelligence
    c. learning disabilities
    d. criminal behavior

12–22. Which of the following traits is usually NOT found in offspring with 45,X monosomy?

    a. short stature
    b. webbing of the neck
    c. coarctation of the aorta
    d. mental retardation

12–23. What deletion is responsible for the cri du chat syndrome?

    a. del (4p)
    b. del (5p)
    c. del (21p)
    d. del (Xp)

12–24. Which specific deletion is associated with Wolf-Hirschorn syndrome?

    a. 2q
    b. 4p
    c. 6q
    d. 8p

12–25. Shprintzen and DiGeorge phenotypes are associated with which karyotype?

    a. 2q11.2
    b. 20q11.2
    c. 22q11.2
    d. 12q11.2

12–26. Which of the following chromosomes is generally NOT involved in Robertsonian translocation?

    a. 1
    b. 13
    c. 14
    d. 21

12–27. In the event of a 14/21 translocation in the father, what is the chance of having a child with Down syndrome?

    a. 1 to 2%
    b. 5%
    c. 15%
    d. 50%

12–28. Approximately what percentage of couples with recurrent pregnancy loss will have either a balanced Robertsonian or reciprocal translocation?

    a. <5
    b. 10
    c. 25
    d. 50

12–29. In which of the following chromosomal inversion types does the inverted segment contain material from only one arm and does not contain the centromere?

    a. pericentric
    b. paracentric
    c. unicentric
    d. monocentric

12–30. Which of the following chromosomes is NOT typically involved with mosaicism resulting from a partial correction of a meiotic error?

    a. 2
    b. 9
    c. 16
    d. 22

12–31. Which of the following is NOT a characteristic of autosomal dominant inheritance?

    a. a single copy of the mutant gene is present
    b. horizontal transmission
    c. no skipped generations
    d. 50% chance of transmission to the offspring

12–32. What is the mechanism by which some autosomal dominant diseases appear to occur at earlier ages with subsequent generations?

    a. penetrance
    b. imprinting
    c. variable expressivity
    d. anticipation

12–33. Which of the following conditions is NOT inherited in an autosomal dominant fashion?

    a. achondroplasia
    b. adult polycystic kidney disease
    c. Marfan syndrome
    d. cystic fibrosis

12–34. Which of the following is NOT an autosomal recessive disease?

    a. Tay-Sachs disease
    b. congenital adrenal hyperplasia
    c. myotonic dystrophy
    d. sickle-cell anemia

12–35. Which of the following is an X-linked disease?

    a. von Willebrand disease
    b. neurofibromatosis
    c. Fabry disease
    d. Tay-Sachs disease

12–36. Mothers with phenylketonuria (PKU) are at increased risk of having children with which of the following disorders?

    a. hydrocephaly
    b. spina bifida
    c. skeletal dysplasia
    d. mental retardation

12–37. What proportion of genes do first cousins share?

    a. 1/2
    b. 1/4
    c. 1/8
    d. 1/16

12–38. What is the risk of having anomalous children result from incest (brother-sister or parent-child)?

    a. 1 to 5%
    b. 10 to 15%
    c. 25 to 30%
    d. 35 to 40%

12–39. Which of the following is an example of an X-linked dominant disorder?

    a. vitamin D-resistant rickets
    b. hemophilia A
    c. hemophilia B
    d. muscular dystrophy

12–40. Which of the following trinucleotide repeats is associated with the fragile X gene (FMR-1)?

    a. CGG
    b. CAG
    c. GCT
    d. GGG

12–41. What percentage of females with full mutations for fragile X syndrome will have some form of mental retardation?

    a. 5
    b. 25
    c. 50
    d. 100

12–42. Which of the following characteristics is NOT a usual manifestation of the fragile X syndrome in affected males?

    a. autism
    b. macro-orchidism
    c. mental retardation
    d. short stature

12–43. What is the best method for detection of both the size of the trinucleotide expansion and methylation of the fragile X gene?

    a. fluorescence in situ hybridization (FISH)
    b. cytogenetic analysis
    c. polymerase chain reaction (PCR)
    d. restriction endonuclease digestion and Southern blot

12–44. Which of the following X-linked conditions is an example of a trinucleotide repeat disorder?

    a. myotonic dystrophy
    b. hemophilia A
    c. hemophilia B
    d. Hunter syndrome

12–45. The gene that contains the unstable trinucleotide repeat (ACG) and is responsible for myotonic dystrophy is located on what chromosome?

    a. X
    b. Y
    c. 9
    d. 21

12–46. What is the mechanism by which the expression of a particular disease is dependent on whether the mutant gene was of paternal or maternal origin?

    a. penetrance
    b. imprinting
    c. uniparental disomy
    d. anticipation

12–47. Angelman and Prader-Willi syndromes are due to imprinting of which chromosome?

    a. 5
    b. 10
    c. 15
    d. 20

12–48. What is the mechanism by which both members of one chromosome pair are inherited from the same parent?

    a. imprinting
    b. variable expressivity
    c. uniparental disomy
    d. anticipation

12–49. Which of the following is a mitochondrial genetic disease?

    a. myoclonic epilepsy with ragged red fibers
    b. Leigh syndrome
    c. pigmentary retinopathy
    d. all of the above

12–50. Which of the following is transmitted via multifactorial inheritance?

    a. Marfan syndrome
    b. Fabry syndrome
    c. neurofibromatosis
    d. neural-tube defect

12–51. Which of the following conditions may be prevented by preconceptional folic acid supplementation?

    a. urogenital defects
    b. cleft lip
    c. fragile X syndrome
    d. neural-tube defects

12–52. Folic acid and 5,10-methylene tetra-hydrofolate reductase (MTHFR) 677 C→T mutations are associated with neural-tube defects AND

    a. renal abnormalities
    b. gastrointestinal defects
    c. cardiac disease
    d. musculoskeletal defects

12–53. What is the approximate number of base pairs in the human genome?

    a. 1 million
    b. 3 million
    c. 1 billion
    d. 3 billion

12–54. Approximately what percentage of the genome encodes genes?

    a. <1
    b. 10
    c. 25
    d. 50

12–55. What are the multiple coding sequences within a gene called?

    a. exons
    b. introns
    c. promoters
    d. demoters

12–56. Which of the following diseases is caused by a single mutation?

    a. cystic fibrosis
    b. myotonic dystrophy
    c. diabetes mellitus
    d. sickle-cell anemia

12–57. Fluorescence in situ hybridization (FISH) is used to detect which of the following?

    a. new mutations
    b. aneuploidy
    c. polyploidy
    d. fragile X syndrome

12–58 Southern blotting is a technique used to identify which of the following?

    a. histones
    b. deoxyribonucleic acid (DNA)
    c. ribonucleic acid (RNA)
    d. proteins

12–59. What in vitro technique is used to synthesize large amounts of specific DNA sequences over a relatively short period of time?

    a. Southern blotting
    b. restriction endonuclease reaction
    c. polymerase chain reaction
    d. allele-specific oligonucleotide reaction

12–60. Approximately how many mutations have been shown to cause cystic fibrosis?

    a. 9
    b. 90
    c. 900
    d. 9000

13

Prenatal Diagnosis and Fetal Therapy

13–1. Which of the following approximates the incidence of major structural or functional abnormalities found in neonates?

    a. <1 %
    b. 2 to 3%
    c. 5 to 8%
    d. 10 to 12%

13–2. Which of the following is NOT currently used for fetal therapy?

    a. cordocentesis
    b. fetal tissue biopsy
    c. stem cell transplantation
    d. vesicoamnionic shunting

13–3. In women with no obstetrical or family history of aneuploidy, which of the following is the most powerful maternal predictor of aneuploidy?

    a. age
    b. race
    c. parity
    d. socioeconomic status

13–4. Approximately what percentage of all conceptuses are aneuploid?

    a. 5
    b. 10
    c. 25
    d. 50

13–5. What percentage of stillbirths and neonatal deaths are attributable to chromosomal abnormalities?

    a. 1 to 3
    b. 5 to 7
    c. 10 to 12
    d. 15 to 20

13–6. Your patient has just spontaneously aborted a 7-week gestation. You counsel her that aneuploidy accounts for approximately what percentage of first-trimester abortion?

    a. 30
    b. 50
    c. 70
    d. 90

13–7. The fetal death rate following amniocentesis approximates which of the following?

    a. 1:100
    b. 1:200
    c. 1:400
    d. 1:500

13–8. Women with which of the following characteristics should be offered amniocentesis for fetal karyotyping?

    a. previous child was 47,XYY
    b. twin gestation regardless of maternal age
    c. will be 35 years or older at time of delivery
    d. prior history of 3 first-trimester spontaneous abortions

13–9. At term, what is the risk of delivering an aneuploid fetus in a 35-year-old woman?

    a. 1:50
    b. 1:100
    c. 1:200
    d. 1:400

13–10. What is the recurrence risk of trisomy, either the same involved chromosome or different, in a young mother who had a previous pregnancy complicated by an autosomal trisomy?

    a. 1%
    b. 3%
    c. 5%
    d. 10%

13–11. What is the approximate recurrence risk of structural abnormalities that are multifactorial in etiology?

    a. 0.5%
    b. 1%
    c. 2 to 3%
    d. 10 to 15%

13–12. Your 25-year-old newly pregnant patient informs you that her cousin was born with anencephaly, which has a multifactorial etiology. How do you counsel her regarding her fetus' risk for this abnormality?

    a. is greater than that of the general population
    b. warrants pregnancy termination
    c. warrants amniocentesis at 14 to 16 weeks
    d. warrants MSAFP level measurement at 16 weeks

13–13. Isolated fetal structural defects are most commonly found in which of the following organs?

    a. liver
    b. heart
    c. bladder
    d. neural tube

13–14. Your patient's first child had an atrioventricular defect. You counsel her that the risk of recurrence of the same defect in future pregnancies is which of the following?

    a. 20%
    b. 40%
    c. 60%
    d. 80%

13–15. Additionally, you counsel the patient in Question 14 that fetal ultrasonography and echocardiography should be performed in future pregnancies at what gestational age?

    a. 6 to 8 weeks
    b. 10 to 12 weeks
    c. 20 to 22 weeks
    d. 26 to 28 weeks

13–16. Your newly pregnant patient informs you that her sister was born with spina bifida. You counsel her which of the following regarding her fetus' risk for this abnormality?

   a. risk is 10 to 15%
   b. risk equals that of the general population
   c. warrants maternal serum alpha-fetoprotein (MSAFP) level measurement
   d. warrants MSAFP level measurement plus fetal ultrasonographic examination

13–17. Which of the following has NOT been associated with an increased risk of fetal neural-tube defects?

   a. concurrent trisomy 13
   b. poorly controlled diabetes
   c. first-trimester acetaminophen use
   d. high maternal fever early in gestation

13–18. Exposure to which of the following drugs is associated with an increased risk of fetal neural-tube defects?

   a. carbamazepine
   b. isotretinoin
   c. valproic acid
   d. all of the above

13–19. The most common hemoglobinopathy in the U.S. is found among persons belonging to which ethnic or geographic background?

   a. Mediterranean
   b. Middle Eastern
   c. Southeast Asian
   d. African American

13–20. Individuals of Jewish ancestry are at increased risk for which of the following diseases?

   a. Canavan
   b. Gaucher
   c. Tay-Sachs
   d. all of the above

13–21. Which of the following fetal structures is NOT involved in the synthesis of alpha-fetoprotein (AFP)?

   a. liver
   b. yolk sac
   c. bone marrow
   d. gastrointestinal tract

13–22. AFP can be found in which of the following body fluids?

   a. fetal urine
   b. fetal serum
   c. maternal serum
   d. all of the above

13–23. At which gestational age is the highest level of amnionic fluid AFP observed?

   a. 7 weeks
   b. 11 weeks
   c. 13 weeks
   d. 17 weeks

13–24. At which gestational age is the highest level of MSAFP observed?

   a. 10 weeks
   b. 14 weeks
   c. 18 weeks
   d. 22 weeks

13–25. Levels of MSAFP are influenced by which of the following maternal factors?

   a. race
   b. diabetic status
   c. maternal weight
   d. all of the above

13–26. In screening your patient's fetus for neural-tube defects at 16 weeks gestation, you obtain an MSAFP result which is 3.0 MoM. Your patient has no history indicating an increased risk for this defect. Which of the following is the next best step in her management?

   a. repeat MSAFP level measurement
   b. amniocentesis for fetal karyotyping
   c. amniocentesis for amnionic fluid AFP level measurement
   d. ultrasonography and amniocentesis for amnionic AFP level measurement

13–27. Which of the following accounts for the largest portion of elevated MSAFP levels in the absence of fetal anomaly?

   a. fetal death
   b. maternal obesity
   c. multiple gestation
   d. incorrect gestational dating

13–28. Which of the following is NOT a condition associated with an elevated MSAFP level?

   a. omphalocoele
   b. cloacal extrophy
   c. oligohydramnios
   d. complete molar pregnancy

13–29. In screening your patient's fetus for neural-tube defects at 16 weeks gestation, you obtain an MSAFP result that is 4.0 MoM. Your patient has no history indicating an increased risk for this defect. Which of the following is the next best step in her management?

   a. ultrasonographic examination
   b. repeat MSAFP measurement
   c. amniocentesis for fetal karyotyping
   d. amniocentesis for amnionic fluid AFP level measurement

13–30. Which of the following fetal cranial ultrasonographic findings is NOT associated with neural-tube defects?

   a. lemon sign
   b. banana sign
   c. cabbage sign
   d. ventriculomegaly

13–31. Open spine defects are associated with specific cranial lesions in what percentage of cases?

   a. 5
   b. 33
   c. 67
   d. 99

13–32. In screening your patient's fetus for neural-tube defects at 17 weeks gestation, you obtain an MSAFP result of 5.0 MoM. Your patient has no history that points to an increased risk for this defect. Ultrasonography reveals a viable singleton gestation with no structural anomalies, normal amnionic fluid index, and fetal measurements consistent with gestational age. Which of the following is the next best step in her management?

   a. reassurance
   b. repeat MSAFP level measurement
   c. amniocentesis for fetal karyotyping
   d. amniocentesis for amnionic fluid AFP level measurement

13–33. In a woman with an elevated MSAFP level and elevated amnionic fluid AFP, what further testing should be performed on the amnionic fluid?

   a. Δ OD 450
   b. fetal fibronectin assay
   c. C-reactive protein assay
   d. acetylcholinesterase assay

13–34. Unexplained elevated abnormal AFP levels are associated with which of the following complications?

   a. fetal death
   b. low birthweight

   c. preterm rupture of membranes
   d. all of the above

13–35. Which of the following maternal serum analytes is NOT included in the "triple screen" for Down syndrome?

   a. AFP
   b. placental lactogen
   c. unconjugated estriol
   d. chorionic gonadotropin

13–36. What percentage of fetuses with Down syndrome can be detected in women older than 35 years using the triple screen?

   a. 50 to 55
   b. 65 to 70
   c. 75 to 80
   d. 90 to 95

13–37. Which of the following is a maternal serum marker used in first-trimester Down syndrome screening?

   a. placental lactogen
   b. acetylcholinesterase
   c. pregnancy-associated plasma protein A
   d. all of the above

13–38. Ultrasonographic measurement of which of the following is commonly used in first-trimester Down syndrome screening protocols?

   a. femur length
   b. intraorbital distance
   c. nuchal translucency
   d. placental sonolucencies

13–39. Cystic fibrosis is inherited via which genetic transmission pattern?

   a. imprinting
   b. X-linked
   c. autosomal recessive
   d. autosomal dominant

13–40. Antenatal cystic fibrosis screening should be offered when both members of a couple are from which of the following ethnic groups?

   a. Southeast Asian
   b. Ashkenazi Jewish
   c. African American
   d. Hispanic American

13–41. Which of the following is the most common cause of familial mental retardation?

   a. trisomy 13
   b. Down syndrome
   c. 47,XXY genotype
   d. fragile X syndrome

13–42. Which of the following patients need NOT be offered screening for fragile X syndrome?

a. males with unexplained mental retardation
b. females with unexplained mental retardation
c. first-degree relative of patients with known fragile X syndrome
d. first-degree relatives of patients with unexplained mental retardation

13–43. What is the most rational initial approach when a major fetal malformation is discovered using ultrasonography?

a. MSAFP testing
b. fetal karyotyping
c. parental karyotyping
d. serial ultrasonographic examinations

13–44. What is the most rational initial approach when two minor structural abnormalities are discovered using ultrasonography?

a. MSAFP testing
b. fetal karyotyping
c. parental karyotyping
d. serial ultrasonographic examinations

13–45. Which of the following changes in the fetal nasal bone have been used as a marker for Down syndrome?

a. absence
b. increased size
c. decreased size
d. increased opacification

13–46. Which of the following is a risk associated with second-trimester amniocentesis?

a. chorioamnionitis
b. amnionic fluid leakage
c. fetal needle stick injury
d. all of the above

13–47. Higher rates of which of the following is a disadvantage of early amniocentesis compared with second-trimester amniocentesis?

a. fetal death
b. foot deformities
c. membrane rupture
d. all of the above

13–48. Increased risk of which of the following is associated with chorionic villous sampling performed after 9 weeks gestation?

a. fetal death
b. limb-reduction defects
c. oromandibular defects
d. cavernous hemangiomas

13–49. What is an advantage of transcervical chorionic villous sampling compared with second-trimester amniocentesis?

a. lower fetal death rate
b. test results received at an earlier gestational age
c. able to perform even if vaginal bleeding is present
d. able to perform on an extremely anteverted or retroverted uterus

13–50. Which of the following procedures has the highest fetal death rate?

a. second-trimester amniocentesis
b. transcervical chorionic villus sampling
c. transabdominal chorionic villus sampling
d. all have approximately equivalent rates

13–51. In which of the following situations would cordocentesis be appropriate?

a. red cell alloimmunization
b. nonimmune fetal hydrops
c. suspected primary fetal CMV infection
d. all of the above

13–52. Fetal tissue biopsy has been used for antenatal diagnosis of which of the following diseases?

a. muscular dystrophy
b. epidermolysis bullosa
c. mitochondrial myopathy
d. all of the above

13–53. Preimplantation genetic analysis techniques can use genetic material from which of the following?

a. blastocyst
b. first polar body
c. second polar body
d. all of the above

13–54. Which of the following has NOT been shown to be an effective method for administering medications for fetal medical therapy?

a. injection into fetal buttock
b. injection into amnionic fluid
c. injection into the umbilical cord
d. oral administration to the mother

13–55. Fetal medical therapy is LEAST likely to show beneficial effects in which of the following fetal conditions?

a. cardiac arrhythmias
b. maternal–fetal infection
c. posterior urethral valves
d. congenital adrenal hyperplasia

13–56. In assessing the usefulness of fetal surgery to correct or ameliorate major malformations, which of the following should be considered?

   a. maternal risks
   b. natural history and prognosis of the malformation
   c. associated high incidence of genetic abnormalities
   d. all of the above

13–57. Of the following conditions, which cannot be ameliorated by antepartum vesicoamnionic shunting?

   a. urethral atresia
   b. renal cystic dysplasia
   c. posterior urethral valves
   d. ureteropelvic junction obstruction

13–58. Thoracoamnionic shunting is performed to prevent which of the following?

   a. pectus carinatum
   b. congenital scoliosis
   c. pulmonary hypoplasia
   d. left ventricular hypertrophy

13–59. Which of the following statements in advocacy of antenatal repair of congenital diaphragmatic hernia is true?

   a. Less than 30% of neonates survive postnatal hernia repair.
   b. Antenatal surgery is associated with only a 15% incidence of preterm birth.
   c. Several antenatal repair procedures are associated with improved neonatal survival.
   d. None of the above are true.

13–60. Pulmonary sequestration and congenital cystic adenomatoid does NOT result in which of the following?

   a. fetal hydrops
   b. pleural effusion
   c. oligohydramnios
   d. pulmonary hypoplasia

13–61. Antenatal repair of spina bifida has been shown to be associated with which of the following?

   a. minimal maternal morbidity
   b. improved lower extremity mobility
   c. reduced need for ventriculoperitoneal shunt placement
   d. none of the above

14

Teratology, Drugs, and Other Medications

14–1. What percentage of children in the United States are born with a major structural malformation detectable at birth?

   a. 1
   b. 3
   c. 5
   d. 7

14–2. Approximately what percentage of children have birth defects identified by their teen years?

   a. 5%
   b. 10%
   c. 15%
   d. 25%

14–3. What proportion of patients seeking counseling for birth defects have a genetic condition?

    a. <one third
    b. one half
    c. two thirds
    d. three fourths

14–4. What percentage of congenital anomalies (structural or functional) are caused by teratogens?

    a. 10
    b. 25
    c. 50
    d. 75

14–5. What is the average number of prescriptions, other than for vitamins, received by women during pregnancy in the United States?

    a. 1
    b. 3
    c. 5
    d. 7

14–6. What are identical defects with different etiologies called?

    a. hadegens
    b. parallel dysmorphisms
    c. phenocopies
    d. polymorphisms

14–7. Which of the following represents the embryonic period?

    a. fertilization through week 6
    b. fertilization through week 10
    c. week 2 through week 8
    d. week 1 through week 12

14–8. Which of the following represents the fetal period?

    a. implantation through week 8
    b. implantation through week 12
    c. week 9 until term
    d. week 12 until term

14–9. Damage to a large number of cells during the preimplantation period of development will likely result in which of the following?

    a. cell division to compensate for lost cells
    b. death of the embryo
    c. major structural malformations
    d. none of the above

14–10. Which of the following periods is most critical with regard to structural malformations?

    a. prefertilization
    b. zygote (ovum)
    c. embryonic
    d. fetal

14–11. By how many weeks of gestation is formation of the heart complete?

    a. 8
    b. 10
    c. 12
    d. 14

14–12. To establish teratogenicity, which of the following criteria must be met?

    a. agent must cross the placenta
    b. biologically plausible cause and effect
    c. consistent findings between epidemiological studies
    d. all of the above

14–13. What minimum relative risk supports an epidemiological link between a suspected teratogen and a birth defect?

    a. 1.5
    b. 2.0
    c. 3.0
    d. 4.0

14–14. Disruption of metabolic pathways requiring folic acid cause birth defects in all of the following structural areas EXCEPT

    a. heart
    b. neural tube
    c. lip and palate
    d. reproductive tract

14–15. Periconceptual folate supplementation lowers the rate of birth defects in mothers taking which type of medication?

    a. anticonvulsants
    b. corticosteroids
    c. hypoglycemics including insulin
    d. phenothiazines

14–16. Which of the following enzymes is needed to detoxify the oxidative intermediates of several potentially teratogenic drugs?

    a. areneoxidase
    b. aromatase
    c. epoxide hydrolase
    d. folate dehydrogenase

14–17. Which are the special genes that play an essential role in the establishment of positional identity of structures along the body axis?

   a. chronomorphic genes
   b. homeobox genes
   c. sequential transcription genes
   d. vertebrate morphometric genes

14–18. Paternal exposure to which of the following is associated with an increase in early pregnancy loss?

   a. Agent Orange
   b. atomic radiation
   c. pesticides
   d. recreational drugs

14–19. Approximately how many drugs or substances are suspected or proven teratogens?

   a. 30
   b. 60
   c. 300
   d. 600

14–20. Which of the following is associated with mental retardation, cardiac defects, joint defects, and craniofacial anomalies?

   a. alcohol
   b. amphetamines
   c. lysergic acid
   d. heroin

14–21. What is the safe daily threshold dose of alcohol during pregnancy?

   a. 1 oz
   b. 3 oz
   c. 5 oz
   d. not established

14–22. Fetal alcohol syndrome is reliably diagnosed prenatally by what method?

   a. amniocentesis
   b. cannot be diagnosed prenatally
   c. history of heavy alcohol consumption
   d. ultrasonography

14–23. Which group of defects are seen in infants of epileptic mothers at a rate almost 10 times that of the general population?

   a. facial clefts
   b. digital abnormalities
   c. cardiac anomalies
   d. gastrointestinal strictures

14–24. Anticonvulsant medications are teratogens via what mechanism(s)?

   a. accumulation of free oxide radicals in fetal tissues
   b. lowered fetal folate levels
   c. both of the above
   d. unknown

14–25. What is the estimated risk of spina bifida from first-trimester valproic acid exposure?

   a. 1 to 2%
   b. 5 to 10%
   c. 20 to 25%
   d. 30 to 40%

14–26. Which of the following abnormalities is NOT an effect of fetal warfarin exposure?

   a. midfacial hypoplasia
   b. stippled bone epiphyses
   c. ventral wall defects
   d. cerebral malformations

14–27. Which of the following antihypertensives is associated with congenital hypocalvaria, renal tubular dysgenesis, oligohydramnios, and neonatal hypotension?

   a. sodium nitroprusside
   b. enalapril
   c. clonidine
   d. labetalol

14–28. Which of the following is true of high doses of vitamin A ingested during pregnancy?

   a. It is a potent teratogen.
   b. Supplementation of greater than the recommended daily allowance is not advised.
   c. It increases the early pregnancy loss rate.
   d. It should be given at high doses only to treat related maternal diseases.

14–29. Which craniofacial defect is most strongly associated with use of isotretinoin?

   a. malformed or absent ears
   b. hypotelorism
   c. hypoplastic upper lip
   d. microphthalmia

14–30. Approximately what percentage of fetuses exposed in utero to isotretinoin will have at least one major malformation?

   a. 5
   b. 20
   c. 30
   d. 50

14–31. Which of the following compounds is highly teratogenic and has been detected in serum almost 3 years after cessation of therapy?

    a. isotretinoin
    b. etretinate
    c. tretinoin
    d. vitamin A

14–32. What is the approximate relative risk of birth defects with use of topical tretinoin for acne?

    a. 1
    b. 3
    c. 5
    d. 7

14–33. During what period of gestation can exposure of a female fetus to exogenous androgens cause complete masculinization?

    a. 2 to 5 weeks
    b. 7 to 12 weeks
    c. 14 to 18 weeks
    d. 22 to 24 weeks

14–34. Exposure to which of the following hormones is most likely to cause virilization of the female fetus?

    a. danazol
    b. medroxyprogesterone acetate
    c. norethindrone
    d. norgestimate

14–35. What is the risk of developing vaginal clear-cell adenocarcinoma following in utero exposure to diethylstilbestrol (DES)?

    a. 1 in 10
    b. 1 in 100
    c. 1 in 1000
    d. 1 in 10,000

14–36. In utero exposure to DES causes which of the following?

    a. male infertility
    b. testicular cancer
    c. uterine malformations
    d. vaginal duplication

14–37. Which antineoplastic drug is most commonly associated with missing or hypoplastic digits on the hands and feet?

    a. aminopterin
    b. cyclophosphamide

    c. methotrexate
    d. platinum

14–38. Which antineoplastic agent is associated with severe cranial and limb abnormalities?

    a. bleomycin
    b. tamoxifen citrate
    c. methotrexate
    d. platinum

14–39. What is the most typical problem seen with tetracycline ingestion during the fetal period of gestation?

    a. alopecia
    b. stained deciduous teeth
    c. hypoplastic fingernails and toenails
    d. peeling and discolored skin

14–40. Which of the following antimicrobials given to the mother near delivery may result in significant hyperbilirubinemia in the preterm neonate?

    a. penicillins
    b. cephalosporins
    c. macrolides
    d. sulfonamides

14–41. Which of the following antimicrobials is a folate antagonist but not associated with adverse fetal effects?

    a. trimethoprim
    b. nitrofurantoin
    c. tetracycline
    d. erythromycin

14–42. Which of the following antifungal agents has a possible association with conjoined twins in humans?

    a. nystatin
    b. clotrimazole
    c. amphotericin B
    d. griseofulvin

14–43. Which of the following antiviral drugs, used as an aerosol inhalation agent in intensive care nurseries, consistently produces hydrocephalus and limb abnormalities in rodents?

    a. acyclovir
    b. amantadine
    c. famciclovir
    d. ribavirin

14-44. A 31-year-old gravida 2, para 1 presents for perinatal care at 8 weeks gestation. She is on chloroquine for treatment of systemic lupus erythematosus. How will you counsel her regarding fetal risks from this medication?

    a. Increased risk of cardiac anomalies.
    b. Increased risk of early pregnancy loss.
    c. Increased risk of pulmonary hypoplasia.
    d. Poses increased risk to the fetus.

14-45. There is a clear dose-dependent relationship between tobacco smoking and which of the following?

    a. decreased global intelligence scores
    b. fetal growth restriction
    c. prematurity
    d. pregnancy-induced hypertension

14-46. Fetuses carrying an allele for a rare polymorphism in the transforming growth factor gene are at increased risk of which of the following congenital malformations if their mothers smoke?

    a. cardiac anomalies
    b. cleft lip and/or palate
    c. limb deformities
    d. spina bifida

14-47. According to the Centers for Disease Control and Prevention (CDC), what proportion of pregnancies involve cocaine use?

    a. 1 in 500
    b. 1 in 200
    c. 1 in 50
    d. 1 in 20

14-48. Which of the following complications is increased fourfold with maternal cocaine use?

    a. adult respiratory distress syndrome
    b. HELLP [hemolysis (H), elevated liver enzymes (EL), and low platelets (LP)] syndrome
    c. placental abruption
    d. preeclampsia

14-49. Which of these abnormalities is increased by maternal cocaine abuse?

    a. cardiac anomalies
    b. developmental delay
    c. urinary tract anomalies
    d. all of the above

14-50. The drug thalidomide, notorious for causing severe limb reduction defects, and once again available, was originally used during what years?

    a. 1946 to 1950
    b. 1956 to 1960
    c. 1966 to 1970
    d. 1976 to 1980

14-51. Which of the following fetal malformations is NOT strongly associated with thalidomide exposure?

    a. cardiac abnormalities
    b. duodenal atresia
    c. limb phocomelia
    d. renal agenesis

14-52. In order to limit fetal exposure to mercury, the Food and Drug Administration (FDA) recommends that women limit total fish or shellfish consumption to 12 ounces per week. Limitation of which fish in particular is recommended?

    a. bass
    b. halibut
    c. sturgeon
    d. tuna

14-53. In what percentage of U.S. pregnancies are salicylates and/or acetaminophen used?

    a. 5
    b. 15
    c. 25
    d. 50

14-54. Which nonsteroidal anti-inflammatory drug, when used as a tocolytic agent, can result in constriction of the fetal ductus arteriosus and cause pulmonary hypertension in the neonate?

    a. ibuprofen
    b. indomethacin
    c. naproxen
    d. piroxicam

14-55. Which narcotic analgesic is most likely to be associated with a fetal sinusoidal heart rate pattern?

    a. butorphanol
    b. codeine
    c. meperidine
    d. morphine

14-56. Your patient suffers from migraine headaches. She has a history of irregular menses and used sumatriptan (a vasoconstrictor) on several occasions before realizing she was pregnant. Ultrasonography shows an intrauterine pregnancy of 9 weeks gestation. How do counsel her about risks of this medication?

a. increased risk of spontaneous abortion
b. increased risk of limb reduction deformities
c. decreased amnionic fluid volume with continued regular use
d. no increased risks identified to date

14–57. What is the association between maternal exposure to anesthetic agents and muscle relaxants during surgery and adverse fetal effects?

a. weak increased risk
b. definite increased risk
c. no increased risk
d. no studies have been done

14–58. What is the incidence of deep vein thrombosis or pulmonary embolus in pregnancy, and therefore, fetal exposure to anticoagulants?

a. 1 in 500
b. 1 in 1000
c. 1 in 5000
d. 1 in 10,000

14–59. What is the risk of low-molecular-weight heparin use in pregnancy?

a. fetal malformations
b. low birthweight
c. maternal osteopenia
d. all of the above

14–60. Which of the following antihypertensives could theoretically cause accumulation of cyanide in the fetal liver?

a. labetolol
b. methyldopa
c. nifedipine
d. nitroprusside

14–61. Fetal exposure to calcium-channel antagonists has been inconclusively implicated as a cause of which of the following?

a. anencephaly and spina bifida
b. cardiac malformations
c. limb defects
d. urinary tract agenesis

14–62. Thiazide diuretics are not associated with congenital anomalies but, if given near delivery, may cause what complication in the neonate?

a. apnea
b. hypoglycemia
c. thrombocytopenia
d. seizures

14–63. Which of the following diuretics has a theoretical potential for causing feminization of male fetuses due to its anti-androgenic properties?

a. spironolactone
b. ethacrynic acid
c. acetazolamide
d. hydrochlorothiazide

14–64. Which of the following antimicrobials crosses the placenta minimally to the fetus when given to the mother?

a. penicillin
b. erythromycin
c. cephalosporins
d. tetracyclines

14–65. Which of the following antimicrobials is an apparently safe alternative to aminoglycosides?

a. aztreonam
b. azithromycin
c. sulfonamide
d. clindamycin

14–66. Which of the following antimicrobials reportedly causes irreversible arthropathy in some animals and should therefore be reserved for treatment of multidrug resistant infections?

a. fluoroquinolones
b. vancomycin
c. nitrofurantoin
d. sulfonamides

14–67. In 2001, the American College of Obstetricians and Gynecologists (ACOG) recommended which antibacterial agent for postexposure maternal anthrax prophylaxis?

a. azithromycin
b. ciprofloxacin
c. erythromycin
d. vancomycin

14–68. Which of the following antiviral drugs used to treat HIV infection is teratogenic?

a. amprenavir
b. didanosine (ddI)
c. zidovudine
d. none of the above

14–69. Which antiviral drug, used to prevent or modify influenza, is a teratogen in animals but not yet studied sufficiently in humans?

a. acyclovir
b. amantadine
c. ganciclovir
d. ribavirin

14–70. Which of the following antiparasitic agents was NOT shown to cause increased adverse effects in over 1700 infants exposed in the first trimester (Piper and colleagues, 1993)?

    a. metronidazole
    b. lindane
    c. pyrimethamine
    d. spiramycin

14–71. Which of the following should NOT be used as first-line therapy for pediculosis pubis during pregnancy due to suboptimal efficacy and potential maternal nervous system toxicity with excessive use?

    a. crotamiton
    b. lindane
    c. piperonyl butoxide
    d. pyrethrins

14–72. Which of the following antiasthmatic drugs has been shown to cause adverse fetal effects in humans?

    a. albuterol
    b. cromolyn
    c. corticosteroids
    d. none of the above

14–73. Which antiarrhythmic drug should NOT be used in pregnancy due to the potential for fetal and neonatal hypothyroidism?

    a. amiodarone
    b. bretylium
    c. diltiazem
    d. procainamide

14–74. Which is problematic in assessing the efficacy and safety of herbal remedies?

    a. They are not regulated as prescriptions or over-the-counter drugs.
    b. The identity and quantity of all ingredients is not defined.
    c. There are limited human and animal studies.
    d. All of the above are true.

14–75. Which herbal remedies can increase intraoperative bleeding?

    a. echinacea and ephedra
    b. garlic and ginkgo
    c. kava and valerian
    d. St. John's wort and black cohosh

14–76. Which herbal abortifacient can cause severe liver and renal toxicity, disseminated intravascular coagulation, and maternal death?

    a. chamomile
    b. glycyrrhiza (licorice)
    c. pennyroyal
    d. phytoestrogen

14–77. What is the association between oral contraceptive use during the first trimester and congenital malformations?

    a. slightly increased risk
    b. threefold increased risk
    c. no increased risk
    d. insufficient information available

14–78. Which of the following psychotropic drugs has a possible association with fetal cardiovascular anomalies, particularly Ebstein anomaly?

    a. amitriptyline
    b. imipramine
    c. lithium
    d. chlorpromazine

14–79. Which of the following antidepressants belongs to the selective serotonin re-uptake inhibitor (SSRI) class and appears safe for use in pregnancy?

    a. lithium
    b. nortriptyline
    c. midazolam
    d. fluoxetine

14–80. What percentage of women in the United States use marijuana or hashish?

    a. 2
    b. 5
    c. 10
    d. 15

14–81. Which of the following is NOT more common in the infants and children of narcotic-addicted women?

    a. fetal malformations
    b. smaller-than-average head circumference in children
    c. sudden infant death syndrome
    d. vomiting and diarrhea in neonates

15

Antepartum Assessment

15–1. What is the goal of antepartum fetal surveillance?

    a. prevent fetal deaths
    b. prevent early deliveries
    c. increase fees for obstetricians
    d. delay delivery until lung maturity achieved

15–2. What is the negative-predictive value of antenatal fetal testing?

    a. 10%
    b. 40%
    c. 70%
    d. ~100%

15–3. What is the positive-predictive value of antenatal fetal testing?

    a. <10%
    b. 10 to 40%
    c. 40 to 80%
    d. 80 to ~100%

15–4. At what gestational age does passive, unstimulated movement begin?

    a. 3 weeks
    b. 7 weeks
    c. 11 weeks
    d. 15 weeks

15–5. At which gestational age do fetuses begin to exhibit rest–activity cycles?

    a. <10 weeks
    b. 10 to 20 weeks
    c. 20 to 30 weeks
    d. 30 to 40 weeks

15–6. All of the following have been used to describe fetal behavioral states EXCEPT

    a. breathing
    b. heart rate

    c. eye movements
    d. body movements

15–7. Quiescent sleep is described by which of the following behavioral states?

    a. 1F
    b. 2F
    c. 3F
    d. 4F

15–8. Fetuses spend most of their time in which of the two states?

    a. 1F and 2F
    b. 1F and 4F
    c. 2F and 3F
    d. 3F and 4F

15–9. What is the mean length of the quiet or inactive state for term fetuses (i.e., "sleep cyclicity")?

    a. 11 min
    b. 23 min
    c. 75 min
    d. 105 min

15–10. What is the range of normal weekly counts of fetal movement?

    a. 20 to 600
    b. 50 to 950
    c. 100 to 1000
    d. 200 to 1200

15–11. Using maternal perception to quantify fetal movement, the threshold for fetal well-being at term is which of the following?

    a. 10 movements in 1 hour
    b. 30 movements in 2 hours
    c. 100 movements in 1 day
    d. none of the above

15–12. Which of the following statements regarding fetal movement is true?

    a. Its highest rates are at term.
    b. It is affected by amnionic fluid volume.
    c. Maternal perception of movement generally correlates poorly with instrumental measurement.
    d. All of the above are true.

15–13. All of the following are descriptions of respiratory movements in the fetus EXCEPT

    a. gasping
    b. paradoxical breathing
    c. glossopharyngeal breathing
    d. irregular bursts of breathing

15–14. In normal fetuses, what is the length of time that fetal breathing movements may be totally absent?

    a. 20 min
    b. 60 min
    c. 120 min
    d. 200 min

15–15. Which of the following may affect fetal breathing movement rates?

    a. labor
    b. fetal hypoxia
    c. cigarette smoking
    d. all of the above

15–16. True statements regarding fetal breathing include which of the following?

    a. They are affected by sound.
    b. They are unaffected by maternal eating.
    c. The highest respiratory rates are at term.
    d. They are used in the assessment of the four fetal behavioral states.

15–17. Which of the following fetal activities is monitored during a contraction stress test?

    a. breathing
    b. eye movements
    c. heart rate
    d. body movements

15–18. In a contraction stress test, all of the following may be a source of contractions EXCEPT

    a. oxytocin
    b. fundal massage
    c. nipple stimulation
    d. spontaneous onset

15–19. What controls fetal heart rate acceleration?

    a. autonomic function at brainstem level
    b. aortic baroreceptor reflexes

    c. carotid baroreceptor reflexes
    d. humeral factors such as atrial natriuretic peptide

15–20. Fetal heart rate accelerations during the nonstress test are affected by which of the following?

    a. fetal lie
    b. fetal acidemia
    c. fetal sex
    d. all of the above

15–21. What is the American College of Obstetricians and Gynecologists' (ACOG) definition of a reactive nonstress test (NST)?

    a. 1 acceleration in 20 min
    b. 2 accelerations in 20 min
    c. 8 accelerations in 20 min
    d. 15 accelerations in 20 min

15–22. What is the associated risk of perinatal pathology for a fetus with a nonreactive nonstress test for 90 minutes?

    a. 10%
    b. 25%
    c. 50%
    d. 90%

15–23. Investigators advocate which nonstress testing schedule?

    a. daily
    b. once weekly
    c. twice weekly
    d. all of the above

15–24. Fetal death within 7 days of a normal nonstress test occurs most commonly with which indication for testing?

    a. postterm pregnancy
    b. gestational diabetes
    c. gestational hypertension
    d. fetal growth restriction

15–25. During acoustic stimulation testing, what fetal response is measured?

    a. breathing
    b. heart rate
    c. eye movements
    d. body movements

15–26. Which of the following is NOT a fetal biophysical variable used in the biophysical profile?

    a. heart rate
    b. breathing
    c. eye movement
    d. body movement

15–27. Which of the following best describes a biophysical score of 6?

    a. normal score
    b. acidotic score
    c. equivocal score
    d. abnormal score

15–28. The modified biophysical profile is described by which of the following?

    a. contraction stress test and Doppler umbilical artery velocimetry
    b. acoustic stimulation nonstress test and amnionic fluid index determination
    c. acoustic stimulation nonstress test and Doppler umbilical artery velocimetry
    d. none of the above

15–29. Which of the following results describes abnormal umbilical artery velocimetry?

    a. absent end-diastolic arterial flow
    b. reversed end-diastolic arterial flow
    c. systolic/diastolic ratio greater than the 95th percentile for gestational age
    d. all of the above

15–30. According to the ACOG, Doppler velocimetry may be beneficial in which of the following clinical situations?

    a. gestational diabetes
    b. postterm gestation
    c. fetal growth restriction
    d. antiphospholipid antibody syndrome

15–31. According to the ACOG, which of the following is considered the BEST test to evaluate fetal well-being?

    a. modified biophysical profile
    b. contraction stress test
    c. umbilical artery Doppler velocimetry
    d. none of the above

15–32. The most important consideration in deciding when to begin antepartum testing is which of the following?

    a. prognosis for neonatal survival
    b. type of maternal disease
    c. severity of maternal disease
    d. none of the above

16

Ultrasonography and Doppler

16–1. Abdominal ultrasonography is most commonly performed using transducers that generate which range of sound frequency?

    a. 1 to 3 mHz
    b. 3 to 5 mHz
    c. 5 to 7 mHz
    d. 7 to 9 mHz

16–2. What is the major biological hazard from fetal ultrasonography?

    a. none
    b. chromosomal breakage

    c. impaired neonatal hearing
    d. early spontaneous abortion

16–3. Several studies have shown the utility of fetal ultrasonography for which of the following?

    a. assist in aneuploidy detection
    b. decrease postterm delivery induction rate
    c. determine gestational age more accurately than the last menstrual period
    d. all of the above

16–4. According to the American Institute of Ultrasound in Medicine (AIUM), assessment of fetal anatomy is best performed no earlier than what gestational age?

    a. 14 weeks
    b. 18 weeks
    c. 22 weeks
    d. 26 weeks

16–5. According to AIUM, which of the following should be evaluated during a first-trimester ultrasound?

    a. fetal weight
    b. fetal presentation
    c. placental location
    d. maternal adnexal evaluation

16–6. With transabdominal ultrasonography, the gestational sac is reliably seen in the uterus by which gestational age?

    a. 4 weeks
    b. 5 weeks
    c. 6 weeks
    d. 7 weeks

16–7. With transvaginal ultrasonography, fetal cardiac motion is reliably seen by which gestational age?

    a. 4 weeks
    b. 5 weeks
    c. 6 weeks
    d. 7 weeks

16–8. A standard fetal ultrasonographic examination includes evaluation of which of the following?

    a. gallbladder
    b. large colon
    c. umbilical cord insertion
    d. hand and foot digit count

16–9. In determining gestational age between 14 and 26 weeks, which of the following is the most accurate parameter to measure?

    a. femur length
    b. biparietal diameter
    c. crown-rump length
    d. abdominal circumference

16–10. Which of the following ultrasonographic views is used to measure the biparietal diameter?

    a. transthalamic
    b. transcerebellar
    c. transventricular
    d. transhemispheric

16–11. Which of the following fetal measurements shows the greatest variation?

    a. femur length
    b. biparietal diameter
    c. crown-rump length
    d. abdominal circumference

16–12. During standard ultrasonographic examination, which of the following cranial structures is NOT routinely evaluated?

    a. cisterna magna
    b. pituitary gland
    c. choroid plexus
    d. lateral ventricles

16–13. What is the incidence of neural-tube defects in the United States?

    a. 0.8 per 1000
    b. 1.6 per 1000
    c. 8 per 1000
    d. 16 per 1000

16–14. Encephalocele is usually associated with which of the following?

    a. hepatomegaly
    b. hydrocephalus
    c. normal intelligence
    d. all of the above

16–15. Ultrasonographic findings of spina bifida and the lemon sign are suggestive of which malformation?

    a. anencephaly
    b. Budd-Chiari
    c. Arnold-Chiari I
    d. Arnold-Chiari II

16–16. Which of the following is used to describe an elongation and downward displacement of the cerebellum?

    a. lemon sign
    b. pickle sign
    c. melon sign
    d. banana sign

16–17. What is the average diameter in millimeters of the lateral ventricular atrium at 15 weeks' gestation and older?

    a. 2 to 4
    b. 6 to 8
    c. 10 to 12
    d. 14 to 16

16–18. A free-floating or dangling choroid plexus is suggestive of which of the following?

    a. hydrocephalus
    b. cerebral atrophy
    c. aqueductal stenosis
    d. choroid plexus cyst

16–19. Cystic hygroma is the result of which of the following?

   a. lymphatic obstruction
   b. meningeal herniation
   c. arterial aneurysm formation
   d. cystic degeneration of the sternocleidomastoid muscle

16–20. What percentage of cystic hygromas are associated with aneuploidy?

   a. 20 to 30
   b. 40 to 50
   c. 60 to 70
   d. 80 to 90

16–21. What is the most common chromosomal anomaly associated with cystic hygroma in second- or third-trimester fetuses?

   a. triploidy
   b. trisomy 18
   c. trisomy 21
   d. monosomy X

16–22. The lungs are best visualized beginning at which gestational age?

   a. 16 to 20 weeks
   b. 20 to 25 weeks
   c. 25 to 28 weeks
   d. 28 to 32 weeks

16–23. In greater than 90% of cases, congenital diaphragmatic hernias are located in which of the thoracic quadrants?

   a. left anterior
   b. left posterior
   c. right anterior
   d. right posterior

16–24. Which of the following is a specific ultrasonographic finding in fetuses with diaphragmatic hernia?

   a. cardiac displacement
   b. small abdominal circumference
   c. absence of intra-abdominal stomach bubble
   d. all of the above

16–25. What is the incidence of congenital cardiac malformation in newborns?

   a. 8 per 100
   b. 8 per 1000
   c. 8 per 10,000
   d. 8 per 100,000

16–26. What percentage of congenital heart defects are due to multifactorial or polygenic transmission?

   a. 10
   b. 33
   c. 67
   d. 90

16–27. Ultrasonographic examination identifies a hypoplastic left heart in your patient's fetus at 18 weeks' gestation. The next most appropriate management step includes which of the following?

   a. Doppler aortic arch velocimetry
   b. amniocentesis for fetal karyotyping
   c. cordocentesis to assess level of fetal anemia
   d. amniocentesis for acetylcholinesterase level measurement

16–28. The four-chamber view of the heart is seen transversely at which fetal body level?

   a. 4th rib
   b. T-8 vertebra
   c. immediately above the diaphragm
   d. branching of the main stem bronchus

16–29. Which of the following typically should NOT prompt fetal echocardiography?

   a. fetal arrhythmia
   b. maternal diabetes
   c. first-degree relative with heart defect
   d. elevated maternal serum alpha-fetoprotein level

16–30. Which of the following ultrasonographic findings has been most frequently associated with fetal heart defects?

   a. oligohydramnios
   b. mediastinal shift
   c. left-axis deviation
   d. raised left hemidiaphragm

16–31. The ultrasonographic detection rate of fetal heart defects in a low-risk population approximates which of the following?

   a. 15%
   b. 35%
   c. 65%
   d. 85%

16–32. Nonvisualization of the fetal stomach during an ultrasonographic examination is common in all of the following EXCEPT

   a. anencephaly
   b. esophageal atresia
   c. diaphragmatic hernia
   d. tracheoesophageal fistula

16–33. Which of the following is NOT associated with echogenic bowel seen ultrasonographically?

    a. trisomy 21
    b. cystic fibrosis
    c. thick meconium-stained fluid
    d. swallowed intra-amnionic blood

16–34. Gastroschisis is associated with which of the following?

    a. aneuploidy
    b. other bowel abnormalities
    c. poor postnatal survival
    d. all of the above

16–35. Which of the following is more likely to be associated with aneuploidy?

    a. anal atresia
    b. gastroschisis
    c. omphalocoele
    d. esophageal atresia

16–36. The "double-bubble" sign is an ultrasonographic finding of which of the following anomalies?

    a. cystic hygroma
    b. duodenal atresia
    c. aqueductal stenosis
    d. two-vessel umbilical cord

16–37. What percentage of fetuses with the "double-bubble" sign will have trisomy 21?

    a. 5
    b. 15
    c. 30
    d. 50

16–38. With which of the following anomalies is hydramnios NOT a typical associated finding?

    a. anal atresia
    b. anencephaly
    c. gastroschisis
    d. esophageal atresia

16–39. The fetal kidneys can routinely be visualized by what gestational age (weeks)?

    a. 8
    b. 12
    c. 18
    d. 22

16–40. Which of the following is NOT characteristic of Potter syndrome?

    a. tight skin
    b. abnormal facies
    c. limb deformities
    d. pulmonary hypoplasia

16–41. Which of the following can NOT be reliably diagnosed antenatally?

    a. renal agenesis
    b. obstructive pyelectasis
    c. multicystic dysplastic kidney disease
    d. autosomal dominant polycystic kidney disease

16–42. Which of the following is the most common cause of neonatal hydronephrosis?

    a. posterior urethral valves
    b. multicystic dysplastic kidney
    c. collecting system duplication
    d. ureteropelvic junction obstruction

16–43. Umbilical artery Doppler velocimetry is recommended in the evaluation of which of the following fetal indications?

    a. macrosomia
    b. growth restriction
    c. suspected cyanotic heart lesion
    d. suspected pulmonary hypoplasia

16–44. Doppler evaluation has been used to screen for ductus arteriosus constriction after exposure to which of the following?

    a. heparin
    b. valproic acid
    c. indomethacin
    d. inhalation anesthetics

16–45. Peak velocities of blood flow through the fetal middle cerebral artery have been shown by Doppler velocimetry to be increased in which of the following fetal complications?

    a. anemia
    b. cerebral palsy
    c. fetal alcohol syndrome
    d. congenital HIV infection

Normal Labor and Delivery

17–1. In modern obstetrical management, approximately what percentage of parturients experience spontaneous labor and delivery, i.e., without induction or augmentation of labor?

a. 90
b. 75
c. 50
d. 30

17–2. What is the relationship of the long axis of the fetus to that of the mother called?

a. presentation
b. lie
c. attitude
d. posture

17–3. What is the lie if the fetal and maternal axes cross at a 45-degree angle?

a. longitudinal
b. breech
c. oblique
d. transverse

17–4. What percentage of term labors present with a longitudinal lie?

a. 20
b. 50
c. 70
d. 99

17–5. Which of the following factors is NOT associated with transverse lie?

a. multiparity
b. oligohydramnios
c. placenta previa
d. uterine anomalies

17–6. In which presentation is the fetal head flexed and the occipital fontanel presenting?

a. vertex
b. face
c. brow
d. sinciput

17–7. In which presentation is the fetal neck sharply extended and the back and occiput in contact?

a. vertex
b. face
c. brow
d. sinciput

17–8. In which presentation is the fetal head partially flexed and a large anterior fontanel presenting?

a. vertex
b. face
c. brow
d. sinciput

17–9. In which of the following presentations does the fetal attitude (vertebral column posture) become concave (extended)?

a. face
b. shoulder
c. cephalic
d. breech

17–10. The incidence of breech presentation between 29 and 32 weeks gestation is 14%. What is its incidence at term?

a. 3%
b. 5%
c. 7%
d. 9%

17–11. Approximately what proportion of all vertex presentations are in the left occiput posterior position?

    a. 15%
    b. 33%
    c. 66%
    d. 95%

17–12. Which Leopold maneuver involves fundal palpation to define which fetal pole occupies the fundus?

    a. first
    b. second
    c. third
    d. fourth

17–13. Which Leopold maneuver involves grasping the lower portion of abdomen just above the symphysis?

    a. first
    b. second
    c. third
    d. fourth

17–14. Which Leopold maneuver involves placing the palms of the hands on each side of the abdomen to determine the location of the back and small parts?

    a. first
    b. second
    c. third
    d. fourth

17–15. What is the approximate sensitivity of Leopold maneuvers in the detection of fetal malpresentation?

    a. 30%
    b. 50%
    c. 70%
    d. 90%

17–16. What is the most common position of the fetal vertex as it enters the pelvis?

    a. right occipitoanterior (ROA)
    b. right occipitotransverse (ROT)
    c. left occipitoanterior (LOA)
    d. left occipitotransverse (LOT)

17–17. Posterior presentations are associated more commonly with which of the following?

    a. narrow forepelvis
    b. normal forepelvis

    c. wide forepelvis
    d. no association with forepelvis type

17–18. What are the cardinal movements of labor (in order)?

    a. descent, engagement, flexion, internal rotation, extension, external rotation, expulsion
    b. descent, flexion, engagement, internal rotation, extension, external rotation, expulsion
    c. engagement, descent, flexion, internal rotation, extension, external rotation, expulsion
    d. engagement, flexion, descent, internal rotation, extension, external rotation, expulsion

17–19. What is the mechanism by which the biparietal diameter passes through the pelvic inlet?

    a. flexion
    b. engagement
    c. descent
    d. internal rotation

17–20. Which of the following describes the alignment of the sagittal suture in asynclitism?

    a. parallel to the inlet's transverse axis
    b. midway between the symphysis and sacral promontory
    c. parallel to the inlet's transverse axis, but not aligned midway between the symphysis and sacral promontory
    d. 45 degrees from the inlet's transverse axis

17–21. What part of the fetal anatomy is palpated easily with extreme asynclitism of the vertex?

    a. nose
    b. mouth
    c. ear
    d. shoulder

17–22. Which of the following is NOT one of the four forces of descent?

    a. pressure of amnionic fluid
    b. direct fundal pressure on the breech
    c. flexing of the fetal body
    d. contraction of abdominal muscles

17–23. The chin is brought into intimate contact with the fetal thorax during which cardinal movement of labor?

    a. flexion
    b. extension
    c. engagement
    d. descent

17–24. The anterior shoulder appears under the symphysis during which cardinal movement of labor?

   a. extension
   b. expulsion
   c. external rotation
   d. descent

17–25. During which cardinal movement of labor is the head returned to the oblique position?

   a. internal rotation
   b. extension
   c. external rotation
   d. expulsion

17–26. The base of the occiput is brought into contact with the inferior margin of the symphysis during which cardinal movement of labor?

   a. extension
   b. expulsion
   c. descent
   d. flexion

17–27. During labor in the occiput posterior position, the occiput has to rotate to the symphysis pubis how many degrees?

   a. 45
   b. 90
   c. 135
   d. 180

17–28. Which of the following increases the risk of persistent occiput posterior or transverse position?

   a. epidural anesthesia
   b. incomplete flexion of the fetal head
   c. weak contractions
   d. all of the above

17–29. What is edematous swelling of the fetal scalp during labor?

   a. molding
   b. caput succedaneum
   c. subdural hematoma
   d. erythema nodosum

17–30. What is a change in the fetal head shape from external compressing forces called?

   a. squashing
   b. forming
   c. shaping
   d. molding

17–31. Which of the following characterizes true labor?

   a. painless contractions with rupture of membranes

   b. engagement of the fetal head
   c. progressive cervical dilatation and effacement
   d. rhythmic lower abdominal pain

17–32. As described by Friedman, labor is divided into three functional divisions that include all of the following EXCEPT

   a. preparatory division
   b. dilatational division
   c. pelvic division
   d. expulsive division

17–33. The active phase of labor is divided into three phases. What is the earliest of these phases called?

   a. acceleration phase
   b. phase of maximum slope
   c. latent phase
   d. deceleration phase

17–34. A prolonged latent phase in a nulliparous patient is one lasting longer than how many hours?

   a. 10
   b. 14
   c. 16
   d. 20

17–35. The latent phase of a multipara's labor is considered to be prolonged if it exceeds how many hours?

   a. 10
   b. 12
   c. 14
   d. 20

17–36. Which of the following is NOT a potential contributor to prolonged latent-phase labor?

   a. epidural analgesia
   b. false labor
   c. premature rupture of membranes
   d. sedation

17–37. What percentage of women progress spontaneously to active labor following strong sedation during the latent phase of labor?

   a. 25
   b. 45
   c. 65
   d. 85

17–38. In the presence of uterine contractions, what cervical dilatation reliably represents the onset of active labor?

   a. 0 to 2 cm
   b. 3 to 5 cm
   c. 4 to 6 cm
   d. 6 to 7 cm

17–39. In multiparas, what is the minimum normal rate of cervical dilatation during active phase labor according to the labor curve of Friedman (1972)?

    a. 0.5 cm/hr
    b. 1.0 cm/hr
    c. 1.5 cm/hr
    d. 2.0 cm/hr

17–40. Arrest of dilatation was defined by Friedman as no cervical change for what period of time?

    a. 1 hr
    b. 2 hr
    c. 3 hr
    d. 4 hr

17–41. A study at Parkland Hospital (Alexander and colleagues, 2002) found that epidural analgesia lengthened the active phase of labor by what amount of time?

    a. 30 min
    b. 1 hr
    c. 2 hr
    d. 3 hr

17–42. What is the median duration of the second stage of labor in a nullipara?

    a. 30 min
    b. 50 min
    c. 70 min
    d. 90 min

17–43. What is the median duration of the second stage of labor in a multipara?

    a. 20 min
    b. 40 min
    c. 60 min
    d. 80 min

17–44. Most women, regardless of parity, will delivery within what time frame after hospital admission for spontaneous labor?

    a. 4 hr
    b. 10 hr
    c. 14 hr
    d. 20 hr

17–45. Which of the following is a feature of false labor?

    a. Contraction intensity remains stable.
    b. Effacement and dilatation of the cervix do not occur.
    c. Discomfort is relieved by sedation.
    d. All of the above.

17–46. What is the name of the federal law protecting patients in active labor from being transferred to another hospital due to financial or other considerations?

    a. Act to Protect Underinsured Patients (APUP)
    b. Emergency Medical Treatment and Labor Act (EMTALA)
    c. Pregnant Patient Bill of Rights
    d. There is no such law in effect.

17–47. An analysis of birth registry information from the state of Washington from 1989 to 1997 (Pang and colleagues, 2002) showed intended home births to be associated with which of the following obstetrical complications?

    a. neonatal death
    b. prolonged labor
    c. postpartum bleeding
    d. all of the above

17–48. In which situation should standard vaginal examination be deferred or modified when admitting a woman with a term gestation to the labor unit?

    a. bleeding in excess of a bloody show
    b. maternal fever
    c. patient nervousness
    d. suspected ruptured membranes

17–49. What is the most reliable indicator of rupture of the fetal membranes?

    a. fluid per cervical os visualized
    b. positive nitrazine test
    c. positive ferning
    d. positive fibronectin

17–50. What is the usual pH of amnionic fluid?

    a. 4.5 to 5.5
    b. 5.5 to 6.5
    c. 7.0 to 7.5
    d. 8.0 to 8.5

17–51. The nitrazine test for rupture of membranes may be falsely positive if which of the following is present?

    a. candida
    b. vaginal bleeding
    c. cervical mucus
    d. scant amnionic fluid

17–52. In assessing labor progress, all of the following cervical properties are assessed EXCEPT

    a. dilatation
    b. effacement
    c. firmness
    d. position

17–53. What is the station where the presenting part is at the level of the ischial spines?

    a. −2
    b. −1
    c. 0
    d. +1

17–54. What is the station at which the fetal head is visible at the introitus (based on centimeters)?

    a. +2
    b. +3
    c. +4
    d. +5

17–55. What is the station of the leading part of the fetal head at which engagement (biparietal diameter is past the pelvic inlet) has occurred?

    a. −2
    b. +1
    c. −1
    d. 0

17–56. When should the fetal heart rate be auscultated during labor?

    a. before a contraction
    b. during a contraction
    c. immediately after a contraction
    d. anytime

17–57. How often during the first stage of labor should the fetal heart rate be auscultated in a low-risk pregnancy?

    a. every 5 min
    b. every 15 min
    c. every 30 min
    d. every 45 min

17–58. How often during the first stage of labor should the fetal heart rate be monitored in a high-risk pregnancy?

    a. every 5 min
    b. every 15 min
    c. every 30 min, before a contraction
    d. every 45 min, after a contraction

17–59. How often should the fetal heart rate be auscultated during the second stage of labor in low- and high-risk patients, respectively?

    a. 5 min, 5 min
    b. 10 min, 5 min
    c. 15 min, 5 min
    d. 30 min, 5 min

17–60. For the purpose of administering antimicrobial prophylaxis for group B streptococcus, prolonged membrane rupture is defined as duration greater than how many hours?

    a. 10
    b. 12
    c. 18
    d. 24

17–61. In a 1998 study of over 1000 women (Bloom and colleagues, 1998), walking during labor had what effect?

    a. prolonged first phase of labor
    b. shortened period of latency and second stage of labor
    c. increased incidence of dysfunctional labor, two intrapartum deaths
    d. no effect on active labor; not harmful

17–62. What is the term for encirclement of the largest diameter of the fetal head by the vulvar ring?

    a. Bandl's ring
    b. crowning
    c. molding
    d. vulvar engagement

17–63. Which of the following is true regarding the routine use of episiotomy?

    a. decreases the risk of anal sphincter laceration
    b. increases the risk of anal sphincter laceration
    c. does not affect the risk of urethral lacerations
    d. increases the risk of urethral lacerations

17–64. What is the maneuver used to facilitate delivery of the fetal head over the perineum in a controlled manner?

    a. MacRoberts
    b. Ragu
    c. Ritgen
    d. Woods

17–65. What percentage of deliveries are complicated by a nuchal cord?

    a. 1
    b. 5
    c. 10
    d. 25

17–66. If the umbilical cord is left unclamped for 3 minutes, what volume of blood can be transfused into the newborn, on average?

    a. 10 mL
    b. 30 mL
    c. 50 mL
    d. 80 mL

17–67. During the third stage of labor, which of the following is NOT a sign of placental separation?

    a. a gush of blood
    b. uterus rises in the abdomen
    c. umbilical cord protrudes farther out of the vagina
    d. uterus becomes flaccid

17–68. Which of the following is a complication of the third stage of labor associated with forced placental separation?

    a. endometritis
    b. uterine atony
    c. Asherman syndrome
    d. uterine inversion

17–69. In the absence of excessive bleeding, after how much time should manual removal of the placenta be performed if spontaneous separation does not occur?

    a. 5 min
    b. 15 min
    c. 25 min
    d. undetermined

17–70. The so-called "fourth stage" of labor, during which risk of postpartum hemorrhage is greatest, lasts how long?

    a. 15 min
    b. 1 hr
    c. 2 hr
    d. 4 hr

17–71. What is the primary mechanism of placental site hemostasis?

    a. vasoconstriction by contracted myometrium
    b. prostaglandin secretion
    c. maternal hypotension
    d. decreased cardiac output

17–72. What is the half-life of oxytocin?

    a. 3 min
    b. 30 min
    c. 3 hr
    d. 3 days

17–73. Which deleterious effect is associated with oxytocin when given intravenously as a 10-unit bolus?

    a. cardiac arrhythmia
    b. hypotension
    c. neuromuscular blockade
    d. seizure

17–74. What is a serious potential complication of prolonged oxytocin administration?

    a. disseminated intravascular coagulation
    b. hyperkalemia
    c. myometrial necrosis
    d. water intoxication

17–75. Which of the following is associated with ergonovine and methylergonovine?

    a. seizure
    b. hypertension
    c. oliguria
    d. thrombocytopenia

17–76. What is a laceration involving the skin, mucous membrane, perineal body, anal sphincter, and rectal mucosa called?

    a. first degree
    b. second degree
    c. third degree
    d. fourth degree

17–77. What is a laceration involving only the vaginal epithelium or perineal skin called?

    a. first degree
    b. second degree
    c. third degree
    d. fourth degree

17–78. What is a laceration involving the skin, mucous membrane, perineal body, and anal sphincter called?

    a. first degree
    b. second degree
    c. third degree
    d. fourth degree

17–79. What is the major advantage of a mediolateral episiotomy?

    a. easy surgical repair
    b. less postoperative pain
    c. less blood loss
    d. fewer third- and fourth-degree extensions

17–80. Clinical trials have shown that routine episiotomy decreases the incidence of which of the following?

    a. anterior perineal trauma
    b. fecal and urinary incontinence
    c. third and fourth degree perineal tears
    d. pelvic floor relaxation

17–81. Episiotomy should be most strongly considered for which of the following?

    a. all vaginal deliveries
    b. nulliparous women
    c. occiput anterior presentations
    d. shoulder dystocia

17–82. Which is true regarding third- and fourth-degree perineal tears?

   a. Incidence is 5%.
   b. Postrepair wound disruption occurs in 10%.
   c. They predispose to long-term anal incontinence.
   d. All of the above.

17–83. The active management of labor generally does NOT include which of the following?

   a. amniotomy as needed
   b. commitment to delivery within a prescribed time frame
   c. oxytocin augmentation if cervical dilatation <1 to 2 cm/hr
   d. walking during first stage of labor

Intrapartum Assessment

18–1. Which voltage is most reliably detected and is represented as part of the fetal electrocardiogram?

   a. P wave
   b. QRS complex
   c. R wave
   d. T wave

18–2. What are the usual settings for vertical and horizontal scaling during electronic fetal monitoring?

   a. 30 bpm; 1 cm/min
   b. 30 bpm; 3 cm/min
   c. 60 bpm; 1 cm/min
   d. 60 bpm; 3 cm/min

18–3. With increasing gestational age, the fetal heart rate baseline undergoes which of the following trends?

   a. increases
   b. remains unchanged
   c. variability changes become more closely tied to activity changes
   d. decreases

18–4. The physiological changes in the fetal heart rate baseline seen with increasing gestational age are attributed to which of the following fetal changes?

   a. increasing body mass
   b. maturing parasympathetic system

   c. increasing density of arterial chemoreceptors
   d. decreasing density of myocyte calcium channels

18–5. What is baseline fetal bradycardia?

   a. <90 bpm
   b. <100 bpm
   c. <110 bpm
   d. <120 bpm

18–6. What is baseline fetal tachycardia?

   a. >160 bpm
   b. >170 bpm
   c. >180 bpm
   d. >190 bpm

18–7. Fetal bradycardia typically may result from which of the following?

   a. maternal fever
   b. fetal head compression
   c. maternal atropine use
   d. none of the above

18–8. What is the most common cause of fetal tachycardia?

   a. drug-induced
   b. thyroid storm
   c. maternal fever
   d. cardiac arrhythmia

18–9. Beat-to-beat baseline variability is predominantly regulated by which of the following?

   a. maternal temperature
   b. arterial chemoreceptors
   c. autonomic nervous system
   d. density of myocyte acetylcholine receptors

18–10. Which of the following ranges of heart beats per minute reflect normal beat-to-beat variability?

   a. 10 to 15
   b. 15 to 20
   c. 20 to 25
   d. all of the above

18–11. Beat-to-beat variability increases in which of the following fetal situations?

   a. acidemia
   b. tachycardia
   c. neurological damage
   d. advancing gestational age

18–12. Decreased beat-to beat variability has been unequivocally linked with which of the following?

   a. analgesia use
   b. fetal breathing
   c. magnesium sulfate use
   d. all of the above

18–13. Which of the following fetal heart rate patterns are most commonly associated with fetal arrhythmias?

   a. sinusoidal
   b. wandering baseline
   c. baseline bradycardia
   d. abrupt baseline spiking

18–14. Which of the following reflects the incidence of fetal arrhythmias at term?

   a. 0.03%
   b. 0.3%
   c. 3%
   d. 13%

18–15. Which of the following is true of supraventricular arrhythmias?

   a. most common class of fetal arrhythmias
   b. majority are linked with chromosomal abnormalities
   c. majority are linked with long-term neurological sequelae
   d. none of the above

18–16. A true sinusoidal fetal heart rate pattern is associated with which of the following?

   a. maternal fever
   b. maternal anemia
   c. fetal anemia
   d. fetal head compression

18–17. Which of the following is a characteristic of the sinusoidal fetal heart rate pattern as defined by Modanlou and Freeman?

   a. contains 5 accelerations per 20 min
   b. Heart rate baseline ranges between 90 and 120 bpm.
   c. Short-term variability ranges from 20 to 30 bpm.
   d. Long-term variability frequency ranges from 2 to 5 cycles/min.

18–18. The absence of which of the following defines the difference between sinusoidal and pseudo-sinusoidal fetal heart rate patterns?

   a. accelerations
   b. decelerations
   c. short-term variability
   d. oscillations above and below the fetal heart rate baseline

18–19. Fetal heart rate accelerations are commonly associated with which of the following?

   a. fetal acidemia
   b. fetal movement
   c. fetal head compression
   d. maternal hypotension

18–20. A gradual decrease in the fetal heart rate that coincides with a uterine contraction describes which of the following deceleration types?

   a. late
   b. early
   c. variable
   d. prolonged

18–21. A gradual, smooth deceleration of the fetal heart rate that follows the peak of a contraction describes which of the following deceleration types?

   a. late
   b. early
   c. variable
   d. prolonged

18–22. Which of the following fetal conditions is the suspected cause of early fetal heart rate decelerations?

   a. anemia
   b. hypoxia
   c. acidemia
   d. head compression

18–23. Late fetal heart rate decelerations are commonly seen in which of the following clinical settings?

    a. maternal fever
    b. maternal anemia
    c. fetal head compression
    d. uteroplacental dysfunction

18–24. Which of the following is characteristic of variable fetal heart rate decelerations?

    a. gradual onset
    b. lasts <2 min
    c. consistently begin with the onset of contractions
    d. all of the above

18–25. Variable decelerations are caused by which fetal situation?

    a. hypoxia
    b. acidemia
    c. cord compression
    d. head compression

18–26. Significant variable decelerations are defined by which of the following fetal heart rates and durations?

    a. <90 bpm for >30 sec
    b. <70 bpm for >30 sec
    c. <90 bpm for >60 sec
    d. <70 bpm for >60 sec

18–27. The fetal heart rate baseline of your laboring patient is 130 bpm with good beat-to-beat variability. The electronic monitor tracing next reveals a 3-minute prolonged variable deceleration with a nadir of 100 bpm. The heart rate baseline then increases to 170 bpm and is accompanied by a 2-minute period of late decelerations. Over the next 2 minutes, the heart rate gradually drops to a 160-bpm baseline with an absence of decelerations or accelerations. The next most appropriate management step of this patient includes which of the following?

    a. continue to observe
    b. deliver immediately
    c. begin intravenous antimicrobials
    d. give terbutaline, 0.25 mg intravenously in a single dose

18–28. As the number of variable decelerations to less than 70 bpm during the second stage increases, rates of neonates with which of the following also increases?

    a. cerebral palsy
    b. low Apgar scores
    c. necrotizing enterocolitis
    d. sudden infant death syndrome

18–29. Risks of fetal electrode use in electronic fetal monitoring include which of the following?

    a. osteomyelitis
    b. uterine perforation
    c. puerperal endometritis
    d. all of the above

18–30. According to the American College of Obstetricians and Gynecologists, relative contraindications to internal electronic fetal monitoring include which of the following maternal infections?

    a. gonorrhea
    b. chorioamnionitis
    c. trichomoniasis
    d. herpes simplex virus infection

18–31. Effective forms of intrapartum fetal stimulation include which of the following?

    a. Allis clamp pinching
    b. fontanel compression
    c. uterine fundal percussion
    d. none of the above

18–32. To use fetal pulse oximetry, clinicians place the sensor against which fetal structure?

    a. face
    b. occiput
    c. fontanel
    d. umbilical cord

18–33. With measurements obtained using fetal pulse oximetry, the lower limit for normal fetal oxygen saturation is considered by most to be which of the following?

    a. 30%
    b. 50%
    c. 70%
    d. 90%

18–34. Benefits of fetal electrocardiography include which of the following?

    a. improved neonatal outcome
    b. lower rates of cesarean delivery for fetal distress
    c. detection of fetal cardiac changes earlier than traditional fetal heart rate monitoring
    d. none of the above

18–35. Fetal heart rate patterns are considered to reflect fetal distress if they lack beat-to-beat variability and also contain which of the following patterns?

    a. prolonged lambda
    b. prolonged saltatory
    c. recurrent overshoot
    d. recurrent severe decelerations

18–36. Meconium-stained amnionic fluid is closely associated with which of the following neonatal outcomes?

    a. death
    b. cerebral palsy
    c. necrotizing enterocolitis
    d. none of the above

18–37. Meconium aspiration syndrome is closely associated with which of the following fetal conditions?

    a. anemia
    b. acidemia
    c. transient neonatal myasthenia gravis
    d. congenital cytomegalovirus infection

18–38. Your patient received epidural analgesia 10 minutes ago. The fetal heart rate tracing shows persistent bradycardia to 90 bpm for 3 minutes. According to the American College of Obstetricians and Gynecologists, management of this situation should include which of the following?

    a. prompt cesarean delivery
    b. ultrasonographic examination
    c. cessation of uterine stimulants
    d. administration of intravenous antimicrobials

18–39. In which of the following intrapartum settings is amnioinfusion NOT employed?

    a. chorioamnionitis
    b. variable decelerations
    c. meconium-stained fluid
    d. amnionic fluid index <3

18–40. Which of the following complications is NOT associated with intrapartum amnioinfusion?

    a. maternal seizures
    b. cord prolapse
    c. chorioamnionitis
    d. uterine hypertonus

18–41. What are the current recommendations for frequency of auscultation of fetal heart rate in high-risk pregnancies during the first and second stages of labor, respectively?

    a. every 30 min and every 15 min
    b. every 30 min and every 5 min
    c. every 15 min and every 15 min
    d. every 15 min and every 5 min

18–42. You are monitoring your patient's contraction pattern. During 20 minutes, she has 6 equally spaced contractions. The baseline uterine tone is 10 mm Hg and the peak intensity of each contraction reaches 50 mm Hg. Which of the following number of Montevideo units defines this uterine activity?

    a. 120
    b. 150
    c. 240
    d. 300

18–43. Which of the following ranges reflects the typical length of contractions during labor?

    a. 20 to 40 sec
    b. 40 to 60 sec
    c. 60 to 80 sec
    d. 80 to 100 sec

18–44. At what intensity are uterine contractions associated with pain?

    a. 5 mm Hg
    b. 10 mm Hg
    c. 15 mm Hg
    d. 20 mm Hg

18–45. The dominant uterine "pacemaker" is located in which part of the uterus?

    a. fundus
    b. left cornua
    c. right cornua
    d. lower uterine segment

18–46. Peak contraction pressures are generated in which part of the uterus?

    a. fundus
    b. left cornua
    c. right cornua
    d. lower uterine segment

18–47. Before one decides to perform a cesarean delivery for presumed dystocia, what minimum range of uterine activity, measured in Montevideo units, should be reached?

    a. 75 to 100
    b. 150 to 175
    c. 200 to 225
    d. 325 to 350

19

Obstetrical Anesthesia

19–1. What percentage of pregnancy-related deaths is secondary to anesthesia complications?

 a. 1 to 2
 b. 3 to 4
 c. 6 to 8
 d. 12 to 16

19–2. Which maternal characteristic is NOT an anesthesia risk factor?

 a. anatomic anomaly of the face
 b. asthma
 c. marked obesity
 d. mild hypertension

19–3. Which of the following factors has contributed to improved safety of obstetrical anesthesia?

 a. increased maternal age
 b. increased parity
 c. increased use of regional anesthesia
 d. decreased obesity

19–4. Which of the following characterizes women who receive continuous emotional support during labor?

 a. deliver by cesarean section more often
 b. request epidural analgesia more often
 c. need oxytocin during labor more often
 d. experience less pain

19–5. When does the peak analgesic effect of meperidine given intramuscularly occur?

 a. <5 min
 b. 20 min
 c. 45 min
 d. 60 min

19–6. When does the onset of the analgesia effect of morphine given intravenously occur?

 a. <5 min
 b. 20 min

 c. 45 min
 d. 60 min

19–7. What is the approximate half-life of meperidine in the newborn?

 a. 1 hr
 b. 2 hr
 c. 8 hr
 d. >13 hr

19–8. What dose of butorphanol is comparable to 50 mg of meperidine?

 a. 0.5 mg
 b. 1 to 2 mg
 c. 4 to 5 mg
 d. 10 mg

19–9. Butorphanol administration has been associated with which fetal heart rate abnormality?

 a. repetitive late decelerations
 b. fetal tachycardia
 c. sinusoidal rhythm
 d. saltatory patter

19–10. Which of the following (according to Bricker and Lavender) provides superior pain relief for labor?

 a. meperidine
 b. butorphanol
 c. morphine
 d. epidural analgesia

19–11. What is the mechanism of action of naloxone hydrochloride?

 a. stimulates acetylcholinesterase
 b. displaces narcotic from specific receptors
 c. inhibits muscarinic receptors
 d. blocks β-receptors

19–12. Which nerve roots are predominantly responsible for early first-stage labor pain?

a. T10, T11
b. T11, T12
c. T10, T11, T12, L1
d. S2, S3, S4

19–13. Which nerve roots are responsible for the pain of vaginal delivery?

a. T10, T11
b. T11, T12
c. T10, T11, T12, L1
d. S2, S3, S4

19–14. Which of the following is NOT a sign of central nervous system (CNS) toxicity from local anesthetics?

a. slurred speech
b. tinnitus
c. paresthesia (mouth)
d. chorea

19–15. Which centrally acting agent is used to control convulsions caused by local anesthetic-induced CNS toxicity?

a. succinylcholine
b. thiopental
c. magnesium sulfate
d. phenytoin

19–16. Which of the following is generally true concerning cardiovascular manifestations of local anesthetic toxicity?

a. They develop before CNS toxicity.
b. They develop simultaneously with CNS toxicity.
c. They develop later than CNS toxicity.
d. There are no cardiovascular manifestations from local anesthetic toxicity.

19–17. Which of the following local anesthetics is exceptional in that CNS and cardiovascular toxicities develop simultaneously?

a. tetracaine
b. lidocaine
c. bupivacaine
d. chloroprocaine

19–18. What is the most common complication of paracervical block?

a. maternal hypotension
b. CNS toxicity

c. fetal bradycardia
d. bleeding

19–19. What is the etiology of spinal headaches?

a. puncture of meninges followed by leaking fluid
b. hypotension after spinal block
c. vasodilation of cerebral vessels
d. drug-induced hormonal changes

19–20. What is the most effective treatment for spinal headache is achieved by

a. vigorous hydration
b. caffeine
c. epidural blood patch
d. placing the patient flat on her back for several hours

19–21. Which of the following is an absolute contraindication to spinal analgesia?

a. preeclampsia
b. skin infection at site of needle entry
c. controlled seizure disorder
d. diabetes

19–22. Which of the following nerve blocks would provide complete analgesia for labor pain and vaginal delivery?

a. T8-S2
b. T10-S5
c. T12-S2
d. T8-L4

19–23. What is the most common side effect of epidural anesthesia?

a. maternal hypertension
b. maternal hypotension
c. CNS stimulation
d. ineffective block

19–24. What is the likely cause of intrapartum fever in women with epidurals?

a. dysregulation of body temperature
b. analgesics
c. placental inflammation
d. a and c

19–25. What are the effects of labor epidurals on the cesarean birthrate according to current information?

a. no change
b. slightly decreased
c. slightly increased
d. markedly increased

19–26. What is a major advantage of using combination opiate and local anesthetic for epidural blockade?

    a. denser motor blockade
    b. decreased toxicity
    c. rapid onset of pain relief
    d. decreased urinary retention

19–27. What is a common side effect of combined opiate-epidural analgesia?

    a. urinary incontinence
    b. nausea and vomiting
    c. pruritis
    d. headaches

19–28. What is the estimated case-fatality rate of general anesthesia for cesarean delivery?

    a. 2 per million live births
    b. 4 per million live births
    c. 16 per million live births
    d. 32 per million live births

19–29. Which physiological condition causes pregnant women to become hypoxemic more rapidly during periods of apnea?

    a. increased tidal volume
    b. decreased functional residual capacity
    c. increased residual volume
    d. decreased total lung capacity

19–30. Which of the following anesthetic agents must be used in combination with others because it is associated with newborn depression at high doses?

    a. thiopental
    b. lidocaine
    c. ketamine
    d. halothane

19–31. What is an advantage of ketamine when compared to thiopental?

    a. not associated with hypotension
    b. causes delirium
    c. causes hallucinations
    d. safer for hypertensive patients

19–32. What is pressure on the cricoid cartilage (to occlude the esophagus) called?

    a. Heimlich maneuver
    b. Circus maneuver
    c. Sellick maneuver
    d. Hawaiian maneuver

19–33. During general anesthesia, which agent can provide amnesia and additional analgesia?

    a. halogenated agent
    b. lidocaine
    c. diazepam
    d. morphine

19–34. Which of the following is a rare side effect of halothane anesthesia?

    a. anemia
    b. thrombocytopenia
    c. hypertension
    d. hepatitis

19–35. What is the most common cause of anesthesia-related death in obstetrics?

    a. cardiac arrhythmia
    b. hemorrhage
    c. aspiration pneumonitis
    d. stroke

19–36. Chemical pneumonitis develops if the gastric pH that is aspirated is less than which of the following?

    a. 2.5
    b. 3.0
    c. 4.0
    d. 5.0

19–37. What are the signs of aspiration of acidic liquid?

    a. bradycardia, decreased respiratory rate, hypotension
    b. bradycardia, tachypnea, hypertension
    c. tachycardia, decreased respiratory rate, hypotension
    d. tachycardia, tachypnea, hypotension

20

Dystocia: Abnormal Labor

20–1. What is the approximate incidence of cesarean delivery in the United States?

a. 15%
b. 20%
c. 25%
d. 30%

20–2. Of the following, which is NOT considered a potential component of dystocia?

a. power (force of contractions and expulsive efforts)
b. passenger (fetus)
c. passage (pelvis)
d. pitocin augmentation

20–3. Approximately what percentage of women with a prior history of cephalopelvic disproportion subsequently deliver vaginally?

a. 10
b. 30
c. 50
d. 70

20–4. What is the most common reason for primary cesarean delivery?

a. malpresentation
b. placental abruption
c. prematurity
d. dystocia

20–5. According to the American College of Obstetricians and Gynecologists (ACOG), what is the minimum cervical dilatation required before the diagnosis of dystocia can be made?

a. 2 cm
b. 3 cm
c. 4 cm
d. 5 cm

20–6. Where in the uterus do the contractions of normal labor begin?

a. cornual region
b. lower uterine segment
c. cervix
d. fundus

20–7. What amplitude of uterine contraction is generally necessary to effect cervical dilatation?

a. 5 mm Hg
b. 15 mm Hg
c. 25 mm Hg
d. 50 mm Hg

20–8. In a nullipara, what is the minimum normal rate of cervical dilatation in the active phase of labor?

a. 0.5 cm/hr
b. 1.2 cm/hr
c. 1.5 cm/hr
d. 2.0 cm/hr

20–9. According to Friedman, what is prolongation of the latent phase of labor in a nullipara?

a. >14 hr
b. >20 hr
c. >24 hr
d. >48 hr

20–10. In a multiparous woman, how is prolonged latent phase defined?

a. >6 hr
b. >14 hr
c. >20 hr
d. >24 hr

20–11. In a multiparous woman, secondary arrest of cervical dilatation is defined as no further dilatation for how long?

a. >1 hr
b. >2 hr
c. >3 hr
d. >14 hr

20–12. How are Montevideo units calculated?

a. number of contractions in 10 min × peak amplitude
b. number of contractions in 20 min × peak amplitude
c. number of contractions in 30 min × peak amplitude
d. add the peak amplitude minus the baseline for each contraction in a 10-min period

20–13. According to ACOG guidelines, when is arrest of first-stage labor diagnosed?

a. The active phase of labor exceeds 8 hr.
b. Montevideo units exceed 200 for 2 hr without cervical change.
c. There is no cervical change in 2 hr regardless of contraction strength.
d. The latent phase of labor exceeds 20 hr.

20–14. Differing from ACOG criteria, Rouse and colleagues (1999) suggest that at least how many hours without cervical change are necessary to diagnose active-phase arrest?

a. 2
b. 4
c. 6
d. 8

20–15. In a nulliparous woman, how long is a prolonged deceleration phase?

a. >1 hr
b. >2 hr
c. >3 hr
d. >20 hr

20–16. Which of the following is NOT associated with precipitous labor and delivery?

a. amnionic fluid embolism
b. postpartum hemorrhage
c. increased perinatal mortality and morbidity
d. chorioamnionitis

20–17. Which of the following is the most common postpartum complication of precipitous labor?

a. hemorrhage
b. endometritis
c. poor mother–neonate bonding
d. vulvar hematoma

20–18. In a woman with a contracted pelvic inlet, what is the diagonal conjugate generally less than?

a. 9.5 cm
b. 10.5 cm
c. 11.5 cm
d. 12.5 cm

20–19. What is the average biparietal diameter of term neonates?

a. 8.5 cm
b. 9.0 cm
c. 9.5 cm
d. >10.5 cm

20–20. What is the anteroposterior diameter in the presence of pelvic inlet contracture?

a. <8 cm
b. <9 cm
c. <10 cm
d. <12 cm

20–21. How increased is the incidence of shoulder presentation in women who have a contracted pelvic inlet compared to those whose pelves are normal?

a. twofold
b. threefold
c. fourfold
d. sixfold

20–22. What is the average interspinous measurement?

a. 8.0 cm
b. 9.5 cm
c. 10.0 cm
d. 10.5 cm

20–23. What is the average posterior sagittal diameter?

a. 4 cm
b. 5 cm
c. 6 cm
d. 8 cm

20–24. The midpelvis is likely to be contracted if the sum of the interischial spinous and the posterior sagittal diameters is less than or equal to which of the following?

a. 9.5 cm
b. 11.5 cm
c. 12.5 cm
d. 13.5 cm

20–25. Which of the following factors is amenable to radiographic measurement (x-ray)?

   a. fetal head size
   b. molding of fetal head
   c. size of bony pelvis
   d. amount of amnionic fluid

20–26. What is the mean gonadal radiation exposure to the fetus with conventional radiographic pelvimetry?

   a. ~0.1 rad
   b. ~1.0 rad
   c. ~10.0 rad
   d. ~100.0 rad

20–27. What is a typical fetal radiation dose with computed tomograms?

   a. ~0.1 rad
   b. ~1.0 rad
   c. ~10.0 rad
   d. ~100.0 rad

20–28. Historically, which maneuver during labor was proposed to predict successful vaginal delivery?

   a. Müller-Hillis
   b. Brandt
   c. Zavanelli
   d. Prague

20–29. What is the presenting part with a face presentation?

   a. sinciput
   b. malar eminence
   c. mentum
   d. occiput

20–30. Which of the following presentations precludes a vaginal delivery in term-sized fetuses?

   a. mentum posterior
   b. mentum anterior
   c. mentum transverse
   d. none of the above

20–31. What is the overall incidence of face presentation?

   a. 0.05%
   b. 0.2%
   c. 2.0%
   d. 5.0%

20–32. Which of the following is associated etiologically with a face presentation?

   a. contracted pelvic inlet
   b. oxytocin induction
   c. small for gestational age infant
   d. tight abdominal musculature

20–33. Approximately what percentage of face presentations are associated with inlet contraction?

   a. 5
   b. 20
   c. 40
   d. 65

20–34. In labor, if the presenting part is the sagittal suture midway between the orbital ridge and the anterior fontanelle, what is the presentation?

   a. face
   b. brow
   c. occiput
   d. left occiput anterior

20–35. In which situation is the brow presentation most likely to deliver vaginally?

   a. small fetus, large pelvis
   b. small fetus, small pelvis
   c. large fetus, large pelvis
   d. large fetus, small pelvis

20–36. What bony landmark determines the designation of lie in shoulder presentations?

   a. acromion
   b. brow
   c. breech
   d. occiput

20–37. What is the incidence of transverse lie at term?

   a. 0.003%
   b. 0.03%
   c. 0.3%
   d. 3.0%

20–38. Which of the following is a common cause of transverse lie?

   a. placental abruption
   b. normal uterus
   c. postterm pregnancy
   d. contracted pelvis

20–39. What is the best way to deliver a term transverse lie in labor with ruptured membranes?

   a. low transverse cesarean delivery
   b. vertical cesarean delivery
   c. version to vertex and vaginal delivery
   d. version to breech and vaginal delivery

20–40. A fetus that is compressed with its head forced against the abdomen during labor is called which of the following?

    a. conduplicato corpore
    b. fetal wedge
    c. convoluted compact fetus
    d. gymnastica fetus

20–41. How often is compound presentation identified at Parkland Memorial Hospital?

    a. 1 in 400
    b. 1 in 800
    c. 1 in 1000
    d. 1 in 2000

20–42. Which of the following characterizes the incidence of occiput posterior positions in early term labor compared with that at delivery?

    a. no change
    b. decreased
    c. markedly decreased
    d. increased

20–43. What is the mean head-to-body delivery time in deliveries complicated by shoulder dystocia?

    a. ~40 sec
    b. ~60 sec
    c. ~80 sec
    d. ~100 sec

20–44. Spong and colleagues (1995) diagnose shoulder dystocia when the head-to-body delivery time exceeds which of the following?

    a. 20 sec
    b. 40 sec
    c. 60 sec
    d. 80 sec

20–45. Which of the following is a maternal risk factor for shoulder dystocia?

    a. nulliparity
    b. obesity
    c. advanced maternal age
    d. chronic hypertension

20–46. In which of the following circumstances should a cesarean delivery be considered to prevent shoulder dystocia (ACOG guidelines)?

    a. term labor, estimated fetal weight (EFW) 4000 g by clinical examination
    b. term labor, EFW 4180 g by ultrasound
    c. diabetic (gestational), term, EFW 4200 g by ultrasound
    d. diabetic (gestational), term, EFW 4600 g by ultrasound

20–47. Which of the following is NOT part of the management of shoulder dystocia?

    a. Woods screw maneuver
    b. fundal pressure
    c. McRoberts maneuver
    d. delivery of posterior shoulder

20–48. Of the following methods used for management of shoulder dystocia, which is associated with the highest incidence of orthopedic and neurological damage?

    a. suprapubic pressure
    b. McRoberts maneuver
    c. Hibbard maneuver
    d. Woods screw maneuver

20–49. When is cephalocentesis performed?

    a. transabdominally during latent labor
    b. transabdominally during second stage of labor (3–4 cm)
    c. transvaginally during latent labor
    d. transvaginally during active labor (3–4 cm)

20–50. What is the approximate incidence of breech presentation at term?

    a. 0.5%
    b. 3.0%
    c. 7.0%
    d. 12.0%

20–51. What percentage of vaginal deliveries are complicated by torn anal sphincter?

    a. 0.5 to 1%
    b. 3 to 6%
    c. 9 to 12%
    d. 15 to 18%

20–52. Which of the following scenarios most strongly predisposes to later development of pelvic floor dysfunction in the parturient?

    a. spontaneous vaginal delivery, birthweight 3850 g
    b. first-degree laceration at the time of delivery, birthweight 3850 g
    c. forceps-assisted delivery, birthweight 4000 g
    d. cesarean delivery for dystocia, birthweight 4300 g

20–53. Which of the following has the weakest association with fetal head molding?

    a. multiparity
    b. oxytocin labor stimulation
    c. vacuum extraction delivery
    d. prolonged labor

21

Disorders of Amnionic Fluid Volume

21–1. At which week of gestation does amnionic fluid typically begin to diminish?

   a. 32
   b. 36
   c. 40
   d. 42

21–2. Amnionic fluid index is derived by adding the vertical depth measurements from which of the following?

   a. the deepest pockets of the four uterine quadrants
   b. the smallest pockets of the four uterine quadrants
   c. the deepest pockets of the right and left uterine halves
   d. the smallest pockets of the right and left uterine halves

21–3. Hydramnios is diagnosed by an amnionic fluid index greater than which of the following?

   a. 16 cm
   b. 20 cm
   c. 24 cm
   d. 28 cm

21–4. What is the most common cause of hydramnios?

   a. fetal anomalies
   b. maternal diabetes
   c. multifetal gestation
   d. idiopathic

21–5. Which of the following fetal conditions is NOT associated with hydramnios?

   a. central nervous system anomalies
   b. nonimmune hydrops
   c. chromosomal abnormalities
   d. renal agenesis

21–6. Which of the following maternal conditions is associated with hydramnios?

   a. listeriosis
   b. sickle-cell anemia
   c. diabetes
   d. systemic lupus erythematosus

21–7. Hydramnios has NO effect on the incidence of which of the following?

   a. perinatal mortality
   b. preeclampsia
   c. postpartum hemorrhage
   d. placental abruption

21–8. Idiopathic hydramnios is associated with an increased rate of which of the following?

   a. cesarean delivery
   b. amnionic fluid embolism
   c. uterine rupture
   d. meconium aspiration

21–9. Amnionic fluid volume may be altered by changes in all EXCEPT which of the following?

   a. maternal hematocrit
   b. maternal hydration
   c. fetal swallowing
   d. altitude

21–10. In cases of anencephaly, fetal increases in which of the following is the most likely cause of hydramnios?

   a. swallowing
   b. transudation
   c. inspiration
   d. vasopressin secretion

21–11. A new patient presents for her first prenatal visit at 26 weeks. She is concerned by rapid abdominal growth. Her fundal height measures 42 cm. Ultrasonographic examination reveals fetal size consistent with 26 weeks and an amnionic fluid index of 28 cm. Associated maternal complications classically may include all of the following EXCEPT

  a. dyspnea
  b. lower extremity edema
  c. seizures
  d. mirror syndrome

21–12. Increased perinatal mortality from hydramnios is most commonly caused by which of these complications?

  a. antenatal infection
  b. uterine rupture
  c. meconium aspiration
  d. preterm delivery

21–13. Your patient with hydramnios in labor at 36 weeks experiences spontaneous rupture of membranes. Following this, the fetal heart rate drops to and remains at 80 beats per minute. Cervical exam reveals a cervix 2 to 3 cm dilated with no evidence of cord prolapse. In this clinical setting, which of the following is the most likely cause for this fetal distress?

  a. positional maternal hypotension
  b. true knot in cord
  c. placental abruption
  d. uterine rupture

21–14. Which of the following are effective methods of improving maternal symptoms of hydramnios?

  a. amniocentesis
  b. fluid restriction
  c. salt restriction
  d. diuretic drugs

21–15. Which of the following is the more common complication of amniocentesis performed to relieve maternal distress from hydramnios?

  a. fetal needle injury
  b. placental abruption
  c. meconium staining of fluid
  d. umbilical cord hematoma

21–16. Which medication, when given orally to mothers, decreases fetal urine output?

  a. aspirin
  b. cimetidine

  c. bromocriptine
  d. indomethacin

21–17. Which of the following is a side effect of using indomethacin for the management of hydramnios?

  a. altered neonatal bleeding times
  b. increased amnionic fluid volume
  c. constriction of the fetal ductus arteriosus
  d. premature separation of the placenta

21–18. Oligohydramnios is defined as an amnionic fluid index measuring less than which of the following?

  a. 3 cm
  b. 5 cm
  c. 9 cm
  d. 14 cm

21–19. Oligohydramnios is often seen in which of the following clinical conditions?

  a. maternal diabetes
  b. postterm gestation
  c. fetal esophageal atresia
  d. fetal spina bifida

21–20. Which of the following is typically NOT an underlying cause of oligohydramnios?

  a. chronic severe placental insufficiency
  b. defect and leak from fetal membranes
  c. fetal Lyme disease infection
  d. fetal renal anomalies

21–21. Which class of drugs is strongly associated with oligohydramnios?

  a. angiotensin-converting enzyme inhibitors
  b. α-adrenergic blockers
  c. calcium-channel blocking agents
  d. hydralazine

21–22. An increased risk of which of the following clinical consequences may frequently accompany oligohydramnios?

  a. premature rupture of membranes
  b. mirror syndrome
  c. placental abruption
  d. cord compression

21–23. Which of the following findings in the fetus is NOT associated with oligohydramnios?

  a. club foot
  b. adhesions of amnion to fetus
  c. decreased subcutaneous tissues
  d. pulmonary hypoplasia

21–24. Anomalies of which of the following organ systems is more commonly associated with oligohydramnios?

    a. urinary
    b. cardiovascular
    c. pulmonary
    d. neural tube

21–25. Which of the following is most commonly responsible for the increased rate of cesarean delivery when oligohydramnios is present?

    a. coexistent fetal anomalies
    b. fetal malpresentation
    c. nonreassuring fetal heart rate patterns
    d. uterine dysfunction

21–26. The American College of Obstetricians and Gynecologists supports the use of amnioinfusion to prevent which of the following?

    a. cesarean delivery
    b. fetal meconium aspiration
    c. cord compression
    d. fetal pulmonary hypoplasia

22

Induction of Labor

22–1. According to the National Center for Health Statistics, the incidence of labor induction or augmentation in 2002 approached what percentage?

    a. 10
    b. 20
    c. 30
    d. 40

22–2. Which of the following is increased in nulliparas undergoing elective induction of labor?

    a. preterm delivery
    b. endometritis
    c. chorioamnionitis
    d. cesarean delivery

22–3. Which of the following is most likely to have a successful induction of labor?

    a. primiparous; cervix 2 cm dilated/20% effaced/0 station
    b. primiparous; cervix 2 cm dilated/20% effaced/−1 station
    c. multiparous; cervix 2 cm dilated/80% effaced/−1 station

    d. multiparous; cervix 1 cm dilated/20% effaced/0 station

22–4. What is the most common indication for emergent hysterectomy following primary cesarean delivery?

    a. atony
    b. chorioamnionitis
    c. sterilization
    d. accreta

22–5. Contraindications to induction of labor include all EXCEPT which of the following?

    a. macrosomia
    b. prior classical cesarean delivery
    c. placenta previa
    d. fetal renal anomaly

22–6. Which of the following is NOT a component of the Bishop score?

    a. parity
    b. dilation
    c. effacement
    d. station

22–7. What is the Bishop score cutoff for an unfavorable cervix and a possible indication for cervical ripening?

   a. ≤2
   b. ≤4
   c. ≤6
   d. ≤8

22–8. PGE$_2$ (dinoprostone) has been shown to decrease which of the following?

   a. induction to delivery time
   b. cesarean delivery rate
   c. Bishop score
   d. chorioamnionitis rate

22–9. What is the recommended time interval after PGE$_2$ administration to initiation of oxytocin?

   a. 30 min
   b. 2 hr
   c. 8 hr
   d. 6 to 12 hr

22–10. The FDA has approved misoprostol for which of the following?

   a. cervical ripening
   b. labor induction
   c. gastroesophageal reflux
   d. peptic ulcers

22–11. What is the dosage of misoprostol that the American College of Obstetricians and Gynecologists recommends be used for cervical ripening?

   a. 25 μg
   b. 50 μg
   c. 100 μg
   d. 200 μg

22–12. A 50 μg misoprostol intravaginal dose has been shown to increase which of the following?

   a. tachysystole
   b. meconium passage
   c. cesarean delivery rate
   d. all of the above

22–13. In which of the following ways is balloon catheter cervical ripening superior to intracervical PGE$_2$ gel?

   a. decreases cesarean delivery rate
   b. lowers Bishop score
   c. decreases intervention-to-delivery time
   d. no difference

22–14. What proportion of women who undergo membrane stripping will enter labor spontaneously within 72 hours?

   a. one fourth
   b. one third
   c. one half
   d. two thirds

25–15. In what year was oxytocin first synthesized?

   a. 1920
   b. 1931
   c. 1942
   d. 1953

22–16. What is the mean half-life of oxytocin?

   a. 5 min
   b. 10 min
   c. 20 min
   d. 30 min

22–17. How long does it take oxytocin to reach steady-state levels in the plasma?

   a. 5 min
   b. 10 min
   c. 20 min
   d. 40 min

22–18. At what gestational age does the uterine response to oxytocin increase?

   a. 6 to 10 weeks
   b. 10 to 18 weeks
   c. 20 to 30 weeks
   d. 32 to 36 weeks

22–19. At what dosage of oxytocin is renal-free water clearance decreased?

   a. 10 mU/min
   b. 20 mU/min
   c. 40 mU/min
   d. 60 mU/min

22–20. How are Montevideo units calculated?

   a. number of contractions in 10 min × peak amplitude
   b. number of contractions in 20 min × peak amplitude
   c. number of contractions in 30 min × peak amplitude
   d. add the peak amplitude minus the baseline for each contraction in a 10-min period

22–21. What is the mean spontaneous uterine contraction pattern that results in vaginal delivery?

    a. 100 to 120 Montevideo units
    b. 140 to 150 Montevideo units
    c. 180 to 190 Montevideo units
    d. 220 to 230 Montevideo units

22–22. According to the American College of Obstetricians and Gynecologists guidelines, when is failure to progress diagnosed?

    a. The latent phase of labor has been completed.
    b. Montevideo units exceed 200 for 2 hr.
    c. There is no cervical change in 2 hr.
    d. The latent phase of labor exceeds 20 hr.

23

Forceps Delivery and Vacuum Extraction

23–1. What is the incidence of operative vaginal delivery?

    a. ≤1%
    b. 5 to 10%
    c. 15 to 20%
    d. 25 to 30%

23–2. Which of the following is NOT a basic component of a forceps branch?

    a. blade
    b. handle
    c. lock
    d. seal

23–3. Which type of shank characterizes Tucker-McLane forceps?

    a. crossing shanks
    b. English lock
    c. parallel shanks
    d. sliding lock

23–4. Which forceps has a sliding lock?

    a. Tucker-McLane
    b. Simpson

    c. Kielland
    d. Piper

23–5. Engagement of the fetal head occurs when the occiput reaches what station?

    a. −2
    b. 0
    c. +2
    d. +4

23–6. Which of the following is true of high forceps deliveries?

    a. forceps applied at +1 station
    b. fetal head engaged
    c. indicated for fetal distress
    d. no place in obstetrics today

23–7. Obstetrical practice over the past 20 years has shown which of the following trends?

    a. increased cesarean delivery
    b. decreased forceps delivery
    c. increased vacuum delivery
    d. all of the above

23–8. When forceps are applied to the fetal head with the scalp visible at the introitus and without manual separation of the labia, what type of delivery occurs?

　　a. outlet forceps
　　b. low forceps
　　c. midforceps
　　d. either outlet or low forceps

23–9. What is the classification for any forceps rotation at +2 cm?

　　a. outlet forceps
　　b. low forceps
　　c. midforceps
　　d. high forceps

23–10. When the fetal head is engaged and at a +1 cm station, how would a forceps delivery be classified?

　　a. outlet forceps
　　b. low forceps
　　c. midforceps
　　d. high forceps

23–11. Forceps applied when the fetal head (left occiput anterior position) has reached the pelvic floor and is at the perineum should be classified as what type of delivery?

　　a. outlet forceps
　　b. low forceps
　　c. midforceps
　　d. high forceps

23–12. Which of the following is NOT associated with regional analgesia?

　　a. increased frequency of forceps delivery
　　b. shorter second stage of labor
　　c. increased frequency of occiput posterior positions
　　d. decreased maternal expulsive efforts

23–13. Which of the following forceps is best suited for low forceps delivery of a fetus with a molded head?

　　a. Simpson
　　b. Tucker-McLane
　　c. Kielland
　　d. Chamberlain

23–14. Which of the following forceps is best suited for low forceps delivery of a fetus with a rounded head?

　　a. Simpson
　　b. Tucker-McLane

　　c. Kielland
　　d. Chamberlain

23–15. Which of the following maternal conditions is NOT an indication for termination of labor by forceps?

　　a. heart disease
　　b. exhaustion
　　c. intrapartum infection
　　d. second stage of labor of 1 1/2 hr in nullipara

23–16. When exceeded, which of the following is considered a prolonged second stage of labor for the nulliparous patient?

　　a. 1 hr without regional anesthesia
　　b. 1 hr with regional anesthesia
　　c. 2 hr without regional anesthesia
　　d. 2 hr with regional anesthesia

23–17. Which of the following is a fetal indication for termination of labor by forceps assuming other requisites are present?

　　a. prolapse of umbilical cord
　　b. meconium-stained amnionic fluid
　　c. placenta previa
　　d. reactive fetal heart rate pattern

23–18. When exceeded, which of the following is the most correct definition of a prolonged second stage in the parous patient?

　　a. 1 hr without regional anesthesia
　　b. 1 hr with regional anesthesia
　　c. 2 hr without regional anesthesia
　　d. 3 hr with regional anesthesia

23–19. Forceps delivery should generally NOT be used *electively* until criteria for which type of delivery are fulfilled?

　　a. midforceps
　　b. low forceps
　　c. outlet forceps
　　d. should never be used electively

23–20. With regard to the use of prophylactic forceps, which of the following statements is correct?

　　a. They will prevent episiotomy extension.
　　b. They will reduce the incidence of fetal brain damage from prolonged perineal pressure.
　　c. They are associated with improved neonatal outcome in low-birthweight infants.
　　d. There is no current evidence that they are beneficial in otherwise normal term labor and delivery.

23–21. Which of the following is NOT a prerequisite for forceps application?

　　a. Head must be engaged.
　　b. Fetus must present either by the vertex or by the face with the chin posterior.
　　c. Cervix must be completely dilated.
　　d. Membranes must be ruptured.

23–22. Which of the following analgesia or anesthesia techniques is LEAST adequate for low forceps or midpelvic procedures?

　　a. pudendal block
　　b. spinal block
　　c. epidural block
　　d. ketamine

23–23. Forceps are correctly applied along which diameter of the fetal head?

　　a. biparietal
　　b. occipitomental
　　c. coronophregmatic
　　d. sagittal

23–24. Regarding traction with forceps, which of the following statements is NOT correct?

　　a. Gentle traction should be intermittent.
　　b. The fetal head should be allowed to recede in intervals.
　　c. Delivery should be deliberate and slow.
　　d. Traction should be applied between contractions.

23–25. Which is TRUE with regard to manual rotation of the fetal head during labor?

　　a. disengagement of the fetal head must be avoided
　　b. forceps are always applied immediately after
　　c. has no place in modern obstetrics
　　d. should be attempted before rupture of fetal membranes

23–26. Which type of pelvis most strongly predisposes to occiput posterior presentations and opposed rotations?

　　a. android
　　b. anthropoid
　　c. gynecoid
　　d. platypelloid

23–27. Which of the following is true of occiput posterior deliveries as compared with occiput anterior deliveries?

　　a. Infants have a higher incidence of Erb and facial palsy.
　　b. There are fewer perineal lacerations.
　　c. Episiotomy is performed less often.
　　d. Forceps delivery is not used in current obstetrical practice.

23–28. In which of the following presentations are forceps contraindicated?

　　a. mentum anterior
　　b. mentum posterior
　　c. right occiput oblique
　　d. left occiput transverse

23–29. In which of the following types of delivery is maternal blood transfusion most likely to be needed?

　　a. cesarean delivery
　　b. spontaneous vaginal delivery
　　c. forceps-assisted delivery
　　d. vacuum extraction

23–30. Which of the following has an increased incidence with operative delivery compared to those who have a spontaneous vaginal delivery?

　　a. episiotomy
　　b. fourth-degree perineal laceration
　　c. vaginal lacerations
　　d. all of the above

23–31. Which of the following increases the risk of postpartum (short-term) urinary or fecal incontinence?

　　a. forceps delivery
　　b. perineal lacerations
　　c. spontaneous vaginal delivery
　　d. all of the above

23–32. Which of the following is NOT associated with fecal incontinence in women?

　　a. low parity
　　b. hysterectomy
　　c. irritable bowel syndrome
　　d. menopause

23–33. Which of the following is NOT increased with midforceps versus cesarean delivery?

　　a. facial nerve palsy in the infant
　　b. maternal blood transfusion
　　c. postpartum metritis
　　d. neonatal morbidity

23–34. A 24-year-old G1P0 is in labor at term with epidural analgesia in place. Upon reaching complete cervical dilation, she pushes for 3 hours and 15 minutes. Exam shows occiput transverse presentation at +1 station. There is no evidence of fetal distress or infection. Contemporaneous guidelines would favor which mode of delivery?

a. await spontaneous vaginal delivery
b. cesarean delivery
c. midforceps
d. vacuum extraction

23–35. Which of the following is NOT a theoretical advantage of the vacuum extractor over forceps?

a. not as much vaginal space required
b. ability to rotate the fetal head without impinging upon maternal soft tissues
c. less intracranial pressure during traction
d. can be applied at higher stations than forceps

23–36. What is a chignon?

a. an artificial caput
b. a scalp hematoma
c. an abrasion caused by the metal vacuum cup
c. a soft vacuum cup

23–37. What complication appears to be decreased with the use of soft vacuum cups as compared to rigid metal cups?

a. birth canal injury
b. cephalohematoma
c. episiotomy extension
d. minor scalp injuries

23–38. Which of the following is a relative contraindication for delivery using vacuum extraction?

a. face presentation
b. 35-week gestation
c. chorioamnionitis
d. post-term pregnancy

23–39. With regard to vacuum delivery, what number of cup detachments ("pop-offs") can be tolerated before increased neonatal morbidity is seen?

a. 1
b. 2
c. 4
d. has not been determined

23–40. Which of the following is NOT a direct complication of delivery using vacuum extraction?

a. cephalohematoma
b. intracranial hemorrhage
c. neonatal acidemia
d. retinal hemorrhage

Breech Presentation and Delivery

24–1. What is the approximate incidence of breech presentation at term?

a. <1%
b. 3 to 4%
c. 7 to 8%
d. 12 to 15%

24–2. Which of the following is NOT a risk factor for breech?

a. multiple fetuses
b. hydramnios
c. uterine anomalies
d. low parity

24–3. Which of the following complications is NOT increased with persistent breech presentation?

   a. perinatal morbidity and mortality
   b. macrosomia
   c. prolapsed cord
   d. placenta previa

24–4. Which of the following describes a frank breech presentation?

   a. flexion of the hips and extension of the knees
   b. flexion of the hips and flexion of the knees
   c. extension of the hips and flexion of the knees
   d. extension of the hips and extension of the knees

24–5. Which of the following best describes a complete breech presentation?

   a. lower extremities flexed at the hips and extended at knees
   b. lower extremities flexed at the hips and one or both knees flexed
   c. one or both hips not flexed or both feet or knees below breech
   d. a foot is in the birth canal

24–6. Which of the following best describes the incomplete breech presentation?

   a. lower extremities flexed at the hips and extended at knees
   b. lower extremities flexed at the hips and one or both knees flexed
   c. one or both hips not flexed or both feet or knees below breech
   d. both feet are in the right fundal area

24–7. When examining a woman at term, hearing fetal heart tones loudest above the umbilicus suggests which type of presentation?

   a. cephalic presentation
   b. transverse lie
   c. breech presentation
   d. multiple pregnancy

24–8. Which of the following help to differentiate a frank breech from a cephalic presentation during vaginal examination?

   a. ischial tuberosities and anus form a straight line
   b. ischial tuberosities and anus form a triangle shape
   c. ischial tuberosities and anus form a circular shape
   d. mouth and malar eminences form a straight line

24–9. Cerebral palsy in a breech-presenting fetus is more likely related to which of the following delivery events?

   a. vaginal breech delivery
   b. Piper forceps to aftercoming fetal head
   c. cesarean delivery
   d. not related to mode of delivery

24–10. Up to what percentage of breech deliveries will be complicated by a nuchal arm?

   a. <1
   b. 3
   c. 6
   d. 10

24–11. Which of the following pelvis type(s) are unfavorable configurations for breech vaginal deliveries?

   a. platypelloid
   b. anthropoid
   c. android
   d. a and c

24–12. Approximately what percentage of breech presentations at term will be associated with an extreme hyperextension of the fetal head?

   a. 0.5
   b. 5
   c. 15
   d. 25

24–13. Which of the following is increased in preterm very-low-birthweight breech fetuses delivered vaginally?

   a. intraventricular hemorrhage
   b. neonatal death
   c. both of the above
   d. neither of the above

24–14. In the Hannah randomized controlled trial comparing planned vaginal breech delivery to planned cesarean delivery, which of the following was significantly decreased in the vaginal delivery group?

   a. maternal hemorrhage
   b. maternal sepsis
   c. perinatal mortality
   d. perinatal morbidity

24–15. What is the position of the bitrochanteric diameter during engagement and descent of the breech?

   a. oblique
   b. transverse
   c. anteroposterior
   d. a and then c

24–16. Which of the following characterizes partial breech extraction?

   a. newborn delivers spontaneously to shoulder
   b. newborn delivers spontaneously to umbilicus
   c. newborn's buttocks deliver spontaneously
   d. newborn is extracted entirely by the attendant

24–17. During early labor in a breech presentation the fetal heart rate should be evaluated how often?

   a. every 5 min
   b. every 15 min
   c. every 30 min
   d. continuously

24–18. How should traction in a breech extraction be employed?

   a. gentle and parallel to the floor
   b. marked 30-degree angle pull toward the ceiling
   c. gentle and downward plus 180 degree rotation of fetal pelvis
   d. marked downward pull until the axilla are visible

24–19. In which maneuver are the index and middle finger applied over the maxilla in order to free the head?

   a. Pinard
   b. Bracht
   c. Mauriceau
   d. Zavanelli

24–20. With breech delivery, which maneuver is suggested when there is persistence of the fetal spine directed toward the maternal sacrum?

   a. Prague
   b. Bracht
   c. Pinard
   d. McRoberts

24–21. What is the maneuver that involves intrauterine manual conversion of a frank breech to a footling breech?

   a. Prague
   b. Pinard
   c. Bracht
   d. Lemille

24–22. During a breech delivery, the fetal back rotates toward the maternal vertebral column. If traction occurs in this position, what may happen to the fetal head?

   a. may flex
   b. may assume a military position
   c. may wedge beneath the symphysis
   d. may extend

24–23. According to the American College of Obstetricians and Gynecologists, what is the approximate success rate of external cephalic version for breech presentations late in pregnancy?

   a. 20%
   b. 40%
   c. 60%
   d. 80%

24–24. Which of the following is most strongly associated with successful external cephalic version?

   a. frank breech
   b. anteriorly located fetal spine
   c. ample amnionic fluid
   d. increasing parity

24–25. A 21-year-old, nulliparous D-negative patient at 36 weeks gestation undergoes an external version for breech presentation. Which of the following should be given?

   a. anti-D immunoglobulin
   b. magnesium sulfate
   c. oxytocin
   d. nifedipine

24–26. Which of the following is NOT associated with a successful external cephalic version?

   a. postterm gestation
   b. large amnionic fluid volume
   c. unengaged fetus
   d. high parity

24–27. Using decision analysis, what is the cost-effectiveness of external cephalic versions?

   a. ↓ cost, ↑ cesarean deliveries
   b. ↓ cost, ↓ cesarean deliveries
   c. ↑ cost, ↑ cesarean deliveries
   d. ↑ cost, ↓ cesarean deliveries

25

Cesarean Delivery and Peripartum Hysterectomy

25–1. Who wrote in detail about obstetrics in the 2nd century AD?

    a. Julius Caesar
    b. Numa Pompilius
    c. Hippocrates
    d. Soranus

25–2. What accounted for the decrease in the cesarean delivery rate in the United States from 1989 to 1996?

    a. increase in vaginal breech deliveries
    b. active management of labor
    c. vaginal birth after cesarean delivery
    d. increase in midforceps deliveries

25–3. What was the total cesarean delivery rate in the United States in 2002?

    a. 20 to 21%
    b. 23 to 24%
    c. 26 to 27%
    d. 29 to 30%

25–4. What is the most common indication for a primary cesarean delivery in the United States?

    a. fetal distress
    b. breech presentation
    c. dystocia or failure to progress
    d. prior cesarean delivery

25–5. Use of electronic fetal monitoring has been shown to decrease which of the following?

    a. cesarean delivery rate
    b. incidence of cerebral palsy
    c. incidence of perinatal death
    d. none of the above

25–6. Which of the following is a possible advantage of the transverse skin incision?

    a. allows exposure of uterus and appendages
    b. easy to extend incision rapidly
    c. stronger than a vertical incision
    d. less hematoma formation subfascially

25–7. Which of the following is NOT an advantage of low transverse cesarean deliveries?

    a. easier to repair
    b. less blood loss
    c. fewer problems with adhesions to bowel
    d. ability to safely extend incision laterally

25–8. What type of incision divides the rectus muscles sharply or with electrocautery?

    a. Maylard
    b. Kerr
    c. Krönig
    d. Frank-Letzko

25–9. What is the least common type of cesarean operation?

    a. low vertical
    b. Kerr-Munro
    c. Krönig
    d. classical

25–10. Sharp extension of the uterine incision is most commonly associated with an increase in which of the following?

    a. postpartum endometritis
    b. bleeding
    c. fetal injuries
    d. maternal ileus

25–11. What is a major side effect of oxytocin 10 units IV bolus given postpartum?

    a. respiratory distress
    b. hypertension
    c. hypotension
    d. seizures

25–12. A decrease in which of the following is the major benefit of closing the subcutaneous layer?

   a. blood loss
   b. wound disruption
   c. fascial dehiscence
   d. wound infection

25–13. Which of the following is NOT an indication for a classical cesarean incision?

   a. cannot visualize the lower uterine segment
   b. transverse lie
   c. premature breech
   d. term breech (frank)

25–14. What is the incidence of bladder laceration at the time of cesarean delivery?

   a. 0.3 per 1000
   b. 0.7 per 1000
   c. 1.4 per 1000
   d. 2.8 per 1000

25–15. According to the Maternal–Fetal Medicine Units Network, what is the incidence of peripartum hysterectomy?

   a. 1:100 cesarean deliveries
   b. 1:200 cesarean deliveries
   c. 1:500 cesarean deliveries
   d. 1:1000 cesarean deliveries

25–16. What are the most common indications for peripartum or cesarean hysterectomy?

   a. atony and accreta
   b. atony and infection
   c. rupture of uterus and atony
   d. accreta and infection

25–17. What percentage of women undergoing emergency peripartum hysterectomy receive a blood transfusion?

   a. 30
   b. 50
   c. 70
   d. 90

25–18. What is the average blood loss with an elective cesarean hysterectomy?

   a. 500 mL
   b. 1000 mL
   c. 1500 mL
   d. 3000 mL

25–19. Which of the following prophylactic antimicrobials has been shown to decrease postpartum endometritis?

   a. metronidazole
   b. cephalosporins
   c. tetracycline
   d. azithromycin

26

Prior Cesarean Delivery

26–1. A trial of labor following cesarean delivery has the highest incidence of which of the following?

   a. uterine rupture
   b. perinatal death
   c. maternal death
   d. thromboembolism

26–2. Compared with patients undergoing elective repeat cesarean delivery, women undergoing trial of labor following cesarean delivery have a higher risk of all of the following EXCEPT

   a. endometritis
   b. uterine rupture
   c. thromboembolism
   d. fetal hypoxic ischemic encephalopathy

26–3. What is the rate of uterine rupture in women undergoing a trial of labor following cesarean delivery?

    a. <1%
    b. 5%
    c. 10%
    d. 15%

26–4. What is the rate of fetal death or injury attributable to trial of labor following cesarean delivery?

    a. 1 per 1000
    b. 5 per 1000
    c. 10 per 1000
    d. 15 per 1000

26–5. Which of the following is true of a planned repeat cesarean delivery compared with a trial of labor following cesarean delivery?

    a. lower hospital charges
    b. higher rates of patient fear regarding their route of delivery
    c. lower patient satisfaction regarding their route of delivery
    d. none of the above

26–6. Which of the following criteria reflects fetal maturity?

    a. 30 weeks have passed since a positive urinary hCG test result
    b. fetal heart sounds have been heard for 20 weeks by Doppler
    c. fetal heart sounds have been heard for 10 weeks by non-electronic fetoscope
    d. crown-rump length at 6 to 11 weeks documents a gestational age of 39 weeks

26–7. Your patient presented for initial prenatal care at 22 weeks' gestation by last menstrual period. At her initial visit, fetal heart tones were heard by non-electronic fetoscope. Fundal height measurement was 22 cm. Ultrasonongraphic measurements were consistent with a 22-week gestation. She has selected a repeat planned cesarean delivery rather than a trial of labor. She is currently at 38 weeks gestation. The next step in the management of this patient includes which of the following?

    a. perform amniocentesis to document fetal lung maturity
    b. schedule her repeat cesarean for 39 weeks gestational age

    c. schedule her repeat cesarean for 40 weeks gestational age
    d. repeat ultrasonographic examination to document fetal gestation age and weight

26–8. Selection criteria set forth by the American College of Obstetricians and Gynecologists regarding trial of labor candidacy include which of the following?

    a. delivery at a tertiary care facility
    b. no more than two prior cesarean deliveries
    c. clinician available during latent and active labor phases
    d. prior low transverse or low vertical incisions without extension

26–9. Women with which of the following incision types would be candidates for a trial of labor following cesarean delivery?

    a. classical
    b. T-shaped
    c. low vertical without extension
    d. low transverse in a bicornuate uterus

26–10. Your patient is contemplating a trial of labor following her prior cesarean delivery. She should be counseled that an increased risk of uterine rupture is associated with all of the following EXCEPT

    a. cervical ripening
    b. prior vaginal delivery
    c. oxytocin augmentation
    d. increasing number of prior cesarean deliveries

26–11. Generally, what is the success rate for trial of labor following cesarean delivery?

    a. 20 to 40%
    b. 40 to 60%
    c. 60 to 80%
    d. 80 to 100%

26–12. Which of the following indications for the prior cesarean delivery are associated with the highest success rates in subsequent trials of labor?

    a. fetal distress
    b. breech presentation
    c. dystocia with cervical dilation ≤5 cm
    d. dystocia during the second stage of labor

26–13. Which of the following is associated with an increased risk of uterine rupture?

    a. labor induction
    b. cervical ripening
    c. oxytocin augmentation
    d. all of the above

26–14. Common maternal signs of uterine rupture include which of the following?

    a. severe abdominal pain
    b. cessation of contractions
    c. increased intrauterins catheter pressures
    d. none of the above

26–15. The most common fetal sign of uterine rupture in women undergoing a trial of labor following prior cesarean delivery is which of the following?

    a. change in presenting part
    b. sustained fetal tachycardia
    c. loss of fetal station
    d. fetal heart rate decelerations

26–16. True statements regarding the use of epidural anesthesia in women undergoing trial of labor following prior cesarean delivery includes which of the following?

    a. should be withheld in these patients
    b. increases trial of labor success rates
    c. decreases trial of labor success rates
    d. none of the above

26–17. A uterine dehiscence found during palpation after a successful VBAC requires repair in which of the following situations?

    a. bleeding at dehiscence site
    b. concurrent chorioamnionitis
    c. patient plans future fertility
    d. all of the above

26–18. The greatest percentage of uterine ruptures is associated with which of the following?

    a. external version
    b. prior cesarean delivery
    c. prior uterine trauma from D&C instruments
    d. fundal pressure during the second stage of labor

26–19. In defining the difference between incomplete and complete uterine rupture, which of the following layers is evaluated?

    a. abdominal fascia
    b. parietal peritoneum
    c. visceral peritoneum
    d. external layer of uterine muscle

26–20. Which of the following reflects the rate of fetal survival with uterine rupture and expulsion of the fetus?

    a. 10 to 25%
    b. 25 to 50%
    c. 50 to 75%
    d. 75 to 90%

27

Abnormalities of the Placenta, Umbilical Cord, and Membranes

27–1. What is the name for incomplete division of the placenta into separate lobes with fetal vessels extending from one lobe to the other?

    a. placenta bipartita
    b. placenta succenturiata
    c. placenta membranacea
    d. placenta fenestrata

27–2. Which type of placenta contains small accessory lobes in the fetal membranes distant from the main placenta?

    a. fenestrated placenta
    b. membranaceous placenta
    c. placenta bilobata
    d. placenta succenturiata

27–3. Of the abnormal placentations, which is NOT associated with postpartum hemorrhage?

   a. membranaceous placenta
   b. placenta bipartita
   c. placenta succenturiata
   d. ring-shaped placenta

27–4. Of the abnormal placentas listed, which is associated with fetal growth restriction?

   a. fenestrated placenta
   b. placenta bilobata
   c. placenta succenturiata
   d. ring-shaped placenta

27–5. What name is given to a placenta whose central portion is missing?

   a. fenestrated placenta
   b. membranaceous placenta
   c. placenta accreta
   d. placenta succenturiata

27–6. In which placental type is the chorionic plate smaller than the basal plate?

   a. extrachorial
   b. fenestrated
   c. membranaceous
   d. ring-shaped

27–7. What placental type is associated with antepartum fetal hemorrhage, placental abruption, preterm delivery, and fetal malformations?

   a. circumvallate placenta
   b. fenestrated placenta
   c. placenta bipartita
   d. triplex placenta

27–8. Which of the following are risk factors for the development of placenta accreta, increta, and percreta?

   a. placenta previa
   b. prior cesarean delivery
   c. uterine perforation in prior pregnancy
   d. all of the above

27–9. By mid-third trimester, what percentage of placentas demonstrate calcification?

   a. <1
   b. 10
   c. 25
   d. >50

27–10. Which of the following is the most common placental pathology?

   a. previa
   b. abruption
   c. infarcts
   d. deciduitis

27–11. What is the incidence of placental infarcts in term, uncomplicated pregnancies?

   a. 10%
   b. 25%
   c. 50%
   d. 67%

27–12. What do small placental infarctions commonly formed at term usually result from?

   a. chorioamnionitis
   b. chronic abruption
   c. normal aging
   d. placental insufficiency

27–13. What sequelae are associated with maternal floor placental infarction?

   a. abortion
   b. central nervous system injury in infant
   c. stillbirth
   d. all of the above

27–14. Placental stem (fetal) artery thrombosis is NOT associated with which of the following conditions?

   a. diabetes (maternal)
   b. fetal growth restriction
   c. twin gestation
   d. stillbirth

27–15. Striking enlargement of the chorionic villi is associated with which of these conditions?

   a. fetal hydrops
   b. twin gestation
   c. postterm pregnancy
   d. maternal genital herpes simplex infection

27–16. Which of the following is the only benign placental tumor?

   a. chorioangioma
   b. fibroma
   c. mesenchymal rest cell
   d. placental site tumor

27–17. Which of the following pregnancy complications may be associated with large chorioangiomas?

   a. oligohydramnios
   b. polyhydramnios
   c. abruption
   d. severe hypertension

27–18. Which malignancy is most likely to metastasize to the placenta?

a. breast
b. melanoma
c. lung
d. endometrial

27–19. In what percentage of deliveries is meconium present in amnionic fluid?

a. <5
b. 10 to 20
c. 40 to 50
d. 70 to 80

27–20. Passage of meconium is most common in which gestational age group?

a. all equal beyond 24 weeks
b. postterm (>42 weeks)
c. preterm (<38 weeks)
d. term (38 to 42 weeks)

27–21. Which is true of meconium staining of the fetal membranes?

a. cannot be dated or timed accurately
b. occurs more than 72 hours after meconium passage
c. seen only in postterm pregnancies
d. signifies fetal lung maturity

27–22. Which of the following is generally associated with meconium passage and staining?

a. cesarean delivery
b. perinatal mortality
c. severe fetal acidemia
d. all of the above

27–23. What percentage of infants exposed to meconium develop meconium aspiration syndrome?

a. <1
b. 10
c. 50
d. 90

27–24. What is the mortality rate of meconium aspiration syndrome?

a. <1%
b. 10%
c. 50%
d. 90%

27–25. Leukocytes are maternal in origin in which of the following inflammatory conditions?

a. amnionitis
b. chorioamnionitis

c. funisitis
d. none of the above

27–26. What is the mean length of the umbilical cord reported to be?

a. 17 cm
b. 37 cm
c. 77 cm
d. 107 cm

27–27. Which of the following is NOT associated with excessively long umbilical cords (≥70 cm)?

a. cord entanglement
b. fetal distress
c. funisitis
d. maternal systemic disease

27–28. Which may be a determinant of umbilical cord length?

a. amnionic fluid volume
b. fetal mobility
c. heredity
d. all of the above

27–29. What percentage of infants missing one umbilical artery (2-vessel cord) will have congenital anomalies?

a. 1
b. 25
c. 75
d. 95

27–30. Which of the following is NOT increased in fetuses with hypercoiled cords?

a. chorioamnionitis
b. fetal distress
c. meconium-stained amnionic fluid
d. preterm birth

27–31. What is insertion of the cord at the placental margin called?

a. Battledore placenta
b. furcate insertion
c. vasa previa
d. velamentous insertion

27–32. In what type of cord insertion do the umbilical vessels separate in the membranes some distance from the placental margin?

a. velamentous insertion
b. marginal insertion
c. furcate insertion
d. all of the above

27–33. Vasa previa is associated with which of the following?

    a. fetal exsanguination
    b. low-lying placenta
    c. placenta succenturiata
    d. all of the above

27–34. Which umbilical cord condition results from active fetal movements?

    a. Battledore placenta
    b. false knots
    c. true knots
    d. vasa previa

27–35. What is the rate of stillbirth in the presence of true cord knots?

    a. 0.06%
    b. 6%
    c. 66%
    d. not increased

27–36. What is the incidence of single-loop nuchal cords?

    a. ≤1%
    b. 5%
    c. 10%
    d. ≥20%

27–37. Which of the following is most commonly associated with nuchal cord loops?

    a. fetal anomalies
    b. perinatal mortality
    c. severe fetal acidosis
    d. variable fetal heart rate decelerations

27–38. Which of the following is often seen with cord stricture?

    a. cocaine use
    b. focal deficiency of Wharton jelly
    c. hyperactive fetus
    d. velamentous cord insertion

27–39. What is the etiology of true cysts of the umbilical cord?

    a. excessive maternal progesterone levels
    b. intra-amniotic infection
    c. liquefaction of Wharton's jelly
    d. remnants of the allantois

27–40. What is the etiology of false cysts of the umbilical cord?

    a. excessive levels of maternal progesterone
    b. intra-amniotic infection
    c. liquefaction of Wharton's jelly
    d. remnants of the allantois

27–41. For which situation is the pathological examination of the placenta and umbilical cord considered the LEAST cost-effective and informative?

    a. all obstetrical deliveries
    b. fetal growth restriction
    c. maternal disorders
    d. stillbirths

28

The Newborn Infant

28–1. Which of the following contributes to transient tachypnea of the newborn?

   a. delay in removal of fluid from alveoli
   b. hypoxia
   c. hypercapnea
   d. hypothermia

28–2. In the normal mature infant, the respiratory pressure–volume ratios change to that of adults over what time period?

   a. <1 min
   b. 5 to 10 min
   c. 1 to 5 hr
   d. 1 to 5 days

28–3. What causes respiratory distress syndrome?

   a. decreased alveolar surface tension
   b. decreased alveolar surfactant
   c. increased alveolar fluid
   d. increased mucus plugging

28–4. The American College of Obstetricians and Gynecologists recommends that an attendant be present at delivery for neonatal care who is able to provide which of the following?

   a. neonatal stimulation and suctioning of nares
   b. facilitation of maternal bonding
   c. accurate identification and neonatal banding
   d. resuscitation

28–5. Initially, most neonates respond physiologically to oxygen deprivation with which of the following?

   a. apnea
   b. rapid breathing
   c. hypothermia
   d. hypotonia

28–6. In most neonates, oxygen deprivation lasting 30 to 60 seconds will lead to all of the following EXCEPT

   a. hypotension
   b. hypotonia
   c. hypoglycemia
   d. bradycardia

28–7. Within the first 30 seconds of life, a neonate under your care following a vaginal delivery begins to breathe rapidly and then becomes apneic with heart rate of 70 beats per minute. Resuscitation of this neonate should include all of the following EXCEPT

   a. stimulation
   b. warming
   c. ventilatory assistance
   d. chest compressions

28–8. If chest compressions are not required, the recommended ventilatory resuscitation rates in breaths per minute for an apneic neonate include which of the following?

   a. 10 to 20
   b. 20 to 40
   c. 40 to 60
   d. 60 to 80

28–9. Clinical indicators used to assess the effectiveness of ventilatory resuscitation include all of the following EXCEPT

    a. color of fetal torso
    b. fetal muscle tone
    c. fetal heart rate
    d. chest excursions

28–10. Obstacles to effective neonatal ventilation may include all of the following EXCEPT

    a. fetal hypotonia
    b. fetal pneumothorax
    c. meconium aspiration
    d. poor fetal positioning

28–11. Indications for endotracheal intubation typically include all of the following EXCEPT

    a. congenital diaphragmatic hernia
    b. need for chest compressions
    c. cyanotic fetal extremities
    d. prolonged bag–mask ventilation

28–12. Clinical indicators that reflect correct endotracheal tube placement include which of the following?

    a. breath sounds at the left infracostal margin
    b. breath sounds in each axilla
    c. right chest wall excursions greater than those of the left
    d. left chest wall excursions greater than those of the right

28–13. Regarding neonatal resuscitation, the recommended ratio of chest compressions relative to ventilations per minute include which of the following?

    a. 40 to 20
    b. 60 to 20
    c. 90 to 30
    d. 100 to 60

28–14. You are called to assist in the resuscitation of a term neonate. Ventilation via endotracheal tube and chest compressions for 60 seconds have failed to raise the neonate's heart rate above 40 beats per minute. An appropriate next clinical step includes which of the following?

    a. electrical cardioversion
    b. endotracheal surfactant
    c. intravenous lidocaine
    d. endotracheal epinephrine

28–15. After delivery, a neonate under your care becomes apneic. Resuscitation is begun and investigation into the cause is focused in part on maternal medication exposure. Which of the following group of drugs is most commonly associated with neonatal apnea?

    a. narcotics
    b. anticonvulsants
    c. antitubercular agents
    d. serotonin-reuptake inhibitors

28–16. During neonatal cardiopulmonary arrest, resuscitative efforts that fail to correct asystole within what time period may be halted?

    a. 5 min
    b. 15 min
    c. 45 min
    d. 60 min

28–17. Which of the following is NOT part of the Apgar score?

    a. heart rate
    b. respiratory effort
    c. color
    d. amnionic fluid consistency

28–18. What is the Apgar score of a neonate at 5 minutes of life whose respiratory effort is irregular, pulse is 90 beats per minute, who is floppy and cyanotic, and who only expresses minimal grimaces?

    a. 1
    b. 3
    c. 5
    d. 7

28–19. A low 1-minute Apgar score helps to identify which of the following?

    a. infant with birth asphyxia
    b. normal infant
    c. infant destined to develop neurological problems
    d. infant who requires resuscitation

28–20. The change in 1-minute to 5-minute Apgar scores is useful to assess which of the following?

    a. risk of cerebral palsy
    b. effectiveness of resuscitation
    c. neonatal maturity
    d. incidence of birth asphyxia

28–21. In addition to hypoxia, an Apgar score may also be affected by any of the following factors EXCEPT

    a. fetal anomalies
    b. prematurity
    c. ethnicity
    d. maternal narcotic use

28–22. Which of the following neurological deficits is most clearly related to perinatal asphyxia?

    a. seizures
    b. mental retardation
    c. cerebral palsy
    d. autism

28–23. Postpartum umbilical cord blood sampling assists in the assessment of which of the following?

    a. anemia
    b. aneuploidy
    c. metabolic disturbances
    d. infection

28–24. Which umbilical artery blood gas represents the expected mean in a normal term neonate?

    a. 7.35, pCO_2 49 mm Hg, HCO_3 10 mEq/L
    b. 7.35, pCO_2 60 mm Hg, HCO_3 23 mEq/L
    c. 7.28, pCO_2 60 mm Hg, HCO_3 10 mEq/L
    d. 7.28, pCO_2 49 mm Hg, HCO_3 23 mEq/L

28–25. The lower limits of the normal pH range in neonates at birth include which of the following?

    a. 6.90 to 6.98
    b. 7.00 to 7.10
    c. 7.12 to 7.20
    d. 7.22 to 7.28

28–26. According to the American College of Obstetricians and Gynecologists, metabolic acidemia is defined by which of the following?

    a. umbilical artery blood pH <6.9 and base deficit ≤12
    b. umbilical artery blood pH <7.0 and base deficit ≤10
    c. umbilical artery blood pH <7.1 and base deficit ≤13
    d. umbilical artery blood pH <7.2 and base deficit ≤11

28–27. In term infants, metabolic acidemia is most consistently associated with which of the following sequela?

    a. multiorgan dysfunction
    b. cerebral palsy
    c. autism
    d. deafness

28–28. The most common source of respiratory acidemia in neonates at birth is which of the following?

    a. placental abruption
    b. intrapartum infection
    c. hypotonic uterine contractions
    d. cord compression

28–29. Blood gas analysis from an umbilical artery sampling reveals a pH of 7.1, pCO_2 65 mm Hg; HCO_3 24 mEq/L corresponds to which type of acidosis?

    a. metabolic
    b. mixed
    c. respiratory
    d. normal

28–30. Blood gas analysis from an umbilical artery sampling reveals a pH of 7.1, pCO_2 65 mm Hg; HCO_3 14 mEq/L corresponds to which type of acidosis?

    a. metabolic
    b. mixed
    c. respiratory
    d. normal

28–31. A blood gas analysis from an umbilical artery sampling reveals a pH of 7.1, pCO_2 49 mm Hg; HCO_3 10 mEq/L corresponds to which type of acidosis?

    a. metabolic
    b. mixed
    c. respiratory
    d. normal

28–32. All EXCEPT which of the following are currently acceptable recommendations from the Centers for Disease Control and Prevention for prevention of gonococcal ophthalmic neonatorum?

    a. aqueous silver nitrate (1%)
    b. erythromycin ointment (0.5%)
    c. azithromycin ointment (0.25%)
    d. tetracycline ointment (1%)

28–33. A neonate that you delivered is now 14 days old and presents with a 3-day history of a persistent, bilateral serosanguineous eye drainage and edematous, erythematous eyelids. In the hospital, this neonate received standard care as recommended by the American Academy of Pediatrics. The most likely etiology for these signs is which of the following?

    a. *Neisseria gonorrhoeae*
    b. chemical irritation from silver nitrate solution
    c. *Staphylococcus aureus*
    d. *Chlamydia trachomatis*

28–34. In the United States, all states require mandatory neonatal screening for which of the following?

    a. hypothyroidism
    b. sickle-cell disease
    c. hepatitis B
    d. narcotics

28–35. Which of the following is commonly administered to neonates during their initial hospitalization?

    a. vitamin K
    b. varicella–zoster vaccination
    c. intraophthalmic azithromycin
    d. none of the above

28–36. In a male neonate, all EXCEPT which of the following are important in assessing gestational age?

    a. testes
    b. breasts
    c. ear lobes
    d. fingernails

28–37. You counsel your puerperal patient that separation of her newborn's umbilical cord from the umbilicus usually occurs at what time following delivery?

    a. 3 to 5 days
    b. 2 weeks
    c. 4 weeks
    d. 6 weeks

28–38. Which of the following statements is true regarding normal term neonates if they are properly nourished?

    a. They maintain their birthweight.
    b. They regain their birthweight by the 30th day of life.
    c. They require feedings every 2 to 4 hr.
    d. They lose weight over the first 2 weeks of life.

28–39. Failure of the neonate to pass stool or urine within the first 48 hours suggests which of the following?

    a. neonatal sepsis
    b. congenital defect
    c. inadequate nutrition
    d. birth asphyxia

28–40. Male circumcision will lower the incidence of all of the following EXCEPT

    a. penile cancer
    b. epiphimosis
    c. paraphimosis
    d. balanoposthitis

28–41. Contraindications to neonatal male circumcision include all of the following EXCEPT

    a. hypospadias
    b. low birthweight
    c. abnormal temperature
    d. recent hepatitis B vaccination

28–42. Preferred analgesia for male circumcision includes which of the following?

    a. dorsal nerve block using 1% lidocaine with epinephrine
    b. lidocaine–prilocaine topical cream
    c. ring block using 1% lidocaine
    d. local lidocaine infiltration

28–43. One of the most common reasons for neonates to be readmitted following an early hospital discharge typically involves which of the following?

    a. dehydration
    b. late-onset group B streptococcal infection
    c. bleeding complications of circumcision
    d. umbilical stump infection

29

Diseases and Injuries of the Fetus and Newborn

29–1. What pulmonary cell type produces surfactant?

   a. alveocyte, type A
   b. bronchiolar columnar cell
   c. pneuomocyte, type II
   d. transitional tracheocyte

29–2. Which is NOT a risk factor for neonatal respiratory distress syndrome?

   a. male gender
   b. maternal use of glucocorticoids antepartum
   c. premature birth
   d. white race

29–3. Which of the following is NOT a sign of neonatal hyaline membrane disease (RDS)?

   a. increased respiratory rate
   b. chest wall retraction during inspiration
   c. grunting
   d. systemic hypertension

29–4. A diffuse reticulogranular infiltrate and air bronchogram on chest radiograph is most common in which of the following disorders of the newborn?

   a. hyaline membrane disease
   b. pneumonia
   c. meconium aspiration
   d. heart failure

29–5. The use of postnatal glucocorticoids to prevent ventilator-induced bronchopulmonary dysplasia is no longer recommended because of an increased risk of which of the following?

   a. impaired cognitive development
   b. intraventricular hemorrhage
   c. necrotizing enterocolitis
   d. pulmonary hypertension

29–6. Exogenous surfactant therapy to prevent hyaline membrane disease is enhanced by antepartum maternal treatment with which of the following?

   a. aspirin
   b. glucocorticoids
   c. magnesium sulfate
   d. thyrotropin

29–7. Which of the following is a complication of hyperoxemia?

   a. intraventricular hemorrhage
   b. pneumonitis
   c. pulmonary hemorrhage
   d. retinopathy

29–8. At approximately what gestational week does the concentration of lecithin relative to sphingomyelin (L/S ratio) begin to rise?

   a. 28
   b. 32
   c. 34
   d. 36

29–9. What L/S ratio threshold indicates that fetal lung maturity is likely?

   a. 1
   b. 2
   c. 4
   d. 8

29–10. Which test of fetal lung maturity is NOT affected by contaminants such as blood, meconium, or vaginal secretions?

   a. lecithin–sphingomyelin ratio
   b. phosphatidylglycerol detection
   c. foam stability (shake) test
   d. all of the above

29–11. Which of the following measures the surfactant-albumin ratio in uncentrifuged amnionic fluid?

    a. fluorescent polarization
    b. amnionic fluid absorbance at 650 nm
    c. DPPC
    d. TDx-FLM

29–12. What amnionic fluid test, like L/S ratio and phosphatidylglycerol assay, accurately assesses fetal lung maturity?

    a. foam stability (shake) test
    b. lamellar body count
    c. macrophage count
    d. prostacyclin-thromboxane ratio

29–13. Neonates that develop retinopathy of prematurity are at increased future risk of which of the following?

    a. blindness
    b. early death
    c. neurological disability
    d. all of the above

29–14. Perinatal subdural hemorrhage is likely due to which of the following?

    a. asphyxia
    b. coagulopathy
    c. prematurity
    d. trauma

29–15. Most peri- and intraventricular hemorrhages of the preterm infant develop within what time period following birth?

    a. 1 hr
    b. 12 hr
    c. 3 days
    d. 7 days

29–16. What is the initiating event of periventricular hemorrhage?

    a. germinal matrix capillary damage
    b. periventricular parenchymal brain infarction
    c. microvascular thrombosis
    d. aqueductal ventricular obstruction

29–17. Approximately what percentage of all neonates born before 34 weeks will have evidence of intraventricular hemorrhage?

    a. 2
    b. 10
    c. 20
    d. 50

29–18. What percentage of term neonates will have evidence of ventricular hemorrhage?

    a. <1
    b. 4
    c. 18
    d. 33

29–19. Which grade of intraventricular hemorrhage is defined by ventricular dilatation?

    a. I
    b. II
    c. III
    d. IV

29–20. Which of the following increases the risk of periventricular bleeding and subsequent periventricular leukomalacia?

    a. postnatal heparin administration in neonatal nursery
    b. neonatal infection
    c. ventilator therapy
    d. all of the above

29–21. Administration of which of the following at least 24 hours prior to delivery reduces the risk and severity of intraventricular hemorrhage?

    a. vitamin K
    b. vitamin E
    c. phenobarbital
    d. corticosteroids

29–22. When administered prior to delivery, which corticosteroid appears to be the most effective in reducing both mortality and periventricular leukomalacia following intra- and periventricular hemorrhage?

    a. betamethasone
    b. cortisol
    c. dexamethasone
    d. hydrocortisone

29–23. Which of the following is NOT a common clinical finding in newborns with necrotizing enterocolitis (NEC)?

    a. pneumatosis intestinalis
    b. abdominal distention
    c. meconium stools
    d. ileus

29–24. What virus may be associated with NEC?

    a. picornavirus
    b. coronavirus
    c. herpesvirus
    d. parvovirus

29–25. Which of the following is true regarding the majority of cases of fetal and neonatal brain damage?

a. occur at or near time of birth
b. incidence decreased by cesarean delivery
c. not preventable
d. forceps delivery involved

29–26. What is the primary etiology of cerebral palsy?

a. environmental factors
b. genetic predisposition
c. multifactorial
d. obstetrical events

29–27. The diagnosis of birth asphyxia, as defined by the American College of Obstetricians and Gynecologists (1998), must meet which of the following criteria?

a. Apgar score of 0 to 3 for longer than 5 min
b. arterial umbilical cord blood pH <7.0
c. neonatal dysfunction of a major organ system
d. all of the above

29–28. What is the only type of cerebral palsy caused by an acute intrapartum hypoxic event?

a. ataxic plus learning disorder
b. diplegic
c. hemiparetic
d. spastic quadriplegic

29–29. What percentage of neonatal encephalopathy arises from events prior to the onset of labor?

a. 30
b. 50
c. 70
d. 90

29–30. What fetal heart rate pattern is most consistent with an intrapartum etiology of cerebral palsy?

a. sinusoidal
b. persistent late decelerations
c. severe variable decelerations
d. none of the above

29–31. Approximately what percentage of cerebral palsy cases are associated with mental retardation (IQ <50)?

a. 5
b. 25
c. 45
d. 65

29–32. What is the approximate incidence of cerebral palsy in developed countries?

a. 2 per 100 live births
b. 2 per 1000 live births
c. 2 per 10,000 live births
d. 2 per 100,000 live births

29–33. Which of the following is NOT associated with cerebral palsy?

a. abnormal fetal position
b. birthweight less than 2000 g
c. congenital malformation
d. forceps delivery

29–34. The fivefold increase in the cesarean delivery rate since 1965 has paralleled what trend in the incidence of cerebral palsy?

a. decreased by half
b. decreased slightly
c. no change
d. slight increase

29–35. Low Apgar scores at 1 and 5 minutes are reliable markers for which of the following?

a. need for resuscitation of neonate
b. failure to manage the delivery optimally
c. hypoxia sufficient to cause neurological damage
d. all of the above

29–36. What is the umbilical artery cord pH cutoff for clinically significant acidemia?

a. <7.2
b. <7.0
c. <6.8
d. <6.6

29–37. What is the increased risk of cerebral palsy in low-birthweight newborns with grade III or IV intraventricular hemorrhage compared with that of controls or of those with only a grade I or II hemorrhage?

a. 2-fold
b. 8-fold
c. 16-fold
d. 100-fold

29–38. The etiology of periventricular leukomalacia, the brain lesion associated with cerebral palsy, is most strongly linked to which of the following?

a. infection
b. intraventricular hemorrhage
c. postterm vaginal delivery
d. cerebral venous thrombosis

29–39. Based on the analysis of neuroradiological imaging, what percentage of cerebral palsy cases delivered at term appear to have been caused by a perinatal brain insult?

a. 20 to 25
b. 50 to 55
c. 70 to 75
d. 90 to 95

29–40. Which of the following clinical signs indicates severe neonatal encephalopathy in term infants?

a. coma
b. multiple seizures
c. recurrent apnea
d. all of the above

29–41. What is the incidence of severe mental retardation in children?

a. 3 per 100
b. 3 per 1000
c. 3 per 10,000
d. 3 per 100,000

29–42. Which of the following, when present without other comorbidities in term infants and children, is believed to be caused by perinatal hypoxia?

a. neonatal encephalopathy
b. mental retardation
c. seizures
d. none of the above

29–43. What is the incidence of chronic morbidity in neonates who weighed between 500 and 750 grams at birth?

a. 13%
b. 33%
c. 63%
d. 93%

29–44. What is the approximate mean cord hemoglobin concentration at term?

a. 10 g/dL
b. 13 g/dL
c. 17 g/dL
d. 21 g/dL

29–45. What test detects the presence of D-antigen-positive fetal red cells in the circulation of a D-antigen-negative mother?

a. Giemsa stain
b. Betke test
c. rosette test
d. Wright stain

29–46. What fetal heart rate characteristic is most suggestive of severe fetal anemia?

a. sinusoidal pattern
b. decreased beat-to-beat variability
c. repetitive late decelerations
d. wandering baseline

29–47. Of the following, which is the LEAST likely cause of fetal-to-maternal hemorrhage?

a. amniocentesis
b. chorionic villus sampling
c. cordocentesis
d. placental abruption

29–48. The results of which test are used to calculate the blood volume of fetal hemorrhage into the maternal circulation?

a. Giemsa stain
b. Kleihauer-Betke (KB) stain
c. rosette test
d. quinacrine banding

29–49. Approximately, what is the chance that a D-antigen–negative woman delivered of a D-antigen–positive, ABO-compatible infant will become D-isoimmunized?

a. 5%
b. 15%
c. 33%
d. 66%

29–50. What percentage of infants have ABO maternal blood group incompatibility?

a. 1
b. 10
c. 20
d. 50

29–51. What percentage of ABO incompatibility causes clinical anemia in the neonate?

a. 5
b. 10
c. 20
d. 30

29–52. What is the most common fetal–neonatal consequence of ABO incompatibility with anemia?

a. early death
b. hydrops fetalis
c. hyperbilirubinemia
d. need for exchange transfusions

29–53. Which of the following is NOT a criteria for the diagnosis of ABO incompatibility?

  a. mother is blood group O
  b. fetus is blood group A or B
  c. onset of jaundice after 7 days
  d. varying degrees of anemia, reticulocytosis, and erythroblastosis

29–54. What are the antigens of the rhesus blood group system?

  a. CDE
  b. cCDeE
  c. CDEcde
  d. cDe

29–55. Rh, or D, negativity is predicated upon the absence of which antigen?

  a. C
  b. d
  c. D
  d. e

29–56. The CDE antigens, inherited independently of other blood group antigens, are located on which chromosome?

  a. 1
  b. 6
  c. 12
  d. X

29–57. Which of the following ethnic groups has the highest incidence of D-antigen negativity (34%)?

  a. Basques
  b. Maori aborigines
  c. Native Americans
  d. Scandinavians

29–58. What percentage of pregnant women have atypical red cell antibodies?

  a. 1
  b. 5
  c. 15
  d. 20

29–59. Which of the following red cell antigens does NOT cause hemolytic disease of the newborn?

  a. Duffy
  b. Lewis
  c. Kell
  d. Kidd

29–60. Your patient undergoes early third-trimester amniocentesis due to a red cell antibody discovered by prenatal screening labs. The amnionic fluid bilirubin value is favorable. She presents 8 days later for decreased fetal movement. Fetal heart sounds are absent and sonography confirms fetal demise. Isoimmunization to which red cell antigen is most likely involved?

  a. CDE
  b. Kell
  c. Lewis
  d. MNS

29–61. The severity of ascites seen with hydrops fetalis correlates most directly with which of the following fetal conditions?

  a. degree and severity of anemia
  b. cardiac output
  c. hypoproteinemia
  d. portal hypertension

29–62. What is the fetal hemoglobin level below which hydrops fetalis is consistently seen?

  a. 4 g/dL
  b. 6 g/dL
  c. 8 g/dL
  d. 10 g/dL

29–63. Kernicterus is the result of elevated neonatal blood levels of which of the following?

  a. albumin
  b. bilirubin
  c. erythropoietin
  d. schistocytes

29–64. What test is performed as a standard part of prenatal care to detect abnormal maternal red cell antibodies?

  a. direct Coombs test
  b. enzyme-linked antiglobulin panel
  c. indirect Coombs test
  d. rosette test

29–65. Your patient is Rh-negative. Her husband, a Caucasian, is Rh-positive (D-positive). What is the risk that their fetus is D-positive?

  a. 25%
  b. 50%
  c. 75%
  d. 100%

29–66. Your patient has anti-Kell antibodies (titer 1:8), presumably from a blood transfusion 5 years ago. She has a 16-week gestation. What is your initial management of this high-risk situation?

  a. cordocentesis for fetal blood type
  b. maternal plasmapheresis
  c. paternal Kell antigen status determination
  d. pregnancy termination

29–67. Doppler flow studies of what fetal structure are highly sensitive for detection of fetal anemia?

   a. aorta
   b. middle cerebral artery
   c. renal artery
   d. umbilical artery

29–68. Within what range would the expected hemoglobin be in a fetus whose delta OD values from amniocentesis are in upper zone 3?

   a. <8 g/dL
   b. 8 to 11 g/dL
   c. 11 to 14 g/dL
   d. >14 g/dL

29–69. Using molecular techniques, fetal D-antigen status is most easily determined by analyzing what fetal cell type?

   a. amniocyte
   b. erythrocyte
   c. keratinocyte
   d. leukocyte

29–70. Your pregnant patient is found to have D-isoimmunization. At 32 weeks gestation, the fetal hemoglobin obtained by cord blood sampling is 2 g/dL below the mean for normal fetuses of the same gestational age. What is the recommended next step?

   a. administer intra-amnionic erythropoietin
   b. repeat cord blood sampling in 2 weeks
   c. amniocentesis for optical density determination
   d. begin fetal transfusions

29–71. What type of blood is used for initial exchange transfusion in the anemic newborn?

   a. O, D-negative
   b. O, D-positive
   c. AB, D-positive
   d. AB, D-negative

29–72. Approximately what percentage of D-negative women having elective pregnancy terminations become isoimmunized without the administration of D-immune globulin?

   a. <1
   b. 5
   c. 25
   d. 33

29–73. One 300 μg dose of D-immune globulin will protect the mother against what volume of fetal–maternal hemorrhage?

   a. 5 mL
   b. 30 mL
   c. 90 mL
   d. 150 mL

29–74. In the otherwise normal, term neonate, what is the level of unconjugated bilirubin above which the risk of kernicterus becomes significant?

   a. 3 mg/dL
   b. 6 mg/dL
   c. 12 mg/dL
   d. 18 mg/dL

29–75. Which of the following confers an increased risk of kernicterus?

   a. acidosis
   b. preterm delivery
   c. sepsis
   d. all of the above

29–76. With physiological jaundice, what is the usual level at which serum bilirubin peaks?

   a. 2 mg/dL
   b. 5 mg/dL
   c. 10 mg/dL
   d. 18 mg/dL

29–77. Which of the following is most commonly used to lower elevated serum bilirubin in neonates?

   a. exchange transfusion
   b. fluorescent light
   c. intravenous hydration
   d. vitamin K injection

29–78. Which of the following is NOT a common cause of nonimmune fetal hydrops?

   a. renal agenesis
   b. cardiac anomaly
   c. chromosomal anomaly
   d. twin-to-twin transfusion

29–79. What is the mortality rate of nonimmune hydrops evident before 24 weeks gestation?

   a. 35%
   b. 55%
   c. 75%
   d. 95%

29–80. Which infectious agents can cause nonimmune hydrops?

   a. parvovirus
   b. syphilis
   c. toxoplasmosis
   d. all of the above

29–81. The mirror syndrome involves development of which maternal condition in the presence of nonimmune fetal hydrops?

   a. heart failure
   b. liver dysfunction
   c. preeclampsia
   d. syncope

29–82. Which of the following fetal cardiac arrhythmias is most common and is rarely associated with adverse outcome?

   a. bradycardia (sustained)
   b. congenital heart block
   c. premature atrial contractions
   d. supraventricular tachycardia

29–83. Neonatal administration of which of the following reduces mortality in term neonates but NOT preterm infants (<34 weeks gestation) with respiratory distress syndrome?

   a. glucocorticoids
   b. indomethacin
   c. nitric oxide
   d. oscillatory ventilation

29–84. What is the primary pathophysiological basis of meconium aspiration syndrome?

   a. airway blockage
   b. chemical pneumonitis
   c. pulmonary hypoplasia
   d. unknown

29–85. In approximately what percentage of term pregnancies is the amnionic fluid stained?

   a. 1
   b. 10
   c. 20
   d. 30

29–86. Which of the following heart rate patterns is predictive of meconium aspiration?

   a. variable decelerations
   b. saltatory
   c. late decelerations
   d. none of the above

29–87. Which of the following markers is most likely to be abnormal in the umbilical cord blood of neonates with meconium-aspiration syndrome?

   a. pH
   b. erythropoietin
   c. hypoxanthine
   d. lactate

29–88. Routine neonatal administration of which of the following is effective in preventing hemorrhagic disease of the newborn?

   a. factor VIII
   b. fibrinogen
   c. niacin
   d. vitamin K

29–89. What is the usual management of pregnancies complicated by immune thrombocytopenia (ITP)?

   a. cesarean delivery
   b. corticosteroids intrapartum
   c. immunoglobulin infusions antepartum
   d. vaginal delivery usually allowed

29–90. What is the most likely diagnosis when the neonate has severe thrombocytopenia but the mother has a normal platelet count?

   a. immune thrombocytopenia (ITP)
   b. preeclampsia–eclampsia
   c. alloimmune thrombocytopenia (ATP)
   d. maternal drug ingestion

29–91. What percentage of stillbirths occur before term?

   a. 20
   b. 40
   c. 60
   d. 80

29–92. Autopsy plus review by a team of specialists in pathology, maternal-fetal medicine, genetics, and pediatrics can identify a cause of death for what percentage of stillbirths?

   a. <30
   b. 50
   c. 70
   d. >90

29–93. What is the most common, single, identifiable cause of fetal death?

   a. cord accident
   b. infection
   c. placental abruption
   d. postterm pregnancy

29–94. Which maternal condition does NOT increase the risk of stillbirth?

   a. diabetes
   b. hypertensive disorders
   c. lupus anticoagulant present
   d. multiple sclerosis

29–95. What approximate percentage of stillborn infants are found to have chromosomal abnormalities?

    a. 10
    b. 20
    c. 40
    d. 60

29–96. What maternal blood testing should be done as part of the evaluation of an unexplained stillbirth?

    a. antiphospholipid antibodies
    b. Kleihauer-Betke stain
    c. serum glucose
    d. all of the above

29–97. Which is true of performing complete autopsies on stillborn infants?

    a. cause needless emotional trauma for parents
    b. alter presumed cause of death in >10%
    c. are required by law
    d. should be offered only if parents initiate the discussion

29–98. What is the risk of recurrent stillbirth?

    a. <10%
    b. 15%
    c. 20%
    d. 25%

29–99. Which of the following increases the risk of recurrent stillbirth?

    a. chronic hypertension
    b. hereditary thrombophilia
    c. prior growth-restricted infant
    d. all of the above

29–100. What is the most common clinical setting for fetal or neonatal interventricular hemorrhage?

    a. eclampsia
    b. forceps delivery
    c. maternal alcohol use
    d. preterm delivery

29–101. What is focal swelling of the scalp due to edema fluid overlying the periosteum called?

    a. cephalohematoma
    b. caput succedaneum
    c. periosteal hematoma
    d. caput periosteum

29–102. What is the approximate incidence in term births of brachial plexus injury?

    a. 1 in 12
    b. 1 in 100
    c. 1 in 500
    d. 1 in 3000

29–103. Which brachial plexus injury is typified by flaccid paralysis of both the arm and hand?

    a. Duchenne paralysis
    b. Erb paralysis
    c. Klumpkes paralysis
    d. Horner syndrome

29–104. Facial paralysis is a potential complication of which type of delivery?

    a. cesarean
    b. forceps
    c. spontaneous vaginal
    d. all of the above

29–105. Intrauterine amputation of a fetal digit or extremity is most likely caused by which of the following?

    a. amnionic band syndrome
    b. cord entanglement
    c. maternal trauma
    d. vascular occlusion

29–106. Torticollis is most commonly associated with which of the following delivery modes?

    a. spontaneous vertex
    b. breech extraction
    c. forceps
    d. cesarean

30

The Puerperium

30–1. The commonly used definition of the puerperium describes which of the following time periods?

   a. 2 weeks following delivery
   b. 4 weeks following delivery
   c. 6 weeks following delivery
   d. 12 weeks following delivery

30–2. Typical permanent anatomical characteristics of the cervix following delivery include which of the following?

   a. wider external os
   b. scarred, narrowed external os
   c. cervical length is doubled from prepregnancy
   d. cervical length is halved from prepregnancy

30–3. How many weeks after delivery does it take the uterus to return to its nonpregnant size?

   a. 2
   b. 4
   c. 6
   d. 12

30–4. Which of the following is the term used to formally describe the process in which the uterus contracts and atrophies to its nonpregnant size?

   a. decompression
   b. contracture
   c. reparation
   d. involution

30–5. One typical clinical characteristic of uterine afterpains includes which of the following?

   a. resolve after the 7th day of the puerperium
   b. require analgesic use
   c. relieved by uterine massage
   d. aggravated by breast feeding

30–6. You may correctly counsel your puerperal patient in regard to lochia with which of the following statements?

   a. Lochia will remain red throughout its duration.
   b. Breast feeding will lessen the duration of lochial flow.
   c. Lochial flow may last up to 8 weeks into the puerperium.
   d. Fetal macrosomia will lengthen the duration of lochial flow.

30–7. A common cause of subinvolution includes which of the following?

   a. puerperal pelvic infection
   b. fetal macrosomia
   c. antenatal polyhydramnios
   d. cessation of breast feeding

30–8. Subinvolutional bleeding may be treated by any of the following EXCEPT

   a. ergonovine
   b. tetracycline
   c. oral estrogen
   d. methylergonovine

30–9. Which of the following statements correctly defines the use of curettage in the treatment of late puerperal hemorrhage?

   a. should be used as a first-line treatment
   b. should be used after pharmacological agents fail to halt bleeding
   c. should be used as an effective tool to remove retained placental tissue
   d. should be used for both light and heavy puerperal bleeding

30–10. You counsel your puerperal patient to expect increased urination between which puerperal time period?

    a. first 24 hr
    b. days 2 to 5
    c. days 5 to 7
    d. weeks 1 to 2

30–11. Which of the following are characteristics of the puerperal bladder?

    a. underdistension; complete emptying
    b. underdistension; incomplete emptying
    c. overdistension; complete emptying
    d. overdistension; incomplete emptying

30–12. Which of the following is most commonly associated with urinary retention?

    a. forceps delivery
    b. precipitous delivery
    c. nitrous oxide analgesia use during second stage of labor
    d. puerperal hemorrhage

30–13. Which of the following is NOT typically associated with puerperal stress urinary incontinence?

    a. prolonged second stage
    b. size of the infant's head
    c. cesarean delivery
    d. episiotomy

30–14. Heart rate and cardiac output typically have returned to normal levels by which of the following time periods after delivery?

    a. 2 weeks
    b. 4 weeks
    c. 6 weeks
    d. 8 weeks

30–15. You counsel your puerperal patient that most women return to their prepregnancy weight by which time period following delivery?

    a. 4 months
    b. 6 months
    c. 8 months
    d. 12 months

30–16. Compared to breast milk, colostrum contains more of which of the following?

    a. fat
    b. minerals
    c. sugar
    d. immunoglobulin M

30–17. Which of the following has NOT been identified in human breast milk?

    a. interleukin-6
    b. prolactin
    c. epidermal growth factor
    d. vitamin K

30–18. Essential hormonal changes during the puerperium necessary for breast feeding include all of the following EXCEPT

    a. decreases in progesterone levels
    b. increases in prolactin levels
    c. increases in estrogen levels
    d. increases in oxytocin levels

30–19. Immunoglobulin A, found in breast milk, is purported to lower the risk of which of the following conditions in breast-fed infants as compared with bottle-fed infants?

    a. enteric infections
    b. respiratory infections
    c. otitis media
    d. asthma

30–20. Bromocriptine use for lactation inhibition is not recommended by the FDA because of its association with which of the following?

    a. hepatitis
    b. renal failure
    c. valvular heart disease
    d. stroke

30–21. Correct statements regarding contraception in breast-feeding women include which of the following?

    a. Depo-medroxyprogesterone lowers the quality of breast milk.
    b. Progestin-only birth control pills do not affect the quantity of breast milk.
    c. Estrogen–progestin birth control pills do not affect the quality of breast milk.
    d. Estrogen–progestin birth control pills do not affect the quantity of breast milk.

30–22. Breast feeding is contraindicated with which of the following maternal infections?

    a. hepatitis C
    b. hepatitis B
    c. active, untreated tuberculosis
    d. cytomegalovirus infection

30–23. Agents that should avoided in breast feeding include all of the following EXCEPT

    a. radioactive isotopes
    b. varicella-zoster vaccinations
    c. cytotoxic agents
    d. ergot alkaloids

30–24. A typical clinical finding regarding mastitis includes which of the following?

    a. severe breast pain
    b. bilateral breast involvement
    c. progression to abscess formation
    d. breast skin ulceration

30–25. What is the most common etiological agent for mastitis?

    a. *Staphylococcus aureus*
    b. *Staphylococcus epidermitis*
    c. enterococci
    d. group A streptococcus

30–26. Treatment of mastitis typically includes which of the following?

    a. intravenous antimicrobial therapy
    b. cessation of breast pumping
    c. cessation of breast feeding
    d. antimicrobial therapy for 10 to 14 days

30–27. Which of the following is a confirmed benefit to ambulation early in the puerperium?

    a. hastens episiotomy repair
    b. lessens severity of postpartum blues
    c. decreases constipation
    d. lessens duration of lochia

30–28. Your patient is now 6 hours postpartum. Her vital signs are within normal range. Her uterus is palpated above the level of the umbilicus. She has not voided. The next management step for this patient would include which of the following?

    a. encourage fluid consumption
    b. urinary catheter placement
    c. uterine massage
    d. ice pack to perineum

30–29. Severe episiotomy pain within the first 24 hours after delivery may typically be a warning sign of which of the following problems?

    a. episiotomy infection
    b. urinary retention
    c. perineal hematoma
    d. constipation

30–30. Your patient becomes tearful during your rounds on the day of her discharge from the hospital. Further questioning reveals her fears about caring for a newborn. She has no history of psychiatric illness. The most appropriate management of this patient includes which of the following?

    a. psychiatric consultation
    b. reassure patient that her mood should improve within 2 to 3 days
    c. initiate a selective serotonin reuptake inhibitor (SSRI)
    d. extend her hospital stay to observe for signs of major depression

30–31. Your patient has a peripheral neuropathy secondary to delivery injury. You counsel her that the median duration of symptoms is which of the following?

    a. 1 month
    b. 2 months
    c. 6 months
    d. 12 months

30–32. Which of the following immunizations should NOT be given postpartum?

    a. diphtheria-tetanus
    b. anti-D immune globulin
    c. measles-mumps-rubella vaccination
    d. no restrictions for any of these

30–33. At what point postpartum (weeks) does menstruation normally return in a non–breast-feeding woman?

    a. 4 to 6
    b. 6 to 8
    c. 12 to 14
    d. 16 to 18

31

Puerperal Infection

31-1. Which of the following factors is most responsible for the decline in maternal deaths from puerperal infection?

    a. expanded number of intensive care units
    b. extensive use of bacterial cultures to identify puerperal infection
    c. development of antimicrobials
    d. improved sterile technique at the time of delivery and wound closure

31-2. What is the definition of puerperal morbidity?

    a. temperature of 38.0°C (100.4°F) or greater, exclusive of the first 24 hours of the puerperium, on any 2 days, during the first 10 days postpartum
    b. temperature of 39.0°C (102.2°F) or greater, exclusive of the first 24 hours of the puerperium during the first 5 days postpartum
    c. temperature of 37.5°C (99.5°F) or greater, anytime during the first 10 days of the puerperium
    d. temperature of 39.0°C (102.2°F) or greater anytime during the first 10 days of the puerperium

31-3. Which of the following is the most common cause of persistent puerperal fever?

    a. atelectasis
    b. genital tract infection
    c. pyelonephritis
    d. breast engorgement

31-4. A high-spiking fever which develops within the first 24 hours of the puerperium is most likely caused by which of the following?

    a. breast engorgement
    b. atelectasis
    c. chlamydial pelvic infection
    d. group A streptococcal pelvic infection

31-5. How can atelectasis be prevented?

    a. coughing and deep breathing
    b. deep breathing and aspirin administration
    c. avoiding opioids for postoperative analgesia
    d. prophylactic theophylline administration

31-6. Fever due to breast engorgement is commonly characterized by which of the following?

    a. exceeds 39.0°C
    b. lasts <24 hr
    c. onset within the first 24 hr of the puerperium
    d. lasts >48 hr

31-7. In puerperal women, the first clinical sign of acute pyelonephritis commonly includes which of the following?

    a. headache
    b. fever
    c. adynamic ileus
    d. hematuria

31-8. What is the single most significant risk factor for puerperal metritis?

    a. number of pelvic exams
    b. duration of labor
    c. duration of membrane rupture
    d. route of delivery

31-9. Which of the following is associated with the greatest risk of puerperal metritis after vaginal delivery?

    a. prolonged rupture of membranes
    b. prolonged labor
    c. intrapartum chorioamnionitis
    d. multiple cervical examinations

31-10. Which of the following is NOT considered a risk factor for postpartum metritis after cesarean delivery?

    a. multiple cervical examinations
    b. internal fetal monitoring
    c. cephalopelvic disproportion
    d. labor <8 hr duration

31–11. Which of the following factors have been linked to a higher risk of puerperal metritis after cesarean delivery?

a. poor nutrition
b. maternal anemia
c. obesity
d. higher socioeconomic status

31–12. Heavy colonization of the vaginal tract with which of the following bacteria is associated with puerperal infection?

a. *Streptococcus pyogenes*
b. *Streptococcus pneumoniae*
c. *Streptococcus agalactiae*
d. *Gardnerella vaginalis*

31–13. Which of the following microbiological characteristics are typical of puerperal metritis?

a. Bacteria are indigenous to the female genital tract.
b. Bacteria from a single species are isolated.
c. Bacteria isolated are typically considered to be of high virulence.
d. Bacteria from an aerobic species are solely isolated.

31–14. Which of the following lower genital tract organisms is NOT associated with increased puerperal infection?

a. *Trichomonas vaginalis*
b. group B streptococcus
c. *Gardnerella vaginalis*
d. *Mycoplasma hominis*

31–15. Which of the following has been associated with toxic shock-like syndrome?

a. *Staphylococcus epidermidis*
b. *Escherichia coli*
c. group A β-hemolytic streptococcus
d. *Klebsiella pneumoniae*

31–16. Which of the following organisms is implicated as a cause of late puerperal infection?

a. *Neisseria gonorrhea*
b. *Chlamydia trachomatis*
c. *Trichomonas vaginalis*
d. *Bacteroides bivius*

31–17. Your patient underwent cesarean delivery 2 days ago. Her temperature is 39.0°C. You find uterine tenderness and foul lochia on examination. Her incision appears intact and is without erythema. The routine management of this patient includes which of the following?

a. obtain vaginal cultures
b. obtain blood cultures

c. await culture results to start antimicrobials
d. antimicrobial selection should include anaerobic coverage

31–18. In addition to fever, which of the clinical findings are commonly associated with puerperal metritis?

a. nausea and vomiting
b. parametrial tenderness
c. positive blood cultures
d. vulvar edema

31–19. How long should women with puerperal metritis be treated with antimicrobials?

a. until afebrile for 24 hr
b. 5-day course
c. 10-day course
d. 14-day course

31–20. Complications of puerperal metritis that commonly cause persistent fever include which of the following?

a. antimicrobial-resistant bacteria
b. drug fever
c. pelvic abscess
d. atelectasis

31–21. Which of the following clinical markers is most commonly used to monitor the improvement of puerperal metritis?

a. temperature
b. leukocyte count
c. abdominal pain
d. odor of lochia

31–22. Which of the following antimicrobial regimens is considered the "gold standard" therapy for puerperal metritis?

a. ampicillin plus gentamicin
b. gentamicin plus clindamycin
c. ampicillin plus clindamycin
d. ampicillin plus gentamicin plus clindamycin

31–23. Which of the following is a correct statement regarding the pharmacological properties of gentamicin for the treatment of puerperal metritis?

a. Once-daily dosing with gentamicin results in inadequate serum levels.
b. Once-daily dosing with gentamicin does not alleviate the need for serum drug level measurement.
c. Once-daily dosing with gentamicin plus clindamycin compared with every-q8h dosing has a higher metritis cure rate.
d. Once-daily dosing with gentamicin plus clindamycin compared with q8h dosing has an equal metritis cure rate.

31–24. The pharmacological advantage to adding β-lactamase inhibitors, such as sulbactam, to drugs in the penicillin family is that they reduce which of the following?

    a. need to add a second antimicrobial agent
    b. risk of allergic reaction to penicillins
    c. drug toxicity associated with penicillins
    d. renal clearance of penicillins

31–25. The American College of Obstetricians and Gynecologists recommends which of the following protocols for the prevention of metritis following cesarean delivery?

    a. a single dose of an antimicrobial drug given perioperatively
    b. a multiple-dose antimicrobial drug regimen given during the 24 hr following delivery
    c. antepartum treatment of asymptomatic bacterial vaginosis
    d. topical metronidazole gel applied preoperatively in addition to intravenous antimicrobial prophylaxis

31–26. What percentage of patients with puerperal metritis will respond to antimicrobials within 72 hours?

    a. 25
    b. 50
    c. 75
    d. 90

31–27. Which of the following is NOT a risk factor for wound infection?

    a. hematoma formation
    b. anemia
    c. hyperthyroidism
    d. diabetes

31–28. What is the most common etiology of fascial dehiscence?

    a. poor surgical technique
    b. infection
    c. obesity
    d. coughing

31–29. Which of the following is a common clinical finding associated with fascial dehiscence?

    a. manifestation on the second postoperative day
    b. concurrent atelectasis
    c. serosanguineous drainage from the wound
    d. feculent drainage from the wound

31–30. Which of the following is NOT a risk factor for necrotizing fasciitis?

    a. obesity
    b. hypertension
    c. diabetes
    d. young maternal age

31–31. In addition to intravenous antimicrobials, the treatment of necrotizing fasciitis typically also requires which of the following?

    a. debridement of fascia
    b. daily topical wound application of metronidazole gel
    c. fascial incision reinforcement with synthetic mesh
    d. daily wound irrigation with chlorhexadine

31–32. What is the antimicrobial regimen of choice for necrotizing fasciitis?

    a. second-generation cephalosporin plus gentamicin
    b. β-lactam agent plus clindamycin
    c. gentamicin plus clindamycin
    d. ampicillin plus gentamicin

31–33. Which of the following is commonly seen with puerperal peritonitis?

    a. prominent abdominal rigidity
    b. minimal bowel distention
    c. adynamic ileus
    d. minimal pain

31–34. Classical characteristics of parametrial phlegmon include which of the following?

    a. cellulitis involving the broad ligament unilaterally
    b. cellulitis involving the rectovaginal septum
    c. cellulitis involving the uterosacral ligaments
    d. cellulitis most commonly extending anteriorly

31–35. What is the recommended treatment of a parametrial phlegmon?

    a. hysterectomy
    b. antimicrobial therapy plus heparin
    c. percutaneous drainage
    d. antimicrobial therapy alone

31–36. Puerperal septic pelvic thrombophlebitis commonly extends to involve which of the following structures?

    a. femoral vein
    b. ovarian vein
    c. inferior vena cava
    d. renal vein

31–37. Your patient underwent cesarean delivery 5 days ago. Intravenous gentamicin and clindamycin were begun on the second postoperative day for clinical signs of puerperal metritis. Despite improvement in her abdominal pain and uterine tenderness, she continues to have daily temperature elevations to 39.0°C. The next diagnostic step in evaluation of this patient should include which of the following?

    a. the heparin challenge test
    b. computed tomography
    c. ultrasonography
    d. abdominal radiography

31–38. Which of the following is the clinical pathognomonic feature of a woman with puerperal septic pelvic thrombophlebitis?

    a. enigmatic fever
    b. lower abdominal pain
    c. pelvic mass
    d. abdominal distension

31–39. What is the most common etiology of episiotomy dehiscence?

    a. postpartum anemia
    b. poor nutrition
    c. infection
    d. faulty episiotomy repair

31–40. What is NOT a predisposing factor for episiotomy breakdown?

    a. human papilloma virus
    b. smoking
    c. coagulation disorders
    d. gonorrhea

31–41. Which of the following is NOT a common clinical component of episiotomy dehiscence?

    a. pain
    b. hematochezia
    c. dysuria
    d. fever

31–42. Three days ago your patient underwent vaginal delivery complicated by a fourth-degree laceration. She now complains of perineal pain despite local ice pack treatments and oral analgesics. Her temperature is 38.5°C. Physical examination reveals erythema, induration, and purulent discharge at her episiotomy site. Clinical management of this patient should involve which of the following?

    a. opening of episiotomy plus intravenous antimicrobial therapy
    b. wound observation plus intravenous antimicrobial therapy

    c. opening of episiotomy plus hydrotherapy
    d. opening of episiotomy plus topical broad-spectrum antimicrobial therapy

31–43. Recommended treatment of the episiotomy defect following dehiscence currently includes which of the following?

    a. rectal flap repair approximately 1 week following dehiscence
    b. wound healing through secondary intention
    c. reapproximation repair approximately 1 week following dehiscence
    d. rectal flap repair approximately 3 months following dehiscence

31–44. Which of the following clinical characteristics are typically associated with necrotizing fasciitis that complicates a perineal laceration?

    a. possesses clinical qualities that are distinct from superficial perineal infection
    b. may extend to the thighs
    c. possesses up to a 15% mortality rate despite aggressive treatment
    d. symptoms progress rapidly within the first 24 to 48 hr following delivery

31–45. Which of the following bacteria is responsible for toxic shock syndrome?

    a. *Staphylococcus aureus*
    b. *Staphylococcus epidermidis*
    c. *Streptococcus pyogenes*
    d. *Staphylococcus toxi*

31–46. Clinical findings of toxic shock syndrome in its early stages may include which of the following?

    a. erythematous rash
    b. conjunctivitis
    c. vertigo
    d. herpetiform skin eruptions

31–47. Treatment of toxic shock syndrome typically includes administration of which of the following?

    a. immunoglobulin directed against *S. aureus* exotoxin
    b. immunoglobulin directed against *S. aureus* endotoxin
    c. intravenous fluids alone
    d. intravenous fluids and antimicrobials

31–48. Recovery from toxic shock syndrome classically includes which of the following?

    a. hypothermia
    b. skin desquamation
    c. watery diarrhea
    d. tinnitus

32

Contraception

32–1. What percentage of adolescents would stop using sexual health care services if parental notification was required?

   a. 10
   b. 20
   c. 40
   d. 60

32–2. For which age group does abortion pose an increased risk of death compared with pregnancy?

   a. 15 to 19 years
   b. 25 to 29 years
   c. 40 to 44 years
   d. not true of any age group

32–3. In the absence of contraception, what percentage of fertile, sexually active women will conceive within 1 year?

   a. 90
   b. 75
   c. 50
   d. 40

32–4. As menopause approaches, which reliably predicts cessation of ovulation?

   a. amenorrhea
   b. elevated gonadotropin levels
   c. hot flashes
   d. none of the above

32–5. What contraceptive method is most commonly used by women in the United States (Piccinino & Mosher, 1998)?

   a. female sterilization
   b. intrauterine device
   c. male condom
   d. oral contraceptives

32–6. With typical use, which of the following contraceptive methods has the highest failure rate within the first year of use?

   a. male condom
   b. progestin-only pill
   c. spermicides
   d. withdrawal

32–7. What is the typical failure rate from DEPO-PROVERA (injectable) during the first year of usage?

   a. 0.03%
   b. 0.3%
   c. 1.0%
   d. 3.0%

32–8. What is the mechanism of action of oral contraceptives?

   a. prevent ovulation
   b. impair passage of sperm into the uterus
   c. cause endometrium to be unfavorable to implantation
   d. all of the above

32–9. Which of the following estrogens is used in oral contraceptives?

   a. estrone
   b. ethinyl estradiol
   c. estriol
   d. equilin

32–10. What is the potency of ethinyl estradiol compared to mestranol?

   a. equal potency
   b. 1.2 to 1.5 times more potent
   c. 2.1 to 2.3 times more potent
   d. 0.4 to 0.5 times weaker

32–11. All but one oral contraceptive progestin are derivatives of which steroid?

   a. androstenedione
   b. 17-hydroxytestosterone
   c. 19-nortestosterone
   d. spironolactone

32–12. The progestin component of oral contraceptives has what action?

   a. lowers free testosterone levels
   b. increases 5α-reductase activity
   c. lowers prolactin levels
   d. increases dihydrotestosterone levels

32–13. The lowest acceptable dose of ethinyl estradiol in oral contraceptives is mainly dictated by the incidence of which of the following?

   a. acne
   b. breakthrough bleeding
   c. dysmenorrhea
   d. headaches

32–14. Which two drugs decrease the effectiveness of oral contraceptives?

   a. aspirin and ibuprofen
   b. erythromycin and ceftriaxone
   c. rifampicin and phenytoin
   d. propranolol and isoniazid

32–15. Erratic use of which of the following vitamins increases the likelihood of breakthrough bleeding during oral contraceptive use?

   a. A
   b. B
   c. C
   d. K

32–16. In healthy young women, which of the following activities is LEAST likely to result in a fatality?

   a. driving an automobile
   b. abortion
   c. oral contraceptive use
   d. term pregnancy

32–17. Which of the following is increased by oral contraceptive use?

   a. bone density
   b. endometrial cancer
   c. ovarian cancer
   d. salpingitis

32–18. In a patient taking oral contraceptives, which of the following is increased?

   a. plasma thyroxine
   b. plasma cortisol
   c. transcortin
   d. all of the above

32–19. Oral contraceptives do not cause, but may accelerate, which of the following?

   a. atherosclerosis
   b. cervical neoplasia
   c. gallbladder disease
   d. ovarian cancer

32–20. The risk of invasive cervical cancer increases after how many years of oral contraceptive use?

   a. 1
   b. 3
   c. 5
   d. 10

32–21. What is the relationship between oral contraceptive use and breast cancer?

   a. cancers are more aggressive
   b. increased risk with family history of breast cancer
   c. risk varies with type of progestin used
   d. no clear association

32–22. Which of the following is increased in healthy nonsmokers who take oral contraceptives?

   a. diabetes
   b. myocardial infarction
   c. strokes
   d. venous thrombosis

32–23. Elevated blood pressure associated with oral contraceptive use is likely related to the increased production of which of the following?

   a. angiotensinogen
   b. antidiuretic hormone
   c. endothelin
   d. aldosterone

32–24. The risk of stroke is increased with oral contraceptive use if which of the following co-factors is present?

   a. hypertension
   b. migraines
   c. smoking
   d. all of the above

32–25. Oral contraceptive use shows what relationship to myocardial infarction according to current information?

   a. risk not increased in nonsmokers
   b. risk increased in both smokers and nonsmokers
   c. risk not increased in any group
   d. risk increased in nonsmokers over age 35

32–26. Oral contraceptives are currently thought to cause which of the following congenital defects?

a. limb-reduction defects
b. sexual ambiguity
c. heart defects
d. no association with any defects

32–27. Oral contraceptives have been associated with an increased incidence of which of the following?

a. acne
b. chloasma
c. HIV infection
d. uterine myomas

32–28. Which of the following is a risk factor for resumption of ovulation less than 6 weeks after pregnancy ends?

a. abortion
b. breast feeding
c. multiple gestation
d. stress

32–29. Of the following, which is NOT an absolute contraindication to oral contraceptives?

a. abnormal genital bleeding
b. active liver disease
c. migraine headaches
d. prior thromboembolism

32–30. Which of the following is NOT true of progestin-only contraceptive pills?

a. inhibit ovulation reliably
b. alter cervical mucous
c. alter endometrial maturation
d. increase incidence of ovarian cysts

32–31. Which of the following is an advantage of progestin-only pills as compared with combination oral contraceptives?

a. fewer ovarian cysts
b. less breakthrough bleeding
c. safer if cardiovascular risk factors present
d. lower incidence of ectopic pregnancy if method fails

32–32. What is a strong contraindication to oral progestin-only contraceptive use?

a. cigarette smoking
b. depression
c. mild hypertension
d. unexplained uterine bleeding

32–33. What is the contraceptive dosage of depomedroxyprogesterone?

a. 50 mg every 3 months
b. 100 mg every 3 months
c. 150 mg every 3 months
d. 200 mg every 3 months

32–34. What percentage of women develop amenorrhea after 5 years of depot progestin use?

a. 10
b. 30
c. 50
d. 80

32–35. Injectable progestin contraceptives show what disadvantages?

a. irregular bleeding
b. delayed resumption of fertility
c. need to visit provider for injection
d. all of the above

32–36. Which aspect of injectable progestin use is particularly worrisome in adolescents and young women?

a. decreased bone mineral density
b. increased pelvic infections
c. worsening of acne
d. increased risk of uterine cancer

32–37. Which of the following is the primary reason that progestin implant contraception is no longer available?

a. contraceptive failure rate
b. expense
c. difficulty of insertion and removal
d. litigation

32–38. Which is increased with LUNELLE contraception as compared with depot progestins?

a. breakthrough bleeding
b. cardiovascular complications
c. delayed resumption of fertility
d. frequency of injections

32–39. How often does the MIRENA intrauterine device need to be replaced?

a. every year
b. every 2 years
c. every 5 years
d. every 10 years

32–40. How often does the PARAGARD intrauterine device need to be replaced?

a. yearly
b. every 5 years
c. every 10 years
d. every 20 years

32–41. Which of the following is NOT a component of the MIRENA intrauterine device?

    a. copper
    b. levonorgestrel
    c. polyethylene
    d. polydimethylsiloxane

32–42. Which of the following is NOT a mechanism of action of the copper intrauterine device?

    a. spermicidal action
    b. prevention of ovulation
    c. local inflammatory reaction of endometrium
    d. prevention of fertilization

32–43. The progestin intrauterine device is associated with which of the following?

    a. increased menstrual blood loss
    b. endometrial atrophy
    c. dysmenorrhea
    d. uterine myomas

32–44. What is the rate of uterine perforation during intrauterine device insertion?

    a. 1 in 100
    b. 1 in 1000
    c. 1 in 10,000
    d. 1 in 100,000

32–45. What percentage of women using the Copper-T 380A intrauterine device will have it removed due to menorrhagia?

    a. 2 to 5
    b. 10 to 15
    c. 20 to 25
    d. 30 to 35

32–46. Which of the following characterizes the risk of pelvic infection in intrauterine device users compared with non-users?

    a. increased risk for duration of IUD use
    b. increased risk of infection during first 20 days after insertion
    c. increased risk of infection for first year of IUD use
    d. no increased risk of infection

32–47. What is the incidence of actinomyces-like structures identified on Pap smears in women with intrauterine devices?

    a. 0.7%
    b. 1.0%
    c. 7.0%
    d. 17.0%

32–48. What is the most appropriate therapy for a woman 8 weeks pregnant with the string of a Copper-T 380 A intrauterine device visible at the cervix?

    a. antibiotics
    b. abortion
    c. removal of intrauterine device
    d. no action

32–49. What is the approximate abortion rate if an intrauterine device is left in situ during pregnancy?

    a. 10%
    b. 25%
    c. 50%
    d. 75%

32–50. What is the approximate abortion rate if an intrauterine device in situ early in pregnancy is removed promptly?

    a. 10%
    b. 25%
    c. 50%
    d. 75%

32–51. Which of the following is NOT an absolute contraindication to using an intrauterine device?

    a. active or recent salpingitis
    b. pregnancy
    c. undiagnosed uterine bleeding
    d. previous cesarean delivery

32–52. What contraindication is specific to the progestin intrauterine device?

    a. dysmenorrhea
    b. history of ectopic pregnancy
    c. prior thromboembolism
    d. Wilson disease

32–53. Use of which of the following may compromise the efficacy of the male condom?

    a. intravaginal spermicides
    b. oil-based lubricants
    c. reservoir tips
    d. spermicidal lubricants

32–54. Which is an advantage of polyurethane condoms compared to latex condoms?

    a. decreased breakage rate
    b. fewer allergic reactions
    c. lower failure rate
    d. none of the above

32–55. What is the breakage rate of the female condom?

  a. <1%
  b. 3%
  c. 5%
  d. 9%

32–56. What is the duration of maximal effectiveness of spermicides?

  a. 1 hr
  b. 6 hr
  c. 8 hr
  d. 24 hr

32–57. Of the following, which is increased when spermicides are used?

  a. neural-tube defects
  b. limb-reduction defects
  c. Down syndrome
  d. none of the above

32–58. What is the minimum amount of time after intercourse that a diaphragm should remain in place?

  a. 2 hr
  b. 6 hr
  c. 12 hr
  d. 18 hr

32–59. The incidence of which of the following is slightly increased with use of the diaphragm?

  a. cervicitis
  b. cystocele
  c. pelvic inflammatory disease
  d. urinary tract infection

32–60. Up to how many hours before intercourse can the contraceptive (TODAY) sponge be inserted?

  a. 1 hr
  b. 6 hr
  c. 12 hr
  d. 24 hr

32–61. Which of the following is NOT a variation of periodic abstinence as a family planning method?

  a. calendar rhythm
  b. cervical mucous method

  c. symptothermal
  d. withdrawal

32–62. When do adolescents typically seek contraception in relation to initiation of sexual activity?

  a. a few weeks prior
  b. a few months prior
  c. a few weeks to months after
  d. a year or more after

32–63. What type of contraception offers the most advantages to adolescents?

  a. oral contraceptives
  b. depo-progestins
  c. intrauterine devices
  d. spermicides

32–64. What percentage of pregnancies in women age 40 and older are terminated?

  a. 15
  b. 35
  c. 65
  d. 95

32–65. Which of the following is true of emergency contraception (EC)?

  a. Advanced provision of EC decreases the use of routine contraception.
  b. Combination estrogen-progestin EC is more effective than progestin-only EC.
  c. EC should be taken within 72 hours of unprotected intercourse for optimal efficacy.
  d. EC can harm established pregnancies.

32–66. Emergency contraception decreases the risk of conception by what percentage?

  a. 25
  b. 50
  c. 75
  d. 100

32–67. Mifepristone (RU-486) provides postcoital contraception via what mechanism?

  a. antagonizes progesterone
  b. antiprostaglandin
  c. blocks progesterone production
  d. induces endometrial lysosomal activity

33

Sterilization

33–1. What is the most popular form of contraception in the United States?

    a. condoms
    b. oral contraceptives
    c. intrauterine devices
    d. sterilization

33–2. At least half of tubal sterilization procedures are done in conjunction with which of the following?

    a. cholecystectomy
    b. hysterectomy
    c. obstetrical delivery
    d. vasectomy

33–3. Which puerperal tubal sterilization procedure is least likely to fail but most difficult to perform?

    a. Pomeroy
    b. Irving
    c. Parkland
    d. fimbriectomy

33–4. The success of the Pomeroy procedure relies upon the use of what type of ligature?

    a. chromic gut
    b. plain gut
    c. synthetic polymer
    d. silk

33–5. The failure rate for Parkland type tubal sterilization approximates which of the following?

    a. 1 in 50
    b. 1 in 100
    c. 1 in 200
    d. 1 in 400

33–6. What is the current mortality rate directly related to laparoscopic sterilization?

    a. 1.5 in 100,000
    b. 1.5 in 10,000

    c. 1.5 in 1000
    d. 1.5 in 100

33–7. Which of the following is NOT an established complication of laparoscopic tubal sterilization?

    a. anesthetic complications
    b. chronic pelvic pain
    c. injury of adjacent structures
    d. sterilization failure

33–8. How often is unplanned laparotomy performed with attempted laparoscopic sterilization?

    a. 1 in 10
    b. 1 in 100
    c. 1 in 1000
    d. 1 in 10,000

33–9. Tubal sterilization failures may be due to which of the following?

    a. fistula formation
    b. mechanical devices are not completely occlusive
    c. inadequate coagulation with the bipolar method
    d. all of the above

33–10. Which of the following tubal sterilization techniques has the highest risk of ectopic pregnancy with failure?

    a. clips
    b. electrocoagulation
    c. rings
    d. tubal resection

33–11. Which of the following is most likely to occur following tubal sterilization?

    a. dysmenorrhea, new-onset or increased
    b. intermenstrual bleeding
    c. menorrhagia
    d. unchanged menstrual volume

33–12. Data exist suggesting tubal sterilization may have beneficial effects on which of the following?

   a. ovarian cancer rates
   b. salpingitis risk
   c. sexual satisfaction
   d. all of the above

33–13. What percentage of women express regret following either tubal sterilization or vasectomy of their husbands?

   a. <10
   b. 20
   c. 50
   d. 80

33–14. Following tubal sterilization reversal, what percentage of women will have an ectopic pregnancy?

   a. 15
   b. 10
   c. 50
   d. 90

33–15. Vasectomy bilaterally disrupts what structure?

   a. epididymis
   b. seminal vesicle
   c. vas deferens
   d. Wolffian duct

33–16. Compared with vasectomy, which of the following is higher with female tubal sterilization?

   a. complication rate
   b. cost
   c. failure rate
   d. all of the above

33–17. Which is a disadvantage of vasectomy?

   a. azoospermia
   b. increased impotence
   c. reversal not possible
   d. sterility is not immediate

33–18. What is the approximate success rate of vasectomy reversal?

   a. 15%
   b. 50%
   c. 75%
   d. 90%

33–19. Following a vasectomy, which statement is true?

   a. Antibodies against spermatozoa are frequently identified.
   b. Autoimmune diseases are more common.
   c. Arteriosclerosis is accelerated.
   d. Testicular cancer is increased.

33–20. Which of the following may have a weak association with vasectomy?

   a. bladder cancer
   b. prostatic cancer
   c. renal cell carcinoma
   d. testicular cancer

34

Hypertensive Disorders in Pregnancy

34–1. What percentage of pregnancies are complicated by hypertension?

    a. <1
    b. 3 to 4
    c. 6 to 8
    d. 10 to 12

34–2. How is hypertension in pregnancy defined?

    a. blood pressure 160/100 or greater
    b. blood pressure 140/90 or greater
    c. increased systolic pressure by 30 mm Hg
    d. increased diastolic pressure by 15 mm Hg

34–3. Which Korotkoff phase sound is used to diagnose pregnancy-induced hypertension?

    a. phase III
    b. phase IV
    c. phase V
    d. phase VI

34–4. What percentage of eclamptic women do not have proteinuria?

    a. 0
    b. 5
    c. 10
    d. 20

34–5. With regard to preeclampsia, proteinuria is defined as how much urinary excretion?

    a. >100 mg/24 hr
    b. >200 mg/24 hr
    c. >300 mg/24 hr
    d. >500 mg/24 hr

34–6. With preeclampsia, what is the significance of severe, right upper quadrant pain?

    a. cholecystitis
    b. pancreatitis
    c. tension on Glisson's capsule
    d. Teitze syndrome

34–7. Which of the following is NOT diagnostic of severe preeclampsia?

    a. increased serum creatinine
    b. 1+ proteinuria
    c. thrombocytopenia
    d. elevated liver enzymes

34–8. Which of the following is considered an abnormal 24-hour urinary protein for the diagnosis of severe preeclampsia?

    a. >300 mg in 24 hr
    b. >1 g in 24 hr
    c. >2 g in 24 hr
    d. >4 g in 24 hr

34–9. According to Chames (2002), 25 percent of eclamptic seizures occur

    a. antepartum
    b. intrapartum
    c. immediately postpartum
    d. beyond 48 hr postpartum

34–10. All of the following are examples of end-organ damage due to chronic hypertension EXCEPT

   a. left ventricular hypertrophy
   b. retinal arterial narrowing
   c. blanched fingernail beds
   d. cotton-wool spots

34–11. What is the MOST common cause of chronic hypertension in pregnancy?

   a. essential
   b. obesity
   c. diabetes
   d. renal disease

34–12. In what percentage of pregnancies does superimposed preeclampsia complicate chronic hypertension?

   a. 5%
   b. 10%
   c. 25%
   d. 50%

34–13. What is the incidence of pregnancy-induced hypertension most commonly cited to be?

   a. <1%
   b. 2 to 3%
   c. 5 to 7%
   d. >10%

34–14. Which of the following patients would be MOST likely to develop true preeclampsia?

   a. a 16-year-old primigravida
   b. a 34-year-old gravida 4, para 3
   c. a 25-year-old primigravida
   d. a 35-year-old with essential hypertension

34–15. Which of the following is associated with a decrease in hypertensive diseases in pregnancy?

   a. twins
   b. smoking
   c. obesity
   d. age >35

34–16. How is the pathophysiology of preeclampsia characterized?

   a. vasodilatation
   b. vasospasm
   c. hemodilution
   d. hypervolemia

34–17. The theory of abnormal trophoblastic invasion as a cause of preeclampsia states which of the following?

   a. Trophoblasts invade the decidual vessels.
   b. Trophoblasts invade the myometrial vessels.
   c. Trophoblasts plus macrophages invade the decidual vessels.
   d. Trophoblasts plus macrophages invade the myometrial vessels.

34–18. Which of the following characterizes normotensive pregnant women?

   a. They are refractory to angiotensin II.
   b. They are sensitive to angiotensin II.
   c. They react to angiotensin II in a way similar to nonpregnant women.
   d. They react to angiotensin II in a way similar to men.

34–19. Increased sensitivity to which of the following precedes the onset of gestational hypertension?

   a. angiotensin II
   b. renin
   c. atrial natriuretic peptide
   d. thromboxane

34–20. Which of the following characterizes nitric oxide in hypertension?

   a. increased production
   b. decreased release
   c. decreased production
   d. no change

34–21. Which of the following is characteristic in preeclampsia?

   a. Cardiac output is decreased and peripheral resistance is decreased.
   b. Cardiac output is decreased and peripheral resistance is increased.
   c. Cardiac output is increased and peripheral resistance is increased.
   d. As vascular resistance increases, so does cardiac output.

34–22. Which of the following is true concerning blood volume in eclampsia?

   a. similar to the nonpregnant state
   b. similar to the normal pregnant state
   c. lower than the nonpregnant state
   d. increased compared with the normal pregnant state

34–23. Which of the following characterizes thrombocytopenia in women with preeclampsia?

   a. platelet activation
   b. platelet consumption
   c. increased platelet production
   d. all of the above

34-24. Which of the following is NOT an abnormal erythrocyte finding in severe pregnancy-induced hypertension?

a. discocytes
b. schizocytes
c. spherocytosis
d. echinocytes

34-25. Which of the following is relatively reduced in women with preeclampsia?

a. renin
b. angiotensin II
c. aldosterone
d. all of the above

34-26. What happens to renal plasma flow and glomerular filtration rate in preeclampsia?

a. increase
b. remain the same
c. decrease
d. vary greatly

34-27. Which of the following is the characteristic glomerular lesion of preeclampsia?

a. endotheliosis
b. capillary leaks
c. burst cells
d. clang cells

34-28. In women with preeclampsia, what is the usual cause of acute tubular necrosis?

a. severe hypertension
b. fragmentation hemolysis
c. hemorrhage with inadequate replacement
d. glomerular capillary endotheliosis

34-29. What percentage of women with eclampsia have cerebral edema?

a. 1
b. 5
c. 10
d. 25

34-30. Which is true of blindness occurring in conjunction with severe preeclampsia?

a. likely central in origin
b. often permanent
c. usually unilateral
d. identified in the majority of severe preeclamptics

34-31. What is the mean diameter of the myometrial spiral arterioles in women with preeclampsia?

a. 50 μm
b. 100 μm
c. 200 μm
d. 500 μm

34-32. What is the mean diameter of the myometrial spiral arterioles in normal pregnant women?

a. 50 μm
b. 100 μm
c. 200 μm
d. 500 μm

34-33. What is the positive-predictive value of a "rollover test" for preeclampsia?

a. 5%
b. 10%
c. 25%
d. 33%

34-34. Which of the following has been shown by meta-analysis (not confirmed by randomized trial) to prevent preeclampsia?

a. calcium supplementation
b. low-dose aspirin
c. zinc supplementation
d. none of the above

34-35. Low-dose aspirin given to pregnant women causes which of the following?

a. decreases thromboxane
b. increases prostacyclin
c. increases prostaglandin E_2
d. all of the above

34-36. Which of the following is NOT an indication of severe pregnancy-induced hypertension?

a. upper abdominal pain
b. oliguria
c. creatinine 0.6 mg/dL
d. fetal growth restriction

34-37. Which of the following is increased in preeclamptic women treated with labetolol?

a. fetal growth restriction
b. eclampsia
c. severe preeclampsia
d. all of the above

34–38. Which of the following is a minimum value on urine dipstick for the diagnosis of severe preeclampsia?

a. trace
b. 1+
c. 2+
d. 3+

34–39. How long does fetal bradycardia associated with an eclamptic seizure usually last?

a. <1 min
b. 3 to 5 min
c. 10 to 12 min
d. >20 min

34–40. How is magnesium excreted?

a. lungs
b. liver
c. kidney
d. gastrointestinal tract

34–41. What plasma magnesium level most often prevents seizures?

a. 3 to 4 mEq/L
b. 4 to 7 mEq/L
c. 7 to 10 mEq/L
d. over 10 mEq/L

34–42. At what serum level of magnesium do patellar reflexes disappear?

a. 6 mEq/L
b. 8 mEq/L
c. 10 mEq/L
d. 12 mEq/L

34–43. How is magnesium toxicity treated?

a. calcium gluconate 1 g intravenously
b. calcium gluconate orally
c. calcium gluconate 1 g intravenously and discontinue magnesium
d. dialysis

34–44. With a serum creatinine of 1.3 mg/dL, how should the dose of $MgSO_4$ be managed?

a. increased
b. kept the same
c. reduced by half
d. discontinued

34–45. What is the initial dose of hydralazine used to treat severe hypertension?

a. 100 mg orally
b. 50 mg intramuscularly
c. 5 to 10 mg intravenous bolus
d. all can be safely used

34–46. What intravenous dose of labetolol is used to control severe hypertension?

a. 5 mg
b. 10 to 20 mg
c. 40 to 80 mg
d. 100 mg

34–47. In severe preeclampsia with pulmonary edema, what immediate treatment should be given?

a. furosemide intravenously
b. digoxin
c. hydrochlorothiazide
d. fluid restriction

34–48. What is the recurrence rate of HELLP syndrome?

a. 2%
b. 5%
c. 17%
d. 25%

35

Obstetrical Hemorrhage

35–1. Currently in the United States, what is the approximate percentage of pregnancy-related deaths attributable to maternal hemorrhage?

   a. 20
   b. 40
   c. 60
   d. 80

35–2. Which of the following is NOT among the top four causes of pregnancy-related deaths due to maternal hemorrhage?

   a. uterine atony
   b. coagulopathy
   c. placenta previa
   d. placental abruption

35–3. Supracervical sources of bleeding during labor include all EXCEPT which of the following?

   a. bloody show
   b. placental abruption
   c. placenta previa separation
   d. ruptured vasa previa vessel

35–4. Which of the following is associated with an increased incidence of placental abruption?

   a. young age
   b. alcohol abuse
   c. oligohydramnios
   d. multifetal gestation

35–5. With which of the following is the associated incidence of placental abruption highest?

   a. hypertension
   b. leiomyomata
   c. thrombophilia
   d. cigarette smoking

35–6. Which of the following approximates the incidence of placental abruption per delivery?

   a. 1:200
   b. 1:400
   c. 1:600
   d. 1:800

35–7. Placental abruption is the cause of approximately what percentage of third-trimester stillbirths?

   a. 10
   b. 20
   c. 30
   d. 40

35–8. Your patient, at 37 weeks gestation, fell and struck her abdomen on the pavement. Fetal heart rate is 140 bpm. Her vital signs are stable and she denies pain. Cervical examination reveals no bleeding. Her cervix is 1 to 2 cm dilated and 50 percent effaced. The fetal head is at −1 station. The next most appropriate management of this patient includes which of the following?

   a. cesarean delivery
   b. induction of labor
   c. monitoring in labor and delivery for several hours
   d. discharge home to bed rest for the following 24 hr

35–9. Your newly pregnant patient suffered a placental abruption at 35 weeks during her first pregnancy. Her chronic hypertension is a complicating factor again this pregnancy. Which of the following antepartum fetal assessment tools has been shown to improve fetal outcome in subsequent pregnancies following an initial placental abruption?

   a. nonstress testing
   b. contraction testing
   c. uterine artery Doppler velocimetry
   d. none of the above

35–10. Which of the following signs or symptoms is most commonly seen with placental abruption?

   a. fetal demise
   b. vaginal bleeding
   c. preterm contractions
   d. increased resting uterine tone

35–11. The coagulopathy following placental abruption involves lowering of which of the following maternal serum hematological components?

   a. plasmin
   b. D-dimers
   c. fibrinogen
   d. fibrinogen–fibrin degradation products

35–12. How can acute tubular necrosis following placental abruption best be prevented?

   a. dialysis
   b. cryoprecipitate infusion
   c. furosemide administration
   d. blood and crystalloid replacement

35–13. Extravasation of blood into the uterine musculature is denoted by which of the following eponyms?

   a. Balzac uterus
   b. Voltaire uterus
   c. Couvelaire uterus
   d. Beaumarchais uterus

35–14. Which of the following is the preferred method of delivery for severe abruption with fetal demise?

   a. vaginal delivery
   b. immediate cesarean delivery
   c. cesarean delivery following blood replacement
   d. cesarean delivery following cryoprecipitate replacement

35–15. Your patient at 35 weeks gestation presents with complaints of painful contractions and vaginal bleeding. Fetal heart rate is 130 bpm with no accelerations or decelerations. Ultrasonography reveals a retroplacental density involving approximately one sixth of the placental surface. Cervical exam reveals a cephalic presentation at zero station and 1 cm dilatation with 50 percent effacement. The best management of this patient involves which of the following?

   a. cesarean delivery
   b. tocolysis with magnesium sulfate
   c. amniotomy, followed by oxytocin induction of labor
   d. amniotomy, avoiding oxytocin augmentation of labor

35–16. Which of the following describes a placenta previa that has its edge at the boundary of the internal cervical os?

   a. brimmed
   b. marginal
   c. selvaged
   d. peripheral

35–17. What is the approximate incidence of deliveries complicated by placenta previa in the United States?

   a. 1:100
   b. 1:300
   c. 1:600
   d. 1:900

36–18. Which of the following is associated with an increased incidence of placenta previa?

   a. low parity
   b. young age
   c. singleton gestation
   d. prior cesarean delivery

35–19. Which of the following ultrasonographic modalities may be safely used to identify placenta previa?

   a. transvaginal
   b. transperineal
   c. transabdominal
   d. all of the above

35–20. Your patient at 30 weeks gestation presents with complaints of vaginal bleeding. She is admitted to a labor room for evaluation. Fetal heart rate is 130 bpm with no accelerations or decelerations. Ultrasonography reveals a placenta covering a portion of the internal cervical os. She currently shows no active vaginal bleeding. The best management of this patient involves which of the following?

   a. cesarean delivery
   b. observation in labor and delivery
   c. amniocentesis to assess fetal lung maturity
   d. gentle cervical examination to assess dilatation and amnionic membrane status

35–21. All EXCEPT which of the following techniques may be attempted to halt uterine bleeding from the implantation site of a placenta previa during cesarean delivery?

   a. bilateral internal iliac artery embolization
   b. bilateral uterine artery ligation
   c. GorTex mesh sutured to implantation site
   d. intraoperative uterine packing with postoperative removal

35–22. Pregnancies complicated by placenta previa have an increased incidence of which of the following?

   a. hydramnios
   b. gestational diabetes
   c. amnionic band syndrome
   d. congenital malformations

35–23. For an average-sized woman, the normal pregnancy-induced expansion in blood volume approximates which of the following?

   a. 500 to 1000
   b. 1000 to 1500
   c. 1500 to 2000
   d. 2000 to 2500

35–24. Which type of vaginal delivery should prompt inspection of the cervix and vagina following the delivery?

   a. breech extraction
   b. low forceps delivery
   c. outlet vacuum extraction
   d. all vaginal deliveries

35–25. Following vaginal delivery, bright red bleeding that continues even in the presence of a firmly contracted uterus is most likely due to which of the following?

   a. uterine rupture
   b. retained placenta
   c. vaginal laceration
   d. thrombocytopenia

35–26. Which of the following is characteristic of Sheehan syndrome?

   a. amenorrhea
   b. profuse lactation
   c. hyperthyroidism
   d. renal insufficiency

35–27. Which of the following is the most dangerous consequence of delivering the placenta by cord traction?

   a. endometritis
   b. cord avulsion
   c. uterine inversion
   d. cervical laceration

35–28. Intravenous bolus oxytocin may cause which of the following?

   a. hypotension and headache
   b. hypertension and headache
   c. hypotension and cardiac arrhythmia
   d. hypertension and cardiac arrhythmia

35–29. Predisposing factors for uterine atony include which of the following?

   a. low parity
   b. preeclampsia
   c. precipitous labor
   d. oligohydramnios

35–30. Intravenous bolus methergine may cause which of the following?

   a. seizure
   b. arrhythmia
   c. hypertension
   d. rebound atony

35–31. Intramuscular prostaglandin (PG) is used to treat hemorrhage caused by uterine atony. What is the preferred PG and its dose?

   a. 15-methyl $F_{2\alpha}$, 1.0 g
   b. 15-methyl $F_{2\alpha}$, 0.25 mg
   c. 15-methyl E_2, 1.0 g
   d. 15-methyl E_2, 0.25 mg

35–32. Which of the following is a side effect of carboprost ($PGF_{2\alpha}$)?

   a. fever
   b. ashen color
   c. constipation
   d. hypotension

35–33. Your patient is in the third stage of her labor. The placenta has been delivered and her uterus is flaccid. Bleeding persists despite administration of an oxytocin solution infusion and multiple intramuscular uterine contractants. Which of the following is NOT considered an appropriate next step in this patient's management?

   a. exploratory laparotomy
   b. visual inspection of the genital tract
   c. bimanual compression of the uterus
   d. manual exploration of uterine cavity

35–34. Internal iliac artery ligation increases the future risk of which of the following?

   a. stillbirth
   b. infertility
   c. secondary amenorrhea
   d. none of the above

35–35. Complications seen with uterine packing to control postpartum hemorrhage include all EXCEPT which of the following?

   a. infection
   b. urinary obstruction
   c. concealed bleeding
   d. myometrial pressure necrosis

35–36. Imperfect development of the Nitabuch layer during placental development that results in placental villi penetrating through the myometrium is termed which of the following?

   a. placenta increta
   b. placenta accreta
   c. placenta percreta
   d. placenta diacreta

35–37. Which of the following is the most common cause of postpartum hemorrhage mandating hysterectomy?

   a. uterine atony
   b. placenta previa
   c. placenta accreta
   d. genital tract laceration

35–38. What is the approximate incidence of placenta accreta per delivery?

   a. 1:700
   b. 1:1500
   c. 1:2500
   d. 1:3500

35–39. Which of the following is a risk factor for placenta accreta?

   a. young age
   b. primigravidity
   c. fundal placenta
   d. previous cesarean delivery

35–40. Which of the following modalities has been used to successfully diagnose placenta accreta in high-risk pregnancies?

   a. ultrasonography
   b. fetal fibronectin assay
   c. maternal serum β-hCG levels
   d. maternal serum pregnancy-related protein A levels

35–41. Which of the following is the best management approach to placenta accreta?

   a. observation
   b. hysterectomy
   c. oxytocin administration
   d. hypogastric artery ligation

35–42. Your patient's uterus inverts during delivery of the placenta. The placenta is no longer attached to the uterus. After calling for additional assistance, which of the following is the first best management step?

   a. prompt hysterectomy
   b. prompt oxytocin administration
   c. attempt to manually replace the uterus
   d. administer inhalation anesthetics prior to manual replacement

35–43. Which of the following anesthetics is the most ideal adjunct for replacement of an inverted uterus?

   a. enflurane
   b. thiopental
   c. succinylcholine
   d. spinal analgesia

35–44. Risk factors for puerperal hematoma include all EXCEPT which of the following?

   a. nulliparity
   b. episiotomy
   c. forceps delivery
   d. advanced maternal age

35–45. What is the most common presenting complaint with a vulvar hematoma?

   a. pain
   b. fever
   c. hemorrhage
   d. urinary retention

35–46. In the recovery room, 1 hour after an outlet forceps delivery, your patient is found to have an 8 × 5 cm expanding, bluish, tense, painful right labia majora. The most appropriate management of this patient includes which of the following?

   a. vaginal pack
   b. incision and drainage
   c. exploratory laparotomy
   d. observation, ice pack, and analgesia

35–47. What is the most common cause of uterine rupture?

   a. excessive oxytocin
   b. manual manipulation
   c. previous uterine perforation
   d. previous cesarean section scar

35–48. A woman with an anatomically normal uterus and with no prior uterine surgeries may be at increased risk of uterine rupture during labor due to which of the following?

   a. low parity
   b. oligohydramnios
   c. multifetal gestation
   d. advanced maternal age

35–49. Which of the following is one of the early compensatory changes that occurs with hemorrhagic blood loss?

  a. slowed heart rate
  b. venular constriction
  c. arteriolar vasodilatation
  d. all of the above

35–50. What is the best way to replace fluid loss in hypovolemic shock?

  a. colloid alone
  b. crystalloid alone
  c. crystalloid plus blood
  d. crystalloid plus albumin

35–51. During an episode of acute, significant hemorrhage, which of the following characteristics is true of the hematocrit?

  a. The highest value is found 2 hr following the onset of bleeding.
  b. The highest value is found 30 min following the onset of bleeding.
  c. The laboratory value mirrors true blood loss throughout the bleeding event.
  d. None of the above are true.

35–52. During hemorrhage, what minimum rate of urine flow should be maintained to prevent renal tubular necrosis?

  a. 10 cc/hr
  b. 30 cc/hr
  c. 100 cc/hr
  d. 200 cc/hr

35–53. In an isovolemic patient, at what hemoglobin level does cardiac output begin to increase significantly?

  a. 3 g/dL
  b. 5 g/dL
  c. 7 g/dL
  d. 9 g/dL

35–54. What will the increase in hematocrit be after the transfusion of 1 unit of whole blood?

  a. 1 to 2%
  b. 3 to 4%
  c. 5 to 6%
  d. 7 to 8%

35–55. Adverse effects associated with autologous blood transfusion harvested by a cell saver during cesarean delivery include which of the following?

  a. fever
  b. respiratory distress

  c. amnionic fluid embolism
  d. none of the above

35–56. What is the most common coagulation defect found in women with multiple transfusions following acute severe hemorrhage?

  a. thrombocytopenia
  b. prolonged bleeding time
  c. antithrombin III deficiency
  d. prolonged prothrombin time

35–57. In an actively bleeding patient, the platelet count should be kept above what level?

  a. 50,000
  b. 75,000
  c. 100,000
  d. 125,000

35–58. Below what fibrinogen level can one expect to see impaired coagulation?

  a. 25 mg/dL
  b. 50 mg/dL
  c. 100 mg/dL
  d. 150 mg/dL

35–59. Crossmatching compared with typing and screening lowers the risk of antibody reaction between the patient and transfused donor blood by what approximate percentage?

  a. 0.05
  b. 0.5
  c. 5
  d. 10

35–60. What is the increase in hematocrit following transfusion of 1 unit of packed red blood cells?

  a. 1 to 2%
  b. 3 to 4%
  c. 5 to 6%
  d. 7 to 8%

35–61. What is the increase in platelet count following transfusion of 1 unit of platelets?

  a. 2500/μL
  b. 5000/μL
  c. 7500/μL
  d. 10,000/μL

35–62. Which of the following factors is NOT a component of cryoprecipitate?

  a. fibrinogen
  b. factor VIII:C
  c. fetal fibronectin
  d. factor VIII:von Willebrand factor

35–63. Which of the following is among the most common sequelae of blood transfusion?

 a. HIV infection
 b. D-isoimmunization
 c. ABO-incompatibility reaction
 d. *Yersinia enterocolitica* infection

35–64. Which of the following signs are commonly associated with hemolytic transfusion reaction?

 a. dyspnea
 b. bradycardia
 c. somnolence
 d. hypertension

35–65. What is the current risk of HIV infection following the transfusion of 1 unit of blood?

 a. 1:200,000
 b. 1:500,000
 c. 1:2 million
 d. 1:5 million

35–66. Inciting agents of disseminated intravascular coagulopathy (DIC) include which of the following?

 a. exotoxins
 b. proteases
 c. thromboplastin
 d. all of the above

35–67. What is the most common cause of DIC in pregnancy?

 a. sepsis
 b. fetal demise
 c. placenta previa
 d. placental abruption

35–68. Which of the following have been shown to be effective in the treatment of active hemorrhage and DIC?

 a. heparin
 b. epsilon-aminocaproic acid
 c. liposome-encapsulated hemoglobin
 d. none of the above

35–69. What is the time interval between fetal death and delivery before which DIC rarely develops?

 a. 2 weeks
 b. 4 weeks
 c. 6 weeks
 d. 8 weeks

35–70. Which of the following most closely approximates the incidence of amnionic fluid embolism per delivery?

 a. 1:2000
 b. 1:20,000
 c. 1:200,000
 d. 1:2,000,000

35–71. Which of the following is NOT characteristic of amnionic fluid embolism?

 a. hypoxia
 b. chest pain
 c. hypotension
 d. disseminated intravascular coagulopathy

35–72. After cardiopulmonary resuscitation for amnionic fluid embolism, initiation of which of the following has been shown to improve maternal prognosis?

 a. intravenous heparin
 b. prompt cesarean delivery
 c. intravenous antimicrobials
 d. none of the above

35–73. Commonly associated complications of amnionic fluid embolism include which of the following?

 a. cardiac arrest
 b. maternal death
 c. fetal neurological damage
 d. all of the above

35–74. DIC associated with abortion develops most commonly in which of the following situations?

 a. septic abortion
 b. uterine perforation
 c. elective vacuum aspiration
 d. misoprostol-induced abortion

36

Preterm Birth

36–1. A small-for-gestational age neonate is one whose birthweight falls below what percentile for its gestational age?

    a. 5th
    b. 10th
    c. 15th
    d. 20th

36–2. In the United States in 2001, how many infants died during the first year of life?

    a. 2800
    b. 28,000
    c. 280,000
    d. 2,800,000

36–3. Of the infant deaths in the first year of life, what proportion are contributed to by preterm birth (delivery before 37 weeks gestation)?

    a. one tenth
    b. one third
    c. one half
    d. two thirds

36–4. Which of the leading causes of infant mortality has NOT declined from 1990 to 2000?

    a. birth defects
    b. respiratory distress syndrome
    c. preterm delivery and low birthweight
    d. sudden infant death syndrome

36–5. Preterm births in the United States remain highest in which ethnic group?

    a. Asian or Pacific Islander
    b. African American
    c. Hispanic
    d. Native American

36–6. Neonatal survival is approximately 20 percent at 24 weeks gestation, and increases to what percentage at 25 weeks?

    a. 25
    b. 30

    c. 45
    d. 50

36–7. Neonatal morbidity and mortality are most strongly influenced by which of the following?

    a. birthweight
    b. gestational age
    c. level of neonatal nursery care
    d. maternal medical condition

36–8. What percentage of surviving infants born prior to 27 weeks gestation are totally free of impairment at or beyond the age of 5 years?

    a. 1
    b. 10
    c. 20
    d. 40

36–9. What trend has occurred in the morbidity and mortality of birth at the threshold of viability (24 to 25 weeks gestation) since 1993?

    a. survival has doubled, morbidity decreased
    b. survival has quadrupled, morbidity decreased
    c. survival unchanged, morbidity decreased
    d. no change in either survival or morbidity

36–10. In general, at what gestational age and weight are most obstetricians willing to perform a cesarean delivery for fetal indications?

    a. 24 weeks and 500 g
    b. 24 weeks and 750 g
    c. 26 weeks or 500 g
    d. 26 weeks or 750 g

36–11. In the United States, there is essentially no increase in survival at or beyond what gestational age as compared with delivery at term?

    a. 30 weeks
    b. 32 weeks
    c. 34 weeks
    d. 36 weeks

36–12. Approximately what percentage of preterm singleton births are medically indicated rather than the result of spontaneous labor?

a. 10
b. 30
c. 50
d. 70

36–13. What is the most common cause of indicated preterm birth?

a. fetal distress
b. preeclampsia
c. fetal growth restriction
d. placental abruption

36–14. Which of the following is increased after threatened abortion?

a. placental abruption
b. preterm labor
c. pregnancy loss before 24 weeks
d. all of the above

36–15. Cigarette smoking has NOT been strongly linked to which of the following?

a. ectopic pregnancy
b. placenta previa
c. preeclampsia
d. preterm premature rupture of membranes

36–16. Your patient has delivered her first two infants prematurely, at 29 and 31 weeks gestation. What is the risk of preterm delivery in a subsequent pregnancy?

a. 5 to 10%
b. 10 to 20%
c. 30 to 40%
d. 70 to 80%

36–17. Clinical use of which of the following has been shown to decrease the recurrence rate of preterm delivery?

a. ambulatory uterine contraction testing
b. digital or ultrasonographic serial cervical assessments
c. risk-scoring system
d. none of the above

36–18. Detection of which of the following in cervicovaginal secretions is a powerful clinical predictor of subsequent preterm birth?

a. decidual relaxin
b. fetal fibronectin
c. interleukin-1
d. tumor necrosis factor

36–19. Which of the following vaginal infections is positively associated with preterm birth?

a. bacterial vaginosis
b. *Trichomonas vaginalis*
c. *Candida vaginalis*
d. herpes simplex infection

36–20. Prenatal treatment of which of the following cervicovaginal infections decreases the risk of preterm birth?

a. bacterial vaginosis
b. *Chlamydia trachomatis*
c. *Trichomonas vaginalis*
d. none of the above

36–21. Which of the following strategies to prevent preterm delivery are currently investigational?

a. progesterone "prophylaxis"
b. salivary estriol level measurement
c. periodontal disease detection and treatment
d. all of the above

36–22. Your patient is at 30 weeks gestation and experiences premature membrane rupture. What is the likelihood that she is in spontaneous labor at the time of presentation?

a. 5%
b. 25%
c. 50%
d. 75%

36–23. When preterm premature rupture of membranes occurs, what is the chance that the fetus will be undelivered 48 hours later?

a. 7%
b. 37%
c. 57%
d. 77%

36–24. Which of the following can be concluded from clinical evidence of preterm premature rupture of membranes?

a. Hospitalization until delivery improves outcome.
b. Intentional delivery in the presence of fetal lung maturity decreases perinatal morbidity and mortality.
c. Pulmonary hypoplasia occurs almost exclusively with premature rupture of membranes prior to 24 weeks gestation.
d. Tocolysis improves perinatal outcome.

36–25. What is the most reliable clinical indicator of chorioamnionitis in the management of premature rupture of membranes?

a. fetal tachycardia
b. fever
c. maternal leukocytosis
d. uterine tenderness

36–26. Chorioamnionitis is associated with which of the following adverse outcomes in very-low-birthweight neonates?

a. cerebral palsy
b. periventricular leukomalacia
c. seizures
d. all of the above

36–27. Current recommendations for management of preterm premature rupture of membranes include which of the following (University of Alabama, Parkland Hospital)?

a. broad-spectrum parenteral antimicrobials initially
b. cesarean delivery if spontaneous labor occurs before 35 weeks gestation
c. gelatin sponge plugging in early second trimester
d. serial sonographic measurements of cervical dilatation

36–28. Which of the following strongly suggest the diagnosis of preterm labor?

a. cervical dilatation >1 cm
b. cervical effacement ≥80%
c. contractions (4 in 20 min) with progressive cervical dilatation
d. all of the above

36–29. Clinical strategies for the management of preterm rupture of membranes and preterm labor focus on prolongation of pregnancy until what gestational age is achieved?

a. 32 weeks
b. 34 weeks
c. 36 weeks
d. 38 weeks

36–30. Administration of which of the following is most beneficial to perinatal outcome for pregnancies at risk for preterm delivery?

a. antimicrobials
b. glucocorticoids
c. phenobarbital plus vitamin K
d. thyrotropin-releasing hormone

36–31. Which of the following strategies have shown conclusive benefit to perinatal outcome when managing preterm birth?

a. bed rest
b. emergency cerclage
c. hydration and sedation
d. none of the above

36–32. What is the mechanism of action of β-adrenergic agents?

a. block thymidine kinase
b. activate aromatase
c. block conversion of ATP to cyclic AMP
d. decrease intracellular ionized calcium

36–33. Which of the following was approved by the Food and Drug Administration for tocolysis of preterm labor?

a. indomethacin
b. magnesium sulfate
c. ritodrine
d. terbutaline

36–34. Analyses show tocolysis with ritodrine to have what average effect on preterm labor?

a. increase birthweight
b. prolong pregnancy by 24 hr
c. decrease perinatal morbidity
d. all of the above

36–35. Which of the following is a potential complication of β-adrenergic agonist fusion?

a. hypoglycemia
b. hypokalemia
c. hypocalcemia
d. hyponatremia

36–36. What is the proposed mechanism of action for magnesium sulfate when used for attempted tocolysis?

a. blocks cyclic AMP
b. increases intracellular calcium
c. calcium antagonist
d. stimulates β-receptors

36–37. Which of the following is being studied as possibly protective against cerebral palsy and other neurological deficits in the offspring of women treated for preterm labor?

a. indomethacin
b. magnesium sulfate
c. ritodrine
d. terbutaline

36–38. Which of the following tocolytics is associated with reversible oligohydramnios?

    a. indomethacin
    b. magnesium sulfate
    c. ritodrine
    d. terbutaline

36–39. Which tocolytic agent enhances the toxicity of magnesium in producing neuromuscular blockade?

    a. nifedipine
    b. ritodrine
    c. indomethacin
    d. ethanol

36–40. Which of the following tocolytics is a competitive oxytocin antagonist?

    a. magnesium
    b. ritodrine
    c. atosiban
    d. nifedipine

36–41. Based on current clinical opinion, management of labor prior to 34 weeks of gestation should include which of the following?

    a. corticosteroid administration
    b. consideration of tocolytics to delay delivery briefly
    c. antimicrobial prophylaxis to prevent group B streptococcus infection
    d. all of the above

37

Postterm Pregnancy

37–1. According to the American College of Obstetricians and Gynecologists, a prolonged or postterm pregnancy is one that extends beyond what gestational age?

    a. 37 weeks
    b. 40 weeks
    c. 42 weeks
    d. 44 weeks

37–2. Postterm pregnancy is defined as greater than or equal to how many days gestation?

    a. 280
    b. 287
    c. 294
    d. 300

37–3. What is the estimated incidence of postterm pregnancy in the United States?

    a. 1%
    b. 4%
    c. 7%
    d. 10%

37–4. What happens to perinatal mortality after 42 weeks gestation?

    a. markedly decreased
    b. slightly decreased
    c. no change
    d. increased

37–5. What is the likelihood of a subsequent postterm birth if the first birth was postterm?

    a. 5%
    b. 10%
    c. 18%
    d. 27%

37–6. Which of the following fetal factors are NOT associated with postterm pregnancy?

    a. renal agenesis
    b. X-linked placental sulfatase deficiency
    c. adrenal hypoplasia
    d. anencephaly

37–7. What is the incidence of neonatal seizures in a posterm fetus (Alexander and colleagues)?

a. 1 per 1000
b. 2 per 1000
c. 4 per 1000
d. 8 per 1000

37–8. Which of the following is NOT a description associated with the postmature infant?

a. smooth skinned
b. patchy peeling skin
c. long, thin body
d. worried-looking faces

37–9. What happens to placental apoptosis (programmed cell death) after 41 weeks gestation?

a. no change
b. decreases
c. increases
d. unknown

37–10. What happens to cord plasma erythropoietin levels at 41 weeks or greater compared with those at 37 to 38 weeks?

a. slightly decreased
b. significantly decreased
c. slightly increased
d. significantly increased

37–11. Which of the following is the principal reason for increased fetal risks in the posterm pregnancy?

a. placental insufficiency
b. cord compression with oligohydramnios
c. decreased umbilical cord diameter
d. meconium-stained amnionic fluid

37–12. In a woman with a favorable cervix and an estimated fetal weight of 3850 g, what is the most common management at 42 weeks gestation?

a. labor induction
b. fetal surveillance started
c. amniocentesis performed for lung maturation studies
d. cesarean delivery scheduled

37–13. In a woman with an unfavorable cervix and an estimated fetal weight of 3800 g, which is the most appropriate management at 42 weeks gestation?

a. sonography to redate pregnancy
b. cesarean delivery
c. hospitalization with bedrest
d. cervical ripening, then labor induction

37–14. How does membrane stripping or sweeping at 38 to 40 weeks gestation affect the frequency of posterm pregnancy (meta-analysis of Boulvain)?

a. decreases
b. no change
c. increases
d. unknown

37–15. What is the incidence of cesarean delivery in nulliparas whose fetal station is −2 at the start of labor induction?

a. 6%
b. 20%
c. 43%
d. 77%

37–16. What is the approximate cost difference (per patient) of fetal testing compared with induction of labor at 41 weeks gestation?

a. $1000 less
b. $200 more
c. $1000 more
d. $4000 more

37–17. A 27-year-old G_3 P_2 at 42 weeks presents in early labor. At amniotomy there is thick meconium. You counsel the patient concerning amnioinfusion. She agrees. The fetal benefits of amnioinfusion include a decrease in which of the following?

a. NICU admissions
b. meconium aspiration syndrome
c. meconium below the vocal cords
d. postmaturity syndrome

38

Fetal Growth Disorders

38–1. How is very-low-birthweight defined?

    a. <1500 g
    b. <2000 g
    c. <2500 g
    d. <3000 g

38–2. How is macrosomia defined?

    a. >3800 g
    b. >4000 g
    c. >4200 g
    d. >4500 g

38–3. What is the incidence of macrosomia?

    a. <1%
    b. 5%
    c. 10%
    d. 25%

38–4. The human brain has increased in size during the last 500,000 years by approximately what percent?

    a. 0
    b. 10
    c. 20
    d. 100

38–5. Which of the following cell growth phases occurs during the first 16 weeks of gestation?

    a. cellular hyperplasia and hypertrophy
    b. cellular hyperplasia
    c. cellular hypertrophy
    d. apoptosis

38–6. What is characteristic of the third phase of fetal growth?

    a. cellular death
    b. cellular swelling
    c. cellular hyperplasia
    d. cellular hypertrophy

38–7. At 34 weeks, the fetus will gain how many grams per day?

    a. 5 to 10
    b. 15 to 20
    c. 30 to 35
    d. 45 to 50

38–8. Cord serum levels of which of the following correlates best with low birthweight?

    a. insulin-like growth factor I (IGF-I)
    b. insulin-like growth factor II (IGF-II)
    c. leptin
    d. insulin growth factor binding protein

38–9. What is the incidence of fetal growth restriction?

    a. <1%
    b. 3 to 10%
    c. 15 to 20%
    d. ~25%

38–10. How are small-for-gestational-age newborns defined?

    a. below 2500 g
    b. below 2000 g
    c. below the 10th percentile for gestational age
    d. below the 20th percentile for gestational age

38–11. Which of the following is NOT a determinant of a newborn's birthweight?

    a. ethnicity
    b. parity
    c. maternal weight
    d. >30-lb maternal weight gain during pregnancy

38–12. Which of the following metabolic abnormalities is associated with growth-restricted fetuses?

    a. hyperinsulinemia
    b. hypertriglyceridemia
    c. hyperglycemia
    d. hypocapnia

38–13. Evaluations of which of the following compounds have been described in the plasma of growth restricted fetuses?

a. prostacyclin
b. placental atrial natriuretic peptide
c. interleukin-1
d. epidermal growth factor

38–14. Which perinatal complication is NOT associated with fetal growth restriction?

a. birth asphyxia
b. sepsis
c. hypoglycemia
d. hypothermia

38–15. How is symmetrical growth restriction characterized?

a. reduction in head size
b. reduction in body size
c. reduction in both body and head size
d. reduction in body and femur length

38–16. What is the brain-to-liver weight ratio in a severely growth-restricted newborn?

a. 1 to 2
b. 2 to 1
c. 3 to 1
d. 5 to 1

38–17. Which of the following is NOT a risk factor for severe fetal growth restriction?

a. maternal weight <100 lb
b. fetal infections
c. trisomy 21
d. smoking

38–18. Which of the following infections is NOT associated with fetal growth restriction?

a. toxoplasmosis infection
b. cytomegalovirus infection
c. congenital rubella
d. human papillomavirus

38–19. Which of the following chromosomal disorders is NOT associated with fetal growth restriction?

a. 45,X
b. trisomy 18
c. trisomy 13
d. trisomy 16

38–20. Which trisomy is responsible for confirmed placental mosaicism and many cases of previously unexplained fetal growth restriction?

a. 13
b. 16

c. 18
d. 21

38–21. Which of the following placental abnormalities is NOT associated with growth restriction?

a. circumvallate placenta
b. placenta previa
c. acute abruption
d. velamentous cord insertion

38–22. Which of the following patients is MOST likely to deliver a growth-restricted newborn?

a. 29 y/o G1 with mononucleosis
b. 29 y/o G2 with gestational diabetes
c. 29 y/o G1 with lupus anticoagulant
d. 29 y/o G2 with a history of acute pyelonephritis at 24 weeks gestation

38–23. Which of the following ultrasound measurements is the most reliable index of fetal size?

a. biparietal diameter
b. abdominal circumference
c. femur length
d. intrathoracic ratio

38–24. What percentage of growth-restricted fetuses can be detected by ultrasound if done within 4 weeks of delivery?

a. 30
b. 50
c. 70
d. 90

38–25. Which sonographic measurement in a growth-restricted fetus correlates best with significant perinatal mortality?

a. biparietal diameter
b. abdominal circumference
c. femur length
d. oligohydramnios

38–26. Which test of fetal well-being correlates with fetal metabolic acidosis at birth?

a. reactive nonstress test
b. negative contraction stress test
c. biophysical profile of 8/10
d. reversed end-diastolic umbilical artery velocimetry

38–27. What is the birthweight threshold for macrosomia if defined as 2 standard deviations above the mean at 39 weeks?

a. 4000 g
b. 4250 g
c. 4500 g
d. 5000 g

38–28. Which of the following is NOT a risk factor for macrosomia?

    a. diabetes
    b. female fetus
    c. maternal obesity
    d. gestational age >42 weeks

38–29. How is fetal weight accurately assessed prior to delivery?

    a. ultrasound
    b. x-ray pelvimetry

    c. Leopold's maneuvers
    d. not possible

38–30. A primary cesarean delivery may be justified in a diabetic pregnancy at what estimated fetal weight?

    a. >4000 g
    b. >4250 g
    c. >4500 g
    d. not justified on estimated weight alone

39

Multifetal Gestation

39–1. What percentage of pregnancies are multifetal?

    a. 1
    b. 3
    c. 5
    d. 7

39–2. Fetuses born of multifetal gestations compared with singleton gestations are at increased risk for which of the following?

    a. death
    b. low birthweight
    c. congenital malformation
    d. all of the above

39–3. Women carrying multifetal gestations compared with those carrying singletons are at increased risk for which of the following?

    a. death
    b. preeclampsia
    c. postpartum hemorrhage
    d. all of the above

39–4. A multifetal gestation resulting from the division of a single ovum is termed which of the following?

    a. dizygotic
    b. fraternal

    c. identical
    d. superfecundal

39–5. Around the time of conception, use of which of the following is thought to increase the risk of monozygotic twinning?

    a. licorice
    b. alcohol
    c. theophylline
    d. oral contraceptive pills

39–6. Zygotic division to form dichorionic, diamnionic twins occurs during which of the following time periods following fertilization?

    a. ≤72 hr
    b. >72 and ≤120 hr
    c. >120 and ≤240 hr
    d. >264 hr

39–7. Division of a monozygote between the fourth and eighth day following fertilization creates which of the following?

    a. conjoined twins
    b. diamnionic, dichorionic
    c. diamnionic, monochorionic
    d. monoamnionic, monochorionic

39–8. Spontaneous fertilization of two ova within the same menstrual cycle but not at the same coitus is termed which of the following?

   a. superfetation
   b. superfertilization
   c. superfecundation
   d. superinsemination

39–9. The incidence of monozygotic splitting is increased by which of the following?

   a. tobacco use
   b. increasing age
   c. ovulation-induction therapy
   d. all of the above

39–10. The incidence of dizygotic twinning is increased by which of the following maternal characteristics?

   a. decreasing age
   b. increasing parity
   c. decreasing FSH levels
   d. increasing cocaine abuse

39–11. Women who are members of which of the following ethnicities have the highest rates of twinning?

   a. Nigerian
   b. Japanese
   c. Asian Indian
   d. African American

39–12. The rates of higher-order multiple gestations resulting from superovulation therapy with human menopausal gonadotropin (hMG) has recently declined due to which of the following?

   a. lowering of hMG drug dosages
   b. increased use of selective fetal reduction
   c. cancelling of cycles with multifollicular ovaries
   d. higher associated rates of "vanishing" twin syndrome with hMG use

39–13. To reduce the incidence of higher-order multiple gestations, which of the following number of embryos is advocated for transfer during assisted reproductive technology (ART) procedures?

   a. 1
   b. 2
   c. 3
   d. 4

39–14. What happens to the incidence of male fetuses in multifetal gestations?

   a. decreases with increasing number of fetuses
   b. increases with increasing number of fetuses
   c. decreases for twins, increases for triplets or greater
   d. increases for twins, decreases for triplets or greater

39–15. Monozygotic twins, compared with dizygotic twins, have greater risks of which of the following?

   a. perinatal mortality
   b. first-trimester abortion
   c. fetal growth restriction
   d. all of the above

39–16. Ultrasonographic evidence pointing to the diagnosis of monochorionicity includes which of the following?

   a. "T" sign
   b. two separate placentas
   c. twins with different gender
   d. dividing membrane >2 mm thick

39–17. Of the following, which is the more sensitive tool for diagnosing multifetal gestation?

   a. radiography
   b. ultrasonography
   c. maternal serum alpha-fetoprotein (MSAFP) measurement
   d. serum human chorionic gonadotropin (hCG) measurement

39–18. Maternal physiological changes with a twin gestation compared with those of a singleton gestation include which of the following?

   a. equivalent cardiac output
   b. lower pulmonary functional residual capacity
   c. greater rise in blood pressure during pregnancy
   d. equivalent severity of pregnancy-related nausea and vomiting

39–19. What is the average blood loss during vaginal delivery of a twin gestation?

   a. 500 mL
   b. 750 mL
   c. 1000 mL
   d. 1500 mL

39–20. With regard to fetal growth restriction in multifetal gestation, which of the following is generally true?

    a. incidence is equivalent between twin and triplet gestations

    b. incidence is equivalent between monozygotic and dizygotic twins

    c. birthweights of twins born after 28 weeks increasingly lag behind those of singletons

    d. estimated fetal weights of twins lag behind that of singletons beginning at 16 weeks gestation

39–21. What percentage of twin gestations are complicated by fetal growth restriction?

    a. 10
    b. 25
    c. 33
    d. 67

39–22. What is the mean duration in weeks of a twin gestation?

    a. 32
    b. 34
    c. 36
    d. 38

39–23. Approximately, what percentage of twin gestations deliver preterm?

    a. 20
    b. 40
    c. 60
    d. 80

39–24. The major cause of neonatal morbidity and mortality results from which of the following?

    a. preterm birth
    b. cerebral palsy
    c. perinatal infection
    d. congenital malformation

39–25. What percentage of monozygotic twins are monoamnionic?

    a. 0.1
    b. 1
    c. 10
    d. 20

39–26. You are evaluating first-trimester bleeding in your pregnant patient. Using ultrasonography, you diagnose twins at 12 weeks gestation. You also identify a single, fused placenta; a "T" sign; and a separating membrane that measures 1 mm in thickness. You counsel your patient that, unlike most twin gestations, this pregnancy has an increased risk of which of the following unique complications?

    a. preeclampsia
    b. cord intertwining
    c. growth discordancy
    d. meconium aspiration syndrome

39–27. Because of increased risk for the unique complication described in question 26, management of this patient should include which of the following at 34 weeks gestation?

    a. strict bed rest
    b. scheduled delivery
    c. assessment of fetal lung maturity
    d. labor induction with amnioinfusion

39–28. Which of the following is the most common type of conjoined twins?

    a. pygopagus
    b. ischiopagus
    c. craniopagus
    d. thoracopagus

39–29. Which of the following is appropriate management of twin reversed-arterial-perfusion (TRAP) sequence?

    a. expectant management
    b. umbilical cord ligation
    c. umbilical cord cauterization
    d. all of the above

39–30. Twin-to-twin transfusion syndrome may result in increased rates of which of the following sequela?

    a. kernicterus in donor twin
    b. cerebral palsy in recipient twin
    c. necrotizing enterocolitis in the recipient twin
    d. meconium aspiration syndrome in donor twin

39–31. The most likely etiology for the neurological damage seen in twin-to-twin transfusion syndrome is which of the following?

    a. vasospasm
    b. hypotension
    c. embolic occlusion
    d. none of the above

39–32. Which of the following is NOT a diagnostic criterion for twin-to-twin transfusion syndrome?

    a. presence of placental vascular connections
    b. oligohydramnios associated with the larger twin
    c. birthweight differences >20% between twins
    d. hemoglobin differences >5 g/dL between twins

39–33. Which of the following is NOT an accepted therapy for twin-to-twin transfusion syndrome?

  a. selective feticide
  b. serial amniocenteses
  c. amnioperitoneal shunting
  d. amnionic membrane septostomy

39–34. A common method to calculate weight discordancy in twins uses which of the following formulas?

  a. $\dfrac{\text{wt of larger twin } - \text{ wt of smaller twin}}{\text{wt of larger twin}}$

  b. $\dfrac{\text{wt of larger twin } - \text{ wt of smaller twin}}{\text{wt of smaller twin}}$

  c. $\dfrac{\text{wt of larger twin}}{\text{wt of larger twin } - \text{ wt of smaller twin}}$

  d. $\dfrac{\text{wt of smaller twin}}{\text{wt of larger twin } - \text{ wt of smaller twin}}$

39–35. In twins, which of the following is the threshold percentage weight discordancy above which there is an increase in adverse perinatal outcome?

  a. 15 to 20
  b. 25 to 30
  c. 35 to 40
  d. 45 to 50

39–36. Increasing weight discordancy between twins is associated with which of the following complications?

  a. fetal death
  b. necrotizing enterocolitis
  c. congenital malformations
  d. all of the above

39–37. One of the twins that your patient is carrying dies at 32 weeks' gestation. This was the donor twin in a pregnancy complicated by twin-to-twin transfusion syndrome. The surviving twin displays reassuring signs such as a biophysical profile score of 8 and a reactive nonstress test. Appropriate management of this pregnancy includes which of the following?

  a. expectant management
  b. prompt heparin administration and expectant management
  c. prompt delivery to avoid maternal coagulopathy
  d. prompt delivery to avoid neurological damage in the surviving twin

39–38. What is the daily recommendation for supplemental folic acid in women with twins or higher-order multiple gestations?

  a. 0.1 mg
  b. 0.4 mg
  c. 1 mg
  d. 4 mg

39–39. Use of which of the following antepartum tests of fetal well-being has been shown to lower stillbirth rates in twin gestations?

  a. nonstress test
  b. biophysical profile
  c. Doppler velocimetry
  d. none of the above

39–40. Which of the following has been shown to decrease the rates of adverse perinatal outcome in twin gestations?

  a. bed rest
  b. tocolytic therapy
  c. routine hospitalization
  d. none of the above

39–41. Which of the following is a valuable tool to predict preterm delivery in twin gestations?

  a. risk-scoring system
  b. salivary estriol assay
  c. fetal fibronectin assay
  d. Nugent scoring for bacterial vaginosis

39–42. What is the most common intrapartum presentation for twins?

  a. cephalic-cephalic
  b. cephalic-breech
  c. breech-breech
  d. breech-cephalic

39–43. Interlocking twins is associated with which of the following presentations?

  a. cephalic-cephalic
  b. cephalic-breech
  c. breech-breech
  d. breech-cephalic

39–44. According to recommendations from the American College of Obstetricians and Gynecologists, which of the following presentations of a twin gestation may be delivered vaginally?

  a. cephalic-cephalic
  b. cephalic-breech, if the second fetus weighs <1500 g
  c. breech-cephalic, if the second fetus weighs <1500 g
  d. all of the above

39–45. Your patient has just given birth vaginally at 36 weeks to her first twin. Cervical examination reveals a cervix 8 cm dilated, a bulging amnionic sac, and a shoulder positioned above the pelvic inlet. Electronic fetal monitoring reveals an adequate contraction pattern and a reassuring fetal heart rate pattern for the second twin. Which of the following would be reasonable next steps in this patient's management?

  a. amniotomy
  b. initiation of pitocin
  c. prompt cesarean delivery
  d. ultrasonographically assisted guidance of the fetal head into the inlet

39–46. According to the American College of Obstetricians and Gynecologists, what maximum time interval should be allowed between delivery of a first twin and the second?

  a. 15 min
  b. 30 min
  c. 60 min
  d. no specific recommendation

39–47. Cesarean delivery is often advocated over vaginal delivery for triplet gestations because of complicating factors. Which of the following in NOT a potential complicating factor in the vaginal delivery of triplet gestations compared with cesarean delivery?

  a. requirement for intrauterine manipulations
  b. cord prolapse
  c. second-stage hemorrhage
  d. worse neonatal outcome

39–48. Transabdominal selective fetal reduction is usually performed during which gestational age range?

  a. 6 to 9 weeks
  b. 10 to 13 weeks
  c. 14 to 17 weeks
  d. 18 to 22 weeks

39–49. With regard to multifetal gestations, which of the following is a common finding associated with selective termination of an abnormal fetus?

  a. abortion of remaining fetuses
  b. maternal infection following procedure
  c. termination of the incorrect (normal) fetus
  d. maternal regret regarding termination decision

40

Abnormalities of the Reproductive Tract

40–1. Which of the following is commonly associated with müllerian duct deformities?

  a. cardiac anomalies
  b. renal anomalies
  c. gastrointestinal tract anomalies
  d. limb anomalies

40–2. The müllerian ducts fuse to form the uterus at what gestational age?

  a. 5 weeks
  b. 10 weeks
  c. 15 weeks
  d. 20 weeks

40–3. Dissolution of the uterine septum to form the uterine cavity is completed by what gestational age?

    a. 5 weeks
    b. 10 weeks
    c. 15 weeks
    d. 20 weeks

40–4. The vagina forms between the müllerian tubercle and which of the following?

    a. mesonephric ducts
    b. ureteral ducts
    c. urogenital sinus
    d. uterus

40–5. The fused müllerian ducts give rise to all of the following structures EXCEPT

    a. cervix
    b. upper two thirds of the vagina
    c. uterine body
    d. vulva

40–6. A transverse vaginal septum and vaginal agenesis are thought to result from which of the following?

    a. defective canalization of the vagina
    b. lack of fusion of the müllerian ducts
    c. unilateral müllerian duct atresia
    d. regional ischemia due to anomalous vascular supply

40–7. What are the müllerian duct fusion anomalies thought to be the result of?

    a. autosomal recessive mutation
    b. local ischemic event during embryogenesis
    c. X-linked dominant mutation
    d. polygenic or multifactorial inheritance

40–8. What is labial fusion most commonly due to?

    a. congenital atresia of the lower vagina and vulva
    b. congenital adrenal hyperplasia
    c. diethylstilbestrol (DES) exposure in utero
    d. oral contraceptive pill use in the first trimester

40–9. Vaginal atresia is seen in which of the following disorders?

    a. androgen insensitivity syndrome
    b. Asherman syndrome
    c. congenital adrenal hyperplasia
    d. 5α-reductase deficiency

40–10. Approximately what percentage of women with vaginal atresia have associated urological abnormalities?

    a. 10
    b. 33
    c. 66
    d. 100

40–11. What is the sensitivity of ultrasound screening for uterine anomalies?

    a. 5%
    b. 20%
    c. 40%
    d. 90%

40–12. What percentage of women with müllerian defects have associated auditory defects?

    a. <1
    b. 15
    c. 33
    d. 55

40–13. Uterine anomalies are associated with what reproductive problems?

    a. abnormal fetal lie
    b. preterm delivery
    c. recurrent miscarriage
    d. all of the above

40–14. Pregnancy outcome in the presence of a unicornuate uterus has what approximate rate of fetal survival for all pregnancies?

    a. 10%
    b. 20%
    c. 40%
    d. 60%

40–15. What percentage of rudimentary uterine horn pregnancies rupture overall?

    a. 10
    b. 25
    c. 50
    d. 100

40–16. When do most rudimentary horn pregnancies rupture?

    a. before the third trimester
    b. during the third trimester
    c. during labor
    d. evenly distributed over trimesters

40–17. What is the rate of breech presentation with uterine didelphys?

    a. 10%
    b. 20%
    c. 40%
    d. 80%

40–18. Which statement is true concerning trial of labor after prior cesarean delivery in the presence of uterine anomalies?

    a. labor curves and vaginal birth rates are equal to normal controls
    b. increased rates of uterine rupture
    c. prolonged first stage of labor in most
    d. pitocin augmentation is safe and effective

40–19. Transabdominal metroplasty is used to repair which uterine anomaly?

    a. arcuate uterus
    b. bicornuate uterus
    c. septate uterus
    d. unicornuate uterus

40–20. Operative hysteroscopy is the best approach for which uterine anomaly?

    a. bicornuate uterus
    b. septate uterus
    c. uterine didelphys
    d. unicornuate uterus

40–21. In utero diethylstilbestrol (DES) exposure is associated with an increased risk of which of the following abnormalities?

    a. cervical neoplasia
    b. vaginal adenosis
    c. vaginal cancer
    d. all of the above

40–22. Up to what percentage of women exposed to DES in utero have identifiable structural variations in the cervix and vagina?

    a. 1
    b. 5
    c. 25
    d. 75

40–23. Which of the following is NOT increased in DES-exposed women?

    a. ectopic pregnancy
    b. multiple gestation
    c. preterm delivery
    d. spontaneous abortion

40–24. DES-exposed women are at increased risk for which obstetrical complication?

    a. cervical incompetence
    b. preeclampsia
    c. gestational diabetes
    d. fetal anomalies

40–25. DES-exposed women are at increased risk of clear-cell adenocarcinoma of which of the following?

    a. breast
    b. cervix
    c. uterus
    d. vagina

40–26. A 26-year-old G2P1 presents for prenatal care at 20 weeks' gestation. An asymptomatic 3 to 4 cm Bartholin cyst is found on physical examination. It does not appear to change over the ensuing months. As delivery approaches, what is the most appropriate management?

    a. drainage and antibiotics
    b. excision of cyst
    c. marsupialization
    d. no treatment needed

40–27. At least how many women have undergone a form of female genital mutilation worldwide?

    a. 80,000
    b. 800,000
    c. 8,000,000
    d. 80,000,000

40–28. What is the form of female genital mutilation that causes the most serious medical and obstetrical complications?

    a. complete clitoridectomy
    b. hymenectomy
    c. infibulation
    d. partial vulvectomy

40–29. In developing countries, what causes the high rate of vesicovaginal fistula formation subsequent to labor?

    a. cesarean delivery under suboptimal conditions
    b. necrotizing fasciitis
    c. untreated urinary tract infections
    d. pressure necrosis from prolonged obstruction of labor

40–30. Cervical stenosis diagnosed during labor is most commonly the result of which of the following?

    a. congenital abnormalities
    b. female genital mutilation
    c. prior conization of the cervix
    d. trauma from prior delivery

40–31. Which of the following is NOT a symptom of an incarcerated uterus?

    a. inability to void
    b. lower abdominal pain
    c. involuntary urinary leakage
    d. fever or chills

40–32. In a woman at term and in labor, an elongated vagina passing above the level of the fetal head most likely represents which of the following?

a. Bandl's ring
b. rupture of the uterus
c. uterine sacculation
d. leiomyoma of the lower uterine segment

40–33. Persistent uterine prolapse during pregnancy is best treated by which of the following?

a. round ligament fixation in the first trimester
b. indwelling bladder catheter
c. pessary
d. sacrospinous uterosacral fixation in the first trimester

40–34. A 34-year-old G4P3 at 26 weeks gestation presents with abdominal pain and low-grade fever. There is point tenderness over the uterine fundus. Degeneration of her previously diagnosed uterine leiomyoma is suspected. What would be the most appropriate initial management?

a. analgesia and observation
b. arterial embolization
c. myomectomy, and then cesarean delivery near term
d. preterm cesarean delivery

40–35. What is the best pregnancy management of a 40-year-old nullipara who has undergone a prior myomectomy during which the endometrial cavity was entered?

a. labor allowed
b. labor allowed, with low forceps delivery to shorten second stage
c. cesarean delivery near term prior to labor
d. oxytocin induction at 38 weeks

40–36. Approximately what percentage of myomas show a significant size change during pregnancy?

a. 25
b. 50

c. 75
d. 100

40–37. During pregnancy, a 7-cm myoma is noted. Its size decreases slightly during the third trimester. This change is likely due to which of the following?

a. carneous degeneration
b. decreased estrogen receptors
c. increased epidermal growth factor
d. increased progesterone receptors

40–38. Which of the following is the most frequent and serious complication of benign ovarian cysts during pregnancy?

a. malignant transformation
b. impaired progesterone production
c. torsion
d. dystocia

40–39. Which of the following ovarian neoplasms is diagnosed most often during pregnancy?

a. benign cystic teratoma
b. endodermal sinus tumor
c. follicular cyst
d. serous cystadenocarcinoma

40–40. What is the best management for a patient with a simple cyst measuring 4.5 cm found on pelvic examination and sonography during the 8th week of pregnancy?

a. immediate laparotomy and cystectomy
b. laparotomy and cystectomy at 16 to 20 weeks
c. observation and serial sonography
d. laparoscopic evaluation with drainage of cyst

40–41. What is the best course of action for a complex 12 cm adnexal mass noted at 18 weeks gestation?

a. observation
b. laparotomy after delivery
c. immediate laparotomy
d. sonographically directed aspiration

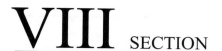

41

General Considerations and Maternal Evaluation

41–1. In general, what is the optimal approach to medical and surgical care of the pregnant woman?

   a. Doing what is best for fetal well-being should dictate care.

   b. Conditions are treated without regard to a woman's pregnant status.

   c. The medical needs of the mother and fetus should be weighed equally.

   d. Care needed by the woman should not be compromised because she is pregnant.

41–2. At what time are most nonobstetrical surgical procedures performed when required during pregnancy?

   a. first trimester

   b. second trimester

   c. third trimester

   d. postpartum

41–3. Which surgical procedure is most commonly performed in the first trimester?

   a. appendectomy

   b. laparoscopy

   c. ovarian cystectomy

   d. tonsillectomy

41–4. Which surgical procedure is most commonly performed in the second trimester?

   a. appendectomy

   b. laparoscopy

   c. ovarian cystectomy

   d. tonsillectomy

41–5. According to a limited number of studies, exposure to general anesthesia during early gestation (4–5 weeks), may increase the risk of which fetal anomalies?

   a. eye anomalies

   b. hydrocephaly

   c. neural-tube defects

   d. all of the above

41–6. What type of anesthesia is most commonly - employed for nonobstetrical surgeries during pregnancy?

   a. epidural

   b. local infiltration

   c. general

   d. regional nerve blocks

41–7. Which of the following neonatal outcomes is significantly increased by nonobstetrical surgery?

   a. birthweight <1500 g

   b. cerebral palsy

   c. congenital malformations

   d. stillbirths

41–8. What appears to be the upper limit of gestational age for performing successful laparoscopic procedures?

   a. 10 to 12 weeks

   b. 16 to 18 weeks

   c. 20 to 22 weeks

   d. 26 to 28 weeks

41–9. What are the effects of laparoscopy on the human fetus?

a. increased congenital anomalies
b. increased spontaneous abortions
c. fetal growth restriction
d. currently unknown

41–10. Compared to x-rays, which of the following characterizes ultrasound?

a. short wavelength, low energy
b. long wavelength, high energy
c. long wavelength, low energy
d. short wavelength, high energy

41–11. What is the relationship between the two units of x-ray dose in common use?

a. 1 Gy = 1 rad
b. 1 Gy = 10 rad
c. 1 Gy = 100 rad
d. 1 Gy = 1000 rad

41–12. During what period of animal development is ionizing radiation most likely to cause a lethal effect?

a. preimplantation
b. first trimester
c. second trimester
d. third trimester

41–13. During what period of gestation does high-dose ionizing radiation exposure pose the most serious risk of mental retardation?

a. 4 to 7 weeks
b. 8 to 15 weeks
c. 20 to 26 weeks
d. 28 weeks to term

41–14. What is the risk of congenital malformations, growth retardation, or abortion from exposure to less than 5 rads of ionizing radiation at 8 to 15 weeks gestation?

a. 1 to 2%
b. 5%
c. 8%
d. not increased

41–15. What is the most common type of anomaly seen in humans as a result of exposure to high-dose (>1–2 Gy) ionizing radiation?

a. central nervous system
b. cardiac
c. limb
d. renal

41–16. What is the approximate fetal exposure from a maternal chest x-ray (two views)?

a. <0.1 mrad
b. 10 mrad
c. 100 mrad
d. 1 rad

41–17. What is the average fetal exposure from a single abdominal radiograph?

a. <0.1 mrad
b. 10 mrad
c. 100 mrad
d. 1 rad

41–18. Computed tomography is useful during pregnancy for evaluation of which of the following conditions?

a. abdominal trauma
b. breech presentation in labor
c. eclampsia
d. all of the above

41–19. What is the approximate dose of radiation to the uterus during a CT scan of the abdomen for trauma evaluation?

a. 3 cGy (rad)
b. 9 cGy (rad)
c. 27 cGy (rad)
d. 36 cGy (rad)

41–20. What is the fetal risk from trace doses of ^{123}I used for thyroid scanning?

a. minimal perinatal morbidity
b. moderate perinatal morbidity
c. severe perinatal morbidity
d. lethal perinatal morbidity

41–21. What are the potential tissue effects of ultrasonography at outputs of greater than those used clinically?

a. agitation
b. cavitation
c. regurgitation
d. vaporization

41–22. For magnetic resonance imaging, the strength of the magnetic field within the bore of the magnet is measured in which units?

a. gray (Gy)
b. tesla (T)
c. curie (Ci)
d. magnorad

41–23. Advantages of magnetic resonance imaging include all EXCEPT which of the following?

    a. ability to characterize tissue
    b. acquisition of images in any plane
    c. high soft-tissue contrast
    d. temporarily immobilizes the fetus

41–24. The protons of which element are used for magnetic resonance imaging?

    a. carbon
    b. hydrogen
    c. oxygen
    d. nitrogen

41–25. Harmful fetal effects of magnetic resonance imaging include which of the following?

    a. fetal heart rate pattern changes
    b. increased spontaneous abortion risk
    c. malformations
    d. no adverse effects have been demonstrated

41–26. For which of the following suspected maternal conditions would magnetic resonance imaging be preferable to computed tomography?

    a. bladder flap hematoma after cesarean delivery
    b. brain tumor
    c. venous thrombosis of pelvic vessels
    d. all of the above

41–27. What is the most common fetal indication for magnetic resonance imaging?

    a. suspected brain abnormalities
    b. malpresentation
    c. oligohydramnios
    d. genetic screening

42

Critical Care and Trauma

42–1. What are the most common reasons for admission to an obstetrical intensive care unit?

    a. gestational diabetes and severe hypertension
    b. obstetrical hemorrhage and severe hypertension
    c. obstetrical hemorrhage and gestational diabetes
    d. sepsis and severe hypertension

42–2. Which of the following conditions is the least likely indication for invasive hemodynamic monitoring?

    a. unexplained pulmonary edema
    b. adult respiratory distress syndrome
    c. peripartum coronary artery disease
    d. asthma

42–3. Which of the following formulas represents systemic vascular resistance?

    a. stroke volume $\times$ body surface area (BSA)
    b. mean systemic arterial pressure (mm Hg) − central venous pressure / cardiac output [(MAP − CVP) / CO] $\times$ 80
    c. mean pulmonary arterial pressure (mm Hg) − mean pulmonary capillary wedge pressure (mm Hg) / cardiac output (MPAP − PCWP) / CO $\times$ 80
    d. CO / BSA

42–4. What is the incidence of acute pulmonary edema complicating pregnancy?

    a. 1 in 50 deliveries
    b. 1 in 100 deliveries
    c. 1 in 500 deliveries
    d. 1 in 5000 deliveries

42–5. What is the mortality rate for acute respiratory failure in pregnant women?

a. <1%
b. 5 to 20%
c. 25 to 40%
d. 50 to 70%

42–6. Which of the following is a criterion for diagnosing the adult respiratory distress syndrome?

a. partial pressure of O_2 (PO_2) >50 mm Hg with fraction of inspired O_2 (FiO_2) >0.6
b. pulmonary capillary wedge pressure >12 mm Hg
c. functional residual capacity increased
d. arterial pressure of O_2 (PaO_2):FiO_2 <200 torr

42–7. How much oxygen is carried by each gram of hemoglobin at 90% saturation?

a. 0.5 mL
b. 1.25 mL
c. 2.5 mL
d. 5.0 mL

42–8. What is the minimum PaO_2 necessary to maintain a 90% oxyhemoglobin saturation?

a. 60 mm Hg
b. 70 mm Hg
c. 80 mm Hg
d. 90 mm Hg

42–9. Which of the following is NOT associated with a rightward shift in the oxyhemoglobin dissociation curve (i.e., decreased hemoglobin affinity for oxygen and increased tissue−capillary interchange)?

a. hypercapnea
b. metabolic acidosis
c. increased body temperature
d. decreased 2,3-diphosphoglycerate

42–10. Which of the following colloid oncotic pressures is characteristic of severe preeclampsia during the antepartum period?

a. 32 mm Hg
b. 24 mm Hg
c. 16 mm Hg
d. 4 mm Hg

42–11. Under normal circumstances, what is the usual colloid oncotic pressure or wedge pressure gradient?

a. 2 mm Hg
b. 4 mm Hg

c. 6 mm Hg
d. ≥8 mm Hg

42–12. Possible therapy for adult respiratory distress syndrome (ARDS) includes all of the following EXCEPT

a. artificial surfactant
b. nitric oxide
c. lipid mediator antagonist
d. interleukin antibodies

42–13. Which of the following is most commonly associated with septic shock?

a. *Enterobacteriaceae*
b. anaerobic streptococci
c. *Bacteroides* species
d. *Clostridium* species

42–14. Which of the following produces an endotoxin as opposed to an exotoxin?

a. *Pseudomonas aeruginosa*
b. *Staphylococcus aureus*
c. group A streptococcus
d. *Escherichia coli*

42–15. Which of the following is directly released upon lysis of the cell wall of gram-negative bacteria?

a. complement
b. kinins
c. lipopolysaccharide
d. tumor necrosis factor

42–16. Of the following, what is NOT characteristic of the "warm phase of septic shock" when treating with intravenous crystalloid?

a. pulmonary hypotension
b. hypovolemia
c. high cardiac output
d. low systemic vascular resistance

42–17. What dose of dopamine causes β-receptor stimulation (i.e., increased vascular resistance and blood pressure)?

a. <2 μg/kg/min
b. 5 to 10 μg/kg/min
c. 10 to 20 μg/kg/min
d. 50 to 60 μg/kg/min

42–18. Which antiinflammatory agent increases mortality in septic shock?

a. ibuprofen
b. methylprednisolone
c. NG-methyl-ʟ-arginine hydrochloride
d. acetaminophen

42–19. What is the incidence of physical trauma in pregnancy?

    a. 1 to 2%
    b. 5 to 7%
    c. 10 to 20%
    d. 30 to 40%

42–20. A 19-year-old at 20 weeks gestation presents to the emergency room with complaints of "being raped." What is included in the treatment protocol for prevention of STDs in this situation?

    a. ceftriaxone plus doxycycline
    b. ceftriaxone plus azithromycin
    c. ceftriaxone plus spectinomycin
    d. ceftriaxone plus cefixime

42–21. What percentage of "minor" maternal injuries are associated with traumatic placental abruptions?

    a. 1 to 6
    b. 10 to 16
    c. 20 to 26
    d. 30 to 36

42–22. Which of the following signs is most useful in predicting the absence of a placental abruption following trauma?

    a. absence of uterine contractions
    b. absence of bleeding
    c. presence of normal fetal heart tones
    d. absence of a tense, painful uterus

42–23. What is the incidence of maternal visceral injuries with penetrating trauma?

    a. <5%
    b. 15 to 40%
    c. 50 to 70%
    d. nearly 100%

42–24. A 27-year-old is involved in a motor vehicle accident during her 7th month of pregnancy. She denies contractions. What is the next step in management?

    a. deflect uterus away from pelvic vessels
    b. administer Rhogam if mother is Rh-negative
    c. fetal heart rate monitoring
    d. all of the above

42–25. What is the best management of a pregnant woman at 38 weeks gestation with burns over 60 percent of her body?

    a. continuous electronic monitoring of the fetus
    b. weekly biophysical profiles
    c. immediate delivery
    d. twice weekly contraction stress tests

42–26. What percentage of infants delivered 12 minutes after maternal cardiopulmonary arrest will be neurologically intact?

    a. 10
    b. 33
    c. 83
    d. 98

43

Obesity

43–1. Obesity in the United States is most correctly described by which term?

    a. endemic
    b. epidemic
    c. pandemic
    d. sporadic

43–2. A recent report (2002) found what percentage of children ages 6 through 11 years to be overweight?

    a. 1
    b. 5
    c. 10
    d. 15

43–3. At present, what portion of the adult U.S. population is either overweight or obese?

    a. 5
    b. 25
    c. 50
    d. 75

43–4. How is the body mass index (BMI) calculated?

    a. weight (kg) / height (m)^2
    b. weight (lb) / waist circumference (in)
    c. percent body fat $\times$ weight (kg)
    d. weight (kg)^2 / abdominal circumference (cm)

43–5. What is a normal BMI?

    a. 18.5 to 24.9
    b. 25 to 29.9
    c. 30.5 to 35.9
    d. 50 to 55.9

43–6. What BMI defines obesity?

    a. $\geq$30
    b. $\geq$35
    c. $\geq$40
    d. $\geq$50

43–7. According to a recent report, which of the following is most predictive of hypertension in women?

    a. BMI $>$30
    b. history of sleep apnea
    c. thigh to waist (circumference) ratio $<$0.25
    d. waist circumference $>$88 cm

43–8. The National Institutes of Health (2001) defined the metabolic syndrome by all of the following EXCEPT

    a. abdominal obesity
    b. elevated high density lipoprotein (HDL)
    c. hypertension
    d. hypertriglyceridemia

43–9. What is the approximate overall prevalence of the metabolic syndrome?

    a. 1%
    b. 5%
    c. 10%
    d. 25%

43–10. Which of the following shows increased mortality rates with increasing obesity?

    a. all causes of death combined
    b. cancer
    c. cardiovascular disease
    d. all of the above

43–11. What is the current weight-related recommendation for pregnant women who are obese?

    a. limit weight gain to $<$15 lbs
    b. laparoscopic stomach banding procedure in first trimester
    c. program to attempt weight loss of up to 30 lbs
    d. no specific recommendations

43–12. Obesity increases the risk of which obstetrical outcome?

    a. failed vaginal delivery after prior cesarean
    b. gestational diabetes
    c. post-cesarean infection
    d. all of the above

43–13. Maternal obesity is a risk factor for all of the following fetal complications EXCEPT

    a. dizygotic twinning
    b. fetal macrosomia
    c. neural-tube defects
    d. stillbirth

43–14. Successful bariatric surgery with resultant weight loss decreases the incidence of which of the following in future pregnancies?

    a. gestational diabetes
    b. hypertensive disorders
    c. fetal macrosomia
    d. all of the above

44

Cardiovascular Disease

44–1. What is the incidence of cardiovascular disease complicating pregnancy?

    a. 0.1%
    b. 1%
    c. 5%
    d. 10%

44–2. During pregnancy, cardiac output is increased by approximately what percentage?

    a. 10
    b. 33
    c. 50
    d. 67

44–3. Cardiac output reaches its maximum at approximately which week of pregnancy?

    a. 12
    b. 20
    c. 28
    d. 36

44–4. In late pregnancy, which of the following contributes to the normal increase in cardiac output?

    a. increased stroke volume
    b. increased resting pulse rate
    c. expanded blood volume
    d. all of the above

44–5. When is heart failure and cardiac-related maternal death most common?

    a. first trimester
    b. second trimester
    c. third trimester
    d. peripartum

44–6. Which of the following symptoms or findings is the most likely indicator of heart disease in a pregnant patient?

    a. nocturia
    b. chest pain
    c. tachycardia
    d. peripheral edema

44–7. Which of the following cardiac signs is NOT a normal finding in pregnancy?

    a. pericardial friction rub
    b. 2/6 midsystolic murmur
    c. brisk and diffuse cardiac apex pulsation
    d. supraclavicular continuous venous hum

44–8. For which of the following procedures is pregnancy an absolute contraindication?

    a. chest radiography
    b. ^{201}Tl SPECT scintigraphy
    c. ^{99}Tc sestamibi perfusion imaging
    d. none of the above

44–9. Which of the following is NOT an electrocardiographic change seen in normal pregnancy?

    a. atrial premature beats
    b. 15-degree left-axis deviation
    c. P wave voltage increase of 50%
    d. mild ST changes in the inferior leads

44–10. Using echocardiography, which of the following is a common pregnancy-induced finding?

    a. aortic insufficiency
    b. mitral valve prolapse
    c. tricuspid regurgitation
    d. right atrial enlargement

44–11. Your patient states that she is comfortable at rest but that walking 40 yards to the mailbox causes shortness of breath and angina? What New York Heart Association classification would you assign to her?

    a. I
    b. II
    c. III
    d. IV

44–12. Which of the following conditions is categorized as a "Group 1-Minimal Risk" for maternal mortality by the New York Heart Association and the American College of Obstetricians and Gynecologists?

    a. ventricular septal defect
    b. pulmonary hypertension
    c. prior myocardial infarction
    d. Marfan syndrome with normal aorta

44–13. What is the approximate incidence of fetal congenital heart disease in the offspring of women born with cardiac anomalies?

    a. 5%
    b. 15%
    c. 25%
    d. 35%

44–14. Your patient has a cardiac lesion which places her at increased risk for heart failure during pregnancy. You counsel her that the most likely first symptom of early heart failure in pregnancy is which of the following?

    a. heartburn
    b. hemoptysis
    c. palpitations
    d. nocturnal cough

44–15. Your pregnant patient has mitral stenosis and is New York Heart Association functional class II. You plan all EXCEPT which of the following - during her pregnancy?

    a. influenza vaccine
    b. pneumococcal vaccine
    c. intrapartum bacterial endocarditis prophylaxis
    d. group B streptococcal vaginal and rectal - culture at 36 weeks

44–16. Which is the preferred intrapartum analgesia in most situations involving maternal heart disease?

    a. paracervical block
    b. intravenous analgesics
    c. continuous epidural analgesia
    d. spinal analgesia (saddle block)

44–17. Which of the following forms of analgesia is contraindicated in women with pulmonary hypertension?

    a. spinal block
    b. pudendal block
    c. general anesthesia
    d. intravenous analgesics

44–18. In general, which of the following is true of pregnancy complicated by a maternal mechanical valve prosthesis?

    a. Fetal loss is rare.
    b. Anticoagulation is mandatory.
    c. Cesarean delivery is recommended for most.
    d. All of the above are true.

44–19. Compared with heparin, warfarin use is associated with high rates of which of the following?

    a. stillbirth
    b. spontaneous abortion
    c. congenital malformation
    d. all of the above

44–20. Disadvantages associated with porcine heart valves include which of the following?

    a. lower durability
    b. mandatory anticoagulation
    c. high rates of thromboembolism
    d. none of the above

44–21. With respect to heparin anticoagulation during pregnancy, which of the following laboratory parameters should be maintained at a level of 1.5 to 2.5 times the baseline value?

    a. bleeding time
    b. thrombin time
    c. prothrombin time
    d. partial thromboplastin time

44–22. Your patient has a mechanical prosthetic heart valve and is receiving heparin anticoagulation therapy. She presents to labor and delivery at 36 weeks' gestation with persistent, heavy vaginal bleeding. Her vital signs are stable. Hemoglobin is 12 g/dL, platelet count is 185,000/μL, and PTT is within the recommended therapeutic range. Sonographic evaluation reveals no evidence of placenta previa or placental abruption. Her cervix is 4 cm dilated with evidence of ruptured membranes. FHTs are 140 bpm with accelerations and no decelerations. What is the most appropriate next step in her care?

    a. platelet transfusion
    b. prompt cesarean delivery
    c. protamine sulfate administration
    d. hypogastric artery angiographic embolization

44–23. How many hours following vaginal delivery should anticoagulation therapy for a mechanical prosthetic valve be reinstated?

    a. 6
    b. 18
    c. 24
    d. 36

44–24. Which of the following surgical treatments for symptomatic mitral stenosis in pregnancy is associated with the lowest maternal and fetal morbidity?

    a. open mitral valvotomy
    b. closed mitral valvotomy
    c. mitral valve replacement
    d. percutaneous balloon mitral valvuloplasty

44–25. Which of the following is currently the most common cause of mitral stenosis in women in the United States?

    a. Lyme disease
    b. Graves disease
    c. rheumatic fever
    d. congenital malformation

44–26. What is the approximate surface area (cm^2) of a normal adult mitral valve?

    a. 1
    b. 2
    c. 3
    d. 4

44–27. Symptoms typically develop when the surface area (cm^2) of a stenotic mitral valve narrows to below what value?

    a. 0.5
    b. 1.5
    c. 2.5
    d. 3.5

44–28. Which of the following is NOT a common symptom of mitral stenosis?

    a. dyspnea
    b. syncope
    c. palpitations
    d. hemoptysis

44–29. Suggested management decisions regarding the labor and delivery of a woman with mitral stenosis and an otherwise uncomplicated pregnancy include which of the following?

    a. epidural analgesia
    b. mandatory cesarean delivery
    c. aggressive hydration prior to epidural analgesia
    d. mandatory antimicrobial bacterial endocarditis prophylaxis

44–30. What is the primary hemodynamic problem associated with severe aortic stenosis?

    a. fixed cardiac output
    b. fixed cardiac preload
    c. ineffectual ventricular contractility
    d. hyperdynamic ventricular contractility

44–31. Suggested management decisions regarding the labor and delivery of a woman with aortic stenosis and an otherwise uncomplicated pregnancy include which of the following?

    a. epidural analgesia
    b. mandatory cesarean delivery
    c. no intravenous hydration prior to epidural analgesia
    d. mandatory antimicrobial bacterial endocarditis prophylaxis

44–32. Which of the following pregnancy-related hemodynamic changes is thought responsible for the negligible effects of aortic and mitral insufficiency during pregnancy?

    a. increased cardiac output
    b. decreased resting heart rate
    c. decreased vascular resistance
    d. increased ventricular contractility

44–33. What is the approximate incidence of congenital heart disease in the United States?

    a. 8 per 100 live births
    b. 8 per 1000 live births
    c. 8 per 10,000 live births
    d. 8 per 100,000 live births

44–34. Which of the following is the most common form of atrial septal defect (ASD)?

    a. ovale type
    b. ostium primum
    c. ostium secundum
    d. sinus venosus

44–35. Which of the following factors most adversely affects the maternal cardiac risk related to atrial septal defect (ASD) and pregnancy?

    a. childhood repair of lesion
    b. concurrent pulmonary hypertension
    c. presence of sinus venosus type ASD
    d. presence of ostium secundum type ASD

44–36. Which of the following is a possible complication of unrepaired ventricular septal defect?

    a. bacterial endocarditis
    b. Eisenmenger syndrome
    c. pulmonary hypertension
    d. all of the above

44–37. What is the incidence of fetal atrial or ventricular septal defect if the mother has such a defect?

    a. 5 to 15%
    b. 15 to 30%
    c. 30 to 45%
    d. 45 to 60%

44–38. Which of the following maternal conditions would most likely prompt the recommendation for pregnancy termination?

    a. atrial septal defect
    b. aortic regurgitation
    c. bacterial endocarditis
    d. Eisenmenger syndrome

44–39. Which of the following cardiac lesions is NOT associated with cyanosis?

    a. mitral stenosis
    b. Fallot tetralogy
    c. Ebstein anomaly
    d. coarctation of the aorta

44–40. Which of the following is NOT an associated finding in Fallot tetralogy?

    a. overriding aorta
    b. pulmonary stenosis
    c. bicuspid aortic valve
    d. right ventricular hypertrophy

44–41. Which of the following is the preferred mode of delivery in a woman with a cyanotic heart lesion?

    a. vaginal delivery with spinal analgesia
    b. vaginal delivery with epidural analgesia
    c. elective cesarean delivery with epidural analgesia
    d. elective cesarean delivery with general anesthesia

44–42. Eisenmenger syndrome may result from which of the following lesions?

    a. atrial septal defect
    b. patent ductus arteriosus
    c. ventricular septal defect
    d. all of the above

44–43. Which of the following is the LEAST common underlying cause of pulmonary hypertension?

    a. atrial septal defect
    b. patent ductus arteriosus
    c. ventricular septal defect
    d. idiopathic primary pulmonary hypertension

44–44. Which drug used for long-term therapy of pulmonary hypertension dilates and lowers pulmonary vascular resistance?

    a. minoxidil
    b. hydralazine
    c. epoprostenol
    d. nitroglycerin

44–45. Mitral valve prolapse most commonly presents with which of the following?

    a. syncope
    b. chest pain
    c. palpitations
    d. no symptoms

44–46. Which of the following statements is true of mitral valve prolapse?

    a. It has a general population incidence of 12 to 15%.
    b. It is commonly associated with other cardiac lesions.
    c. It typically presents with palpitations and syncope.
    d. None of the above are true.

44–47. Which of the following etiological factors has been identified in women with peripartum cardiomyopathy?

    a. mitral stenosis
    b. viral myocarditis
    c. chronic hypertension
    d. all of the above

44–48. Myocardial biopsy in women with presumed idiopathic cardiomyopathy most commonly reveals which of the following?

    a. gummas
    b. myocarditis
    c. caseating granulomas
    d. myxomatous degeneration

44–49. Which of the following conditions carries the highest risk for bacterial endocarditis?

    a. mitral valve prolapse without valvar regurgitation
    b. cardiac pacemaker in place
    c. prior coronary bypass graft surgery
    d. porcine prosthetic cardiac valve in place

44–50. Which of the following is the most common cause of bacterial endocarditis, both acute and subacute forms?

    a. *Streptococcus viridans*
    b. *Streptococcus aureus*
    c. *Neisseria gonorrhoeae*
    d. *Streptococcus pneumoniae*

44–51. Which of the following is a nearly universal characteristic of endocarditis?

    a. fever
    b. syncope
    c. headache
    d. scleral petechiae

44–52. Which of the following antimicrobial combinations is recommended for bacterial endocarditis prophylaxis?

   a. ampicillin plus gentamicin
   b. ampicillin plus doxycycline
   c. penicillin G plus doxycycline
   d. vancomycin plus clindamycin

44–53. Which of the following is contraindicated for the treatment of arrhythmias in pregnancy?

   a. digoxin
   b. cardiac pacemaker
   c. electrical cardioversion
   d. none of the above

44–54. Which of the following is the most commonly seen cardiac arrhythmia?

   a. atrial fibrillation
   b. complete heart block
   c. ventricular tachycardia
   d. paroxysmal supraventricular tachycardia

44–55. Which of the following, if chronic during pregnancy, requires heparin anticoagulation therapy?

   a. atrial fibrillation
   b. ventricular tachycardia
   c. first-degree heart block
   d. paroxysmal supraventricular tachycardia

44–56. A pregnant patient at 32 weeks' gestation is brought to the emergency room following a syncopal episode. She complains of a sudden onset of chest pain that she describes as constant and "ripping" in nature and states that it radiates to her back (pointing to her interscapular area). Her BP is 150/98, pulse is 90, temperature is 98.8°F, and respiratory rate is 14. Neurological examination reveals no abnormalities. Her cardiac examination reveals weak peripheral pulses and a murmur consistent with aortic regurgitation. Your initial questioning should include a search for which of the following possible underlying etiologies?

   a. Turner syndrome
   b. Marfan syndrome
   c. Noonan syndrome
   d. all of the above

44–57. The patient in Question 56 is found to have nonspecific ST changes on ECG. Her chest radiograph shows a widened mediastinum and abnormal aortic arch contour. Which of the following tests is considered definitive for identification of this disorder?

   a. echocardiography
   b. aortic angiography
   c. computed tomography of head
   d. magnetic resonance imaging of chest

44–58. Women are at increased risk for cardiovascular complications during pregnancy with an aortic root diameter greater than which of the following?

   a. 20 mm
   b. 30 mm
   c. 40 mm
   d. 50 mm

44–59. Of the following, which is the most commonly associated complication of aortic coarctation?

   a. aortic rupture
   b. atrial fibrillation
   c. tricuspid regurgitation
   d. pulmonary hypertension

44–60. Women are at greatest mortality risk if a myocardial infarction occurs during which of the following periods?

   a. early first trimester
   b. early second trimester
   c. late second trimester
   d. late third trimester

44–61. The most common cause of nonfamilial left ventricular hypertrophy is which of the following?

   a. diabetes
   b. mitral stenosis
   c. pulmonic stenosis
   d. chronic systemic hypertension

44–62. What is the most common cause of death in women with hypertrophic cardiomyopathy?

   a. stroke
   b. arrhythmia
   c. aortic dissection
   d. vascular occlusion

45

Chronic Hypertension

45–1. Risk factors for the development of chronic hypertension include which of the following?

a. heredity
b. smoking
c. parity >3
d. prior molar pregnancy

45–2. In nonpregnant women, antihypertensive therapy for mild to moderate hypertension has been shown to decrease the incidence of which of the following?

a. infertility
b. mortality
c. diabetes
d. endometrial cancer

45–3. Nonpharmacological interventions to treat hypertension include all EXCEPT which of the following?

a. weight loss
b. high-fat diet
c. physical activity
d. smoking cessation

45–4. Your nonpregnant patient's blood pressure measures 146/94 on several visits and persists despite lifestyle changes. The first-line treatment agent for her should come from which of the following antihypertensive medication groups?

a. thiazide-type diuretics
b. calcium-channel blockers
c. β-adrenergic receptor blocker
d. angiotensin-converting enzyme inhibitors

45–5. Your nonpregnant patient's blood pressure measures 164/98 on two separate visits. The most effective treatment for this patient typically requires which of the following?

a. sodium-lowering diet plus thiazide-type diuretic
b. sodium-lowering diet plus β-adrenergic receptor blocker
c. thiazide-type diuretic plus angiotensin-converting enzyme inhibitor
d. angiotensin-converting enzyme inhibitor plus angiotensin-receptor blocker

45–6. Evaluation of uncomplicated, long-standing, chronic hypertension early in pregnancy includes all EXCEPT which of the following?

a. echocardiography
b. serum creatinine level
c. ophthalmological evaluation
d. serum thyroid-stimulating hormone level

45–7. In hypertensive women, adverse pregnancy outcomes most commonly occur when which of the following is also present?

a. parity >3
b. renal dysfunction
c. prior molar pregnancy
d. prior deep venous thrombosis

45–8. Pregnant women with chronic hypertension are at greatest risk compared with nonhypertensive controls for which of the following adverse events?

a. placental abruption
b. deep venous thrombosis
c. first-trimester abortion
d. postpartum cardiomyopathy

45–9. The development of superimposed preeclampsia in a chronic hypertensive patient is increased proportionately with which of the following?

a. severity of baseline obesity
b. severity of baseline hypertension
c. number of family members with hypertension
d. number of family members with prior preeclampsia

45–10. Low-dose aspirin therapy during pregnancy in women with chronic hypertension has been shown in some studies to decrease the incidence of which of the following?

   a. eclampsia
   b. preterm labor
   c. oligohydramnios
   d. cesarean delivery

45–11. Which adverse pregnancy outcome is NOT increased in pregnancies completed by chronic hypertension?

   a. preterm birth
   b. perinatal death
   c. fetal-growth restriction
   d. spontaneous preterm rupture of membranes

45–12. In chronically hypertensive women, which of the following is most commonly associated with fetal-growth restriction?

   a. maternal obesity
   b. increased maternal age
   c. increased maternal parity
   d. maternal hyperthyroidism

45–13. What is the mechanism of action of alpha-methyldopa?

   a. relaxes arterial smooth muscles
   b. increased sodium and water diuresis
   c. increased peripheral vascular resistance
   d. acts centrally to decrease vascular tone

45–14. Your pregnant patient persistently displays blood pressure readings of 150/104. The most appropriate first-line therapy for this patient includes which of the following?

   a. thiazide-type diuretics
   b. calcium-channel blocker
   c. central-acting anti-adrenergic agents
   d. angiotensin-converting enzyme inhibitors

45–15. Angiotensin-converting enzyme inhibitors are contraindicated in pregnancy due to what fetal effects?

   a. cardiac defects
   b. fetal renal defects
   c. thrombocytopenia
   d. patent ductus arteriosus

45–16. Beta-blockers, in particular atenolol, are associated with which of the following perinatal morbidities?

   a. preterm birth
   b. hyperglycemia
   c. fetal-growth restriction
   d. respiratory distress syndrome

45–17. The criteria that support the diagnosis of superimposed preeclampsia in women with underlying chronic hypertension include all of the following EXCEPT

   a. severe headache
   b. thrombocytopenia
   c. new-onset proteinuria
   d. iron-deficiency anemia

45–18. What is the risk of superimposed pregnancy-induced hypertension in women with chronic hypertension?

   a. <1%
   b. 10%
   c. 25%
   d. 50%

45–19. Regarding delivery of chronically hypertensive patients with superimposed severe preeclampsia, all of the following are acceptable EXCEPT

   a. induction of labor
   b. epidural anesthesia
   c. await delivery at term
   d. vaginal route of delivery

45–20. In the puerperium, women with severe chronic hypertension are at greatest risk for which of the following?

   a. pulmonary edema
   b. deep venous thrombosis
   c. ovarian vein thrombosis
   d. postpartum hemorrhage

Pulmonary Disorders

46–1. What is the incidence of chronic asthma in pregnancy?

    a. 1 to 4%
    b. 6 to 10%
    c. 12 to 16%
    d. 18 to 22%

46–2. Which of the following cannot be measured directly?

    a. tidal volume
    b. residual volume
    c. minute ventilation
    d. expiratory reserve volume

46–3. Which of the following characterizes functional residual capacity during pregnancy?

    a. decreases by approximately 500 mL
    b. stays unchanged compared with nonpregnant values
    c. increases by approximately 500 mL
    d. increases by approximately 1 L

46–4. How much does basal oxygen consumption increase during the last half of pregnancy?

    a. 1 to 5 mL/min
    b. 10 to 15 mL/min
    c. 20 to 40 mL/min
    d. 60 to 80 mL/min

46–5. How much does the tidal volume increase during pregnancy?

    a. 200 mL
    b. 300 mL
    c. 400 mL
    d. 500 mL

46–6. Which of the following organisms is the major cause of adult community-acquired bacterial pneumonia?

    a. *Staphylococcus aureus*
    b. *Chlamydia trachomatis*
    c. *Mycoplasma pneumoniae*
    d. *Streptococcus pneumoniae*

46–7. Which of the following is a risk factor for lung colonization with *Legionella*?

    a. smoking
    b. diabetes
    c. asthma
    d. alcohol in moderation

46–8. What is the incidence of pneumonia complicating pregnancy?

    a. 1 in 100
    b. 1 in 300
    c. 1 in 600
    d. 1 in 1000

46–9. A 27-year-old woman at 32 weeks gestation presents complaining of cough, fever, chest pain, and dyspnea. Which of the following tests would be most helpful in making a diagnosis?

    a. complete blood cell count
    b. mycoplasma-specific immunoglobulin G
    c. urinalysis for pneumococcal antigen
    d. chest x-ray

46–10. Which of the following factors is NOT an indication for hospitalization of a woman with pneumonia?

    a. altered mental status
    b. hypertension
    c. hypothermia
    d. respiratory rate >30 per min

46–11. What is first-line therapy in a pregnant woman with uncomplicated community-acquired pneumonia?

    a. dicloxicillin
    b. clindamycin
    c. ampicillin
    d. erythromycin

46–12. What is the approximate percentage of penicillin-resistant pneumococcus?

    a. 2
    b. 5
    c. 10
    d. 20

46–13. Which of the following perinatal complications is associated with bacterial pneumonia?

    a. fetal growth retardation
    b. preterm labor
    c. persistent fetal circulation
    d. cerebral palsy

46–14. Pneumococcal vaccine should be given for which of the following conditions?

    a. sickle-cell disease
    b. gestational diabetes
    c. pregnancy-induced hypertension
    d. all pregnancies

46–15. Pregnant women with which condition should be vaccinated against influenza no matter what stage of pregnancy?

    a. allergic rhinitis
    b. hyperthyroidism
    c. insulin-dependent diabetes
    d. all pregnancies

46–16. What are the current Centers for Disease Control and Prevention recommendations for influenza vaccine (not Flumist) in pregnancy?

    a. vaccinate only high-risk women
    b. vaccinate only if epidemic is expected
    c. vaccinate only if a new virus is expected
    d. all should be vaccinated

46–17. What is the treatment of choice for chemoprophylaxis and treatment of influenza in pregnancy?

    a. oseltamivir
    b. amantadine
    c. acyclovir
    d. ganciclovir

46–18. Which of the following may be associated with in utero exposure to influenza A infection at mid-pregnancy?

    a. hallucinations
    b. bipolar disorder
    c. schizophrenia
    d. depression

46–19. Primary infection with varicella leads to pneumonia in what percentage of adults?

    a. 10
    b. 20
    c. 30
    d. 40

46–20. In a seronegative individual who is exposed to active infection, what is the attack rate of varicella?

    a. 30%
    b. 50%
    c. 70%
    d. 90%

46–21. What is a risk factor for varicella pneumonia in pregnancy?

    a. >100 skin lesions
    b. smoking
    c. no prior infection
    d. all of the above

46–22. Which of the following agents lowers the incidence and severity of varicella pneumonia?

    a. amantadine
    b. varicella-zoster immunoglobulin
    c. gamma-globulin
    d. all of the above

46–23. What was the mortality rate of varicella pneumonia during pregnancy reported by the NIH Maternal–Fetal Medicine Units Network?

    a. <1%
    b. 5 to 15%
    c. 25 to 35%
    d. 50 to 60%

46–24. What is the best management for a susceptible pregnant woman within 96 hours of exposure to varicella?

    a. varicella isoimmunization IM
    b. varivax
    c. varicella-zoster immune globulin
    d. expectant management or observation

46–25. Which of the following treatment regimens is effective for *Pneumocystis carinii* pneumonia?

    a. ampicillin
    b. erythromycin
    c. trimethoprim-sulfamethoxazole
    d. azithromycin

46–26. Pregnant women infected with human immunodeficiency virus (HIV) should receive aerosolized pentamidine or oral trimethoprim-sulfamethoxazole to prevent pneumocystic infection in which of the following situations?

a. $CD4^+$ count T-lymphocyte $<200/\mu L$
b. $CD4^+$ count T-lymphocyte $<500/\mu L$
c. $CD4^+$ count T-lymphocyte $<750/\mu L$
d. administer to all HIV-positive women

46–27. In pregnant women with coccidioidomycosis, what finding is associated with a better prognosis?

a. acute infection
b. hypotension
c. erythema nodosum
d. HIV coinfection

46–28. What is the incidence of asthma in the general population?

a. 0.5 to 1.5%
b. 3 to 4%
c. 6 to 8%
d. 10 to 12%

46–29. Airway responsiveness and inflammation in persons with asthma are linked to which of the following chromosomes?

a. 11
b. 5
c. 14
d. all of the above

46–30. What proportion of asthmatics can expect worsening of disease during pregnancy?

a. none
b. one fourth
c. one third
d. one half

46–31. Which of the following pregnancy complications is NOT increased in those with asthma?

a. preterm labor
b. perinatal mortality
c. low-birthweight infants
d. congenital anomalies

46–32. Which of the following findings is associated with the "danger zone" stage of asthma?

a. PO_2 normal; PCO_2 decreased; pH increased
b. PO_2 normal; PCO_2 increased; pH normal
c. PO_2 decreased; PCO_2 normal; pH normal
d. PO_2 decreased; PCO_2 decreased; pH increased

46–33. Which of the FEV_1 (forced expiratory volume in 1 sec) presented, as percentage of predicted values, is associated with respiratory acidosis (stage 4 asthma)?

a. <35
b. 35 to 49

c. 50 to 64
d. 65 to 80

46–34. Which signs most strongly point to a potentially fatal asthmatic attack?

a. use of accessory muscles, labored breathing
b. central cyanosis, labored breathing
c. use of accessory muscles, prolonged expiration
d. central cyanosis, altered consciousness

46–35. Which of the following tests is most useful in monitoring airway obstruction?

a. chest x-ray
b. arterial blood gas
c. FEV_1
d. pulse oximeter

46–36. What is the first-line therapy for mild asthma?

a. antibiotics
b. β-adrenergic agonists
c. methylxanthines
d. cromolyn sodium

46–37. Which of the following agents is used to stabilize mast cell membranes?

a. theophylline
b. cromolyn sulfate
c. corticosteroids
d. epinephrine

46–38. Which of the following analgesics is a nonhistamine-releasing narcotic and therefore should be used for asthmatics?

a. morphine
b. meperidine
c. fentanyl
d. codeine

46–39. Which agent may be used to treat refractory postpartum hemorrhage in women with asthma?

a. prostaglandin E_2
b. prostaglandin $F_{2\alpha}$
c. 15-methyl $PGF_{2\alpha}$
d. none of the above

46–40. Which of the following groups is NOT at particular risk for tuberculosis?

a. pregnant women
b. the elderly
c. urban poor
d. ethnic minorities

46–41. What percentage of tuberculosis is resistant to at least one drug?

a. 3
b. 6
c. 12
d. 18

46-42. How should a pregnant woman who is tuberculin-positive but who has a negative chest radiograph reading be managed?

a. rifampin 10 mg/kg daily for 12 months
b. isoniazid 300 mg daily for 12 months
c. ethambutol 25 mg/kg daily for 12 months
d. observation and treatment after delivery

46-43. How should nonpregnant patients younger than age 35 who are tuberculin-positive but who have negative chest radiographic findings be treated?

a. rifampin for 4 months
b. streptomycin for 12 months
c. isoniazid for 12 months
d. pyridoxine for 12 months

46-44. Which of the following antituberculosis agents is associated with severe congenital deafness if given during pregnancy?

a. streptomycin
b. isoniazid
c. rifampin
d. ethambutol

46-45. Which of the following chest x-ray findings is the hallmark of sarcoidosis?

a. mediastinal widening
b. diffuse infiltrates
c. patchy infiltrates
d. interstitial pneumonitis

46-46. How is symptomatic severe pulmonary sarcoidosis treated?

a. betamethasone 12 mg intramuscularly every day
b. decadron 6 mg orally twice a day

c. prednisone 1 mg/kg/day
d. cyclophosphamide 1 mg/kg/day

46-47. The cystic fibrosis transmembrane conductance receptor regulator (CFTR) is associated with which chromosome?

a. 3p
b. 5q
c. 7q
d. 9p

46-48. Which of the following electrolyte patterns in sweat is associated with cystic fibrosis?

a. ↑ sodium ↓ potassium ↑ chloride
b. ↑ sodium ↑ potassium ↓ chloride
c. ↑ sodium ↓ potassium ↓ chloride
d. ↑ sodium ↑ potassium ↑ chloride

46-49. In patients with cystic fibrosis, colonization with which of the following organisms is associated with a worse prognosis?

a. *Burkholderia cepacia*
b. *Pseudomonas aeruginosa*
c. *Staphylococcus aureus*
d. *Haemophilus influenzae*

46-50. Lung function in women with cystic fibrosis is improved by using which of the following to decrease the viscosity of sputum?

a. recombinant human deoxyribonuclease I
b. acetylcysteine mist
c. bronchodilators
d. diuretics

46-51. Treatment of carbon monoxide poisoning in pregnancy includes which of the following?

a. supportive measures
b. 100% O_2
c. hyperbaric O_2
d. all of the above

47

Thromboembolic Disorders

47–1. What is the estimated incidence of antepartum deep vein thrombosis per 1000 pregnancies?

   a. 0.005
   b. 0.05
   c. 0.5
   d. 5.0

47–2. What is the estimated incidence of pulmonary embolism per 1000 pregnancies?

   a. 1 in 70
   b. 1 in 700
   c. 1 in 7000
   d. 1 in 70,000

47–3. Of the following, which finding is NOT part of Virchow's triad?

   a. infection (local)
   b. trauma (local)
   c. stasis
   d. hypercoagulability

47–4. Which of the following risk factors is associated with an increased likelihood of pulmonary embolism during the puerperium?

   a. cesarean delivery
   b. severe preeclampsia
   c. diabetes
   d. all of the above

47–5. Which thrombophilia is inherited in an autosomal recessive fashion?

   a. factor V Leiden mutation
   b. antithrombin deficiency
   c. protein C deficiency
   d. hyperhomocysteinemia

47–6. Which of the following is the MOST important inhibitor of thrombin in clot formation?

   a. antithrombin
   b. thrombomodulin
   c. protein C
   d. protein S

47–7. In a gravida with protein C deficiency, what is the risk of thromboembolism?

   a. 1%
   b. 10%
   c. 40%
   d. 70%

47–8. The circulating anticoagulant protein S is activated by which of the following?

   a. protein C
   b. protein M
   c. antithrombin
   d. thrombomodulin

47–9. Purpura fulminans is caused by which of the following?

   a. heterozygous protein C deficiency
   b. homozygous protein C deficiency
   c. heterozygous protein S deficiency
   d. combination of protein C and protein S deficiency

47–10. What is the MOST prevalent known thrombophilia?

   a. protein S deficiency
   b. protein C deficiency
   c. factor V Leiden mutation
   d. antithrombin deficiency

47–11. What happens to resistance to activated protein C during pregnancy?

   a. increases after the first trimester
   b. increases after the second trimester
   c. decreases after the first trimester
   d. deceases after the second trimester

47–12. Management of gravidas who are homozygous for the factor V Leiden mutation should include which of the following?

   a. adjusted-dose heparin prophylaxis
   b. full anticoagulation with heparin
   c. low-dose aspirin
   d. full anticoagulation with warfarin

47–13. How is the mutation of 5,10-methylene tetrahydrofolate reductase (MTHFR) that raises homocysteine levels inherited?

a. autosomal recessive
b. autosomal dominant
c. X-linked recessive
d. mitochondrial

47–14. A 28-year-old woman at 6 weeks gestation presents with a history of recurrent pregnancy loss and carries antiphospholipid antibodies. She denies venous or arterial thrombosis. How should she be managed during this pregnancy?

a. careful surveillance
b. low-dose heparin prophylaxis
c. adjusted-dose heparin administration
d. full anticoagulation with heparin

47–15. Phlegmasia alba dolens is clinically suspected in which of the following situations?

a. abrupt onset of leg pain and edema
b. edema of both lower extremities exists
c. red, hot lower extremity is noted
d. none of the above

47–16. What is the procedure of choice to diagnose deep venous thrombosis?

a. impedance plethysmography
b. real-time ultrasonography
c. venography
d. compression ultrasonography plus color Doppler

47–17. Where does thrombosis associated with pulmonary embolism in pregnant women frequently originate?

a. popliteal veins
b. femoral veins
c. iliac veins
d. vena cava

47–18. When is the peak anti-factor Xa activity in a woman taking enoxaparin sodium (Lovenox)?

a. 1 hr prior to dosing
b. 1 hr after dosing
c. 3.5 hr prior to dosing
d. 3.5 hr after dosing

47–19. Low-molecular-weight heparin should not be used in patients with which of the following conditions?

a. mitral valve prolapse
b. ventricle septal defect
c. atrial septal defect
d. prosthetic heart valve

47–20. What is the most serious complication with heparin?

a. hemorrhage
b. thrombosis
c. osteoporosis
d. thrombocytopenia

47–21. A major side effect of heparin is osteoporosis. This is more likely to occur in which of the following situations?

a. less than 20,000 units is given per day for a short time
b. treatment exceeds 7 weeks
c. more than 20,000 units per day are given for 3 months
d. more than 20,000 units per day are given for 6 months

47–22. Which of the following is given to reverse the anticoagulation effects of heparin?

a. protamine sulfate
b. vitamin D
c. vitamin E
d. vitamin K 10 mg intravenously

47–23. What is the treatment for superficial thrombophlebitis?

a. analgesia and coumarin
b. analgesia and rest
c. "mini-dose" heparin
d. full anticoagulation

47–24. A negative ventilation-perfusion scan is associated with pulmonary embolism in what percentage of patients?

a. <1
b. 4
c. 10
d. >15

47–25. In general, for "full" anticoagulation, what should be the total daily dose of heparin?

a. 2000 to 5000 U
b. 10,000 to 12,000 U
c. 15,000 to 20,000 U
d. 25,000 to 40,000 U

47–26. How should a woman with deep venous thrombosis in a previous pregnancy be managed in a current pregnancy?

a. careful observation
b. mini-dose subcutaneous heparin
c. full prophylactic dose subcutaneous heparin
d. low-dose aspirin

48

Renal and Urinary Tract Disorders

48–1. During pregnancy, effective renal plasma flow is increased by what percentage?

    a. 5 to 10
    b. 20 to 30
    c. 40 to 65
    d. 80 to 90

48–2. Which of the following is NOT a change observed in the urinary tract during pregnancy?

    a. dilatation of renal calyces, pelves, and ureters
    b. increased predisposition to infection
    c. increased vesicoureteral reflux
    d. all of the above are observed

48–3. What is the threshold for significant proteinuria during pregnancy?

    a. 50 mg/day
    b. 100 mg/day
    c. 200 mg/day
    d. 300 mg/day

48–4. What is the average daily excretion of albumin during pregnancy?

    a. <50 mg
    b. 100 mg
    c. 200 mg
    d. 500 mg

48–5. Idiopathic hematuria prior to 20 weeks gestation is associated with a twofold increase in the development of which of the following?

    a. chronic renal disease
    b. preterm labor
    c. preeclampsia
    d. pyelonephritis

48–6. Postural (orthostatic) proteinuria is defined as proteinuria in which of the following circumstances?

    a. when ambulatory
    b. secondary to mild renal disease
    c. due to bacteriuria
    d. at night time in a patient with hypertension

48–7. Which of the following enhances the virulence of *Escherichia coli*?

    a. glycoprotein receptors
    b. P-fimbriae
    c. endotoxins
    d. nuclear pili

48–8. What is the prevalence of asymptomatic bacteriuria in pregnancy?

    a. 4%
    b. 2 to 7%
    c. 10 to 12%
    d. 20%

48–9. Which is true of asymptomatic bacteriuria during pregnancy?

    a. It has its highest incidence among affluent Caucasians of low parity.
    b. If not treated, it will develop into an acute symptomatic infection during pregnancy in 25% of women.
    c. It has not been associated with adverse pregnancy outcomes.
    d. It is diagnosed by catheterized specimen containing >100 organisms/mL in asymptomatic women.

48–10. Which of the following is most likely to be associated with covert bacteriuria?

    a. age <20 years
    b. hypertension
    c. sickle-cell trait
    d. lupus

48–11. What is the best time to screen for bacteriuria?

   a. preconceptually
   b. at the first prenatal visit
   c. during the second trimester
   d. at 36 weeks gestation

48–12. Using multivariate analysis, what are the adverse pregnancy outcomes associated with asymptomatic bacteriuria?

   a. low-birthweight infants
   b. preterm delivery
   c. acute antepartum pyelonephritis
   d. all of the above

48–13. What is the most likely diagnosis in a woman with frequency, urgency, pyuria, dysuria, and a sterile urine culture?

   a. *Escherichia coli* cystitis
   b. group B streptococcus cystitis
   c. *Chlamydia trachomatis* urethritis
   d. *Neisseria gonorrhoeae* urethritis

48–14. What is the most common serious medical complication of pregnancy?

   a. thrombophlebitis
   b. pneumonia
   c. pancreatitis
   d. pyelonephritis

48–15. In what percentage of renal infections in pregnancy is *Escherichia coli* isolated from blood or urine?

   a. 10%
   b. 30%
   c. 50%
   d. >70%

48–16. What percentage of women with acute antepartum pyelonephritis have bacteremia?

   a. <1
   b. 5 to 10
   c. 15 to 20
   d. >30

48–17. Which of the following cause alveolar injury, and hence respiratory insufficiency, in women with pyelonephritis?

   a. prostaglandins
   b. cytokines
   c. interferons
   d. endotoxins

48–18. Anemia in women with pyelonephritis is due to which of the following?

   a. hemolysis induced by endotoxin
   b. dilution due to hydration
   c. increased erythropoietin production
   d. cytokine-induced thrombocytopenia

48–19. When can a pregnant woman be discharged home on oral antibiotics following parenteral antibiotic therapy for pyelonephritis?

   a. when she is no longer symptomatic
   b. when she becomes afebrile
   c. when 10 full days of inpatient therapy is complete
   d. when pyuria resolves

48–20. What percentage of renal stones are identified by a plain abdominal radiograph?

   a. 60
   b. 70
   c. 80
   d. 90

48–21. An 18-year-old nulliparous black woman has been on antibiotics for 4 days for pyelonephritis. She continues to have fever ranging from 38.9 to 39.6°C. Work-up reveals a right ureteral obstruction secondary to calculi. What is the next most appropriate step in her management?

   a. change antibiotics
   b. continue present antibiotics
   c. pass a double-J ureteral stent
   d. perform percutaneous nephrostomy

48–22. What is the incidence of bacteriuria in pregnancy after surgical correction of ureteral reflux?

   a. 10%
   b. 30%
   c. 50%
   d. 70%

48–23. What is the composition of the majority of renal stones?

   a. struvite
   b. calcium salts
   c. uric acid
   d. magnesium salts

48–24. What is the most common presenting symptom of renal stones in pregnant women?

   a. flank pain
   b. abdominal discomfort
   c. hematuria
   d. infection

48–25. Which of the following is NOT one of the five major glomerulopathic syndromes?

   a. rapidly progressive glomerulonephritis
   b. chronic pyelonephritis
   c. nephrotic syndrome
   d. acute nephritic syndrome

48–26. Which of the following are signs and symptoms of acute glomerulonephritis?

   a. hematuria, proteinuria, edema, and hypertension
   b. proteinuria and hypertension without edema
   c. hematuria, hypotension, and proteinuria
   d. proteinuria, hypotension, and edema

48–27. Which of the following is NOT a fetal effect of glomerulonephritis?

   a. fetal loss
   b. fetal growth retardation
   c. preterm birth
   d. fetal intraventricular hemorrhage

48–28. What is the incidence of hypertension in pregnancy in women with glomerulonephritis?

   a. 10%
   b. 25%
   c. 50%
   d. 75%

48–29. Which of the following is NOT strongly associated with a poor perinatal prognosis in parturients with glomerulonephritis?

   a. impaired renal function
   b. severe hypertension
   c. anemia
   d. proteinuria >3 g/24 hr

48–30. What are the characteristics of nephrotic syndrome?

   a. proteinuria >3000 mg/d, hyperlipidemia, and edema
   b. proteinuria >3000 mg/d and hypolipidemia
   c. proteinuria >300 mg/d, hyperlipidemia, and edema
   d. proteinuria >300 mg/d and hypolipidemia

48–31. Of the following, which is the most common cause of nephrotic syndrome?

   a. membranous glomerulopathy
   b. minimal change disease
   c. poststreptococcal glomerulonephritis
   d. amyloidosis

48–32. Successful pregnancy outcome can be anticipated despite maternal nephrosis in which of the following circumstances?

   a. The patient is normotensive.
   b. Renal insufficiency is moderate.
   c. Proteinuria is <5 g/d.
   d. Hypertension is controlled with blood pressure medications.

48–33. What is the significance of proteinuria that antedates pregnancy?

   a. benign in most cases
   b. associated with persistent anemia in 25%
   c. chronic hypertension in 70%
   d. preterm delivery in 10%

48–34. What is the mechanism of inheritance in adult polycystic kidney disease?

   a. sporadic
   b. X-linked recessive
   c. autosomal recessive
   d. autosomal dominant

48–35. The majority of cases of polycystic kidney disease are due to which of the following mutations?

   a. PKD_2 gene on chromosome 4
   b. PKD_1 gene on chromosome 16
   c. PKC_2 gene on chromosome 4
   d. PKC_2 gene on chromosome 16

48–36. Which of the following is NOT a symptom of polycystic kidney disease?

   a. flank pain
   b. nocturia
   c. hematuria
   d. malaise

48–37. Which of the following is associated with polycystic kidneys?

   a. hepatic cysts
   b. mitral stenosis
   c. diverticulosis
   d. uterine anomalies

48–38. What is the effect of normotensive maternal polycystic kidney disease on perinatal outcome when compared with normal control pregnancies?

   a. increased spontaneous abortions
   b. increased stillbirths
   c. increased neonatal liver failure
   d. no adverse effects

48–39. What is the most common cause of end-stage renal disease?

   a. diabetes
   b. hypertension
   c. glomerulonephritis
   d. polycystic kidney disease

48–40. What is the average blood volume expansion in pregnant women with mild renal insufficiency?

   a. 10%
   b. 30%
   c. 50%
   d. 70%

48–41. What is the average blood volume expansion in pregnant women with severe renal insufficiency?

   a. 10%
   b. 25%
   c. 35%
   d. 45%

48–42. Which of the following pregnancy complications is most common in women with chronic renal insufficiency?

   a. anemia
   b. fetal growth restriction
   c. preeclampsia
   d. preterm delivery

48–43. Which of the following is a major side effect from recombinant erythropoietin use in pregnancy?

   a. hyperviscosity
   b. hypertension
   c. human immunodeficiency viral transmission
   d. worsening renal function

48–44. What is the effect of pregnancy on the natural history of renal insufficiency (in the absence of superimposed preeclampsia or severe obstetrical hemorrhage)?

   a. accelerated renal insufficiency
   b. complete resolution of renal insufficiency
   c. partial improvement of renal insufficiency
   d. no appreciable effect on progression

48–45. Which of the following is NOT included in the differential diagnosis of renal transplant rejection during pregnancy?

   a. pyelonephritis
   b. preeclampsia
   c. respiratory distress syndrome
   d. recurrent glomerulonephropathy

48–46. Which of the following is most helpful in making the diagnosis of renal transplant rejection during pregnancy?

   a. renal biopsy
   b. clinical symptoms
   c. urinalysis
   d. renal vein laboratory studies

48–47. What is the most common cause of acute renal failure in pregnancy?

   a. drug abuse
   b. systemic lupus erythematosus
   c. preeclampsia or eclampsia
   d. sickle-cell disease

49

Gastrointestinal Disorders

49–1. During endoscopic retrograde cholangiopancreatography (ERCP), what ampulla is cannulated?

   a. Morgagni
   b. Bochdalek
   c. ovale
   d. Vater

49–2. What is the incidence of exploratory laparoscopy or laparotomy during pregnancy?

   a. 1 in 240
   b. 1 in 500
   c. 1 in 1000
   d. 1 in 5000

49–3. What is the incidence of non-obstetrical surgery in pregnancy?

a. 1 in 200
b. 1 in 400
c. 1 in 800
d. 1 in 1600

49–4. Long-term follow-up studies in infants born to mothers who underwent a laparoscopic procedure during pregnancy found an increased incidence of which of the following?

a. mental retardation
b. cerebral palsy
c. growth retardation
d. none of the above (no deleterious effects)

49–5. Why does total parenteral nutrition require catheterization of the jugular or subclavian vein?

a. Thromboembolism occurs if given in a smaller vein.
b. The solution is hyperosmolar and needs to be diluted in a high-flow system.
c. Essential fatty acids block smaller veins.
d. The potassium content causes sclerosis of the smaller veins.

49–6. What is the most common complication associated with peripherally inserted central catheters for hyperalimentation?

a. osmotic diuresis
b. thrombosis
c. electrolyte imbalance
d. infection

49–7. Which of the following findings would be expected in women with hyperemesis gravidarum?

a. hematocrit <30 vol%
b. creatinine 0.3 mg/dL
c. ALT 86 IU/L
d. K^+ 5.8 mEq/L

49–8. Which of the following complications in pregnancy are increased in women with a female fetus?

a. cholelithiasis
b. hepatitis
c. reflux esophagitis
d. hyperemesis gravidarum

49–9. Which of the following vitamin deficiencies is associated with hyperemesis?

a. vitamin A
b. vitamin B
c. vitamin C
d. vitamin K

49–10. What is the etiology of reflux esophagitis in pregnancy?

a. constriction of upper esophageal sphincter
b. relaxation of upper esophageal sphincter
c. constriction of lower esophageal sphincter
d. relaxation of lower esophageal sphincter

49–11. Diaphragmatic hernias are herniations of abdominal contents through which foramen?

a. Morgagni
b. ovale
c. magnum
d. Bochlek

49–12. Which of the following is a motor disorder of esophageal smooth muscle?

a. diaphragmatic hernia
b. hiatal hernia
c. reflux esophagitis
d. achalasia

49–13. Which of the following treatments is NOT indicated in the management of achalasia?

a. soft foods
b. hyperalimentation
c. anticholinergic drugs
d. pneumatic dilatation

49–14. What organism is associated with peptic ulcer disease?

a. *Helicobacter stomachi*
b. *Helicobacter pylori*
c. *Helicobacter acidi*
d. *Helicobacter gastrecti*

49–15. Which of the following is associated with normal pregnancy?

a. decreased mucus secretion
b. increased gastric secretion
c. decreased gastric motility
d. constriction of lower esophageal sphincter

49–16. The majority of pregnancies with upper gastrointestinal bleeding have which of the following?

a. Boerhaave syndrome
b. stomach cancer
c. Mallory-Weiss tears
d. peptic ulceration

49–17. Which of the following is a dangerous complication associated with ulcerative colitis?

a. toxic megacolon
b. bloody diarrhea
c. arthritis
d. erythema nodosum

49–18. Which of the following surgical procedures is protective against the development of ulcerative colitis?

    a. tonsillectomy
    b. adenectomy
    c. appendectomy
    d. cholecystectomy

49–19. Which of the following HLA haplotypes is associated with ulcerative colitis?

    a. HLA-Bw35
    b. HLA-A2
    c. HLA-B3
    d. HLA-A16

49–20. What is the cardinal presenting finding in ulcerative colitis?

    a. lower abdominal pain
    b. bloody diarrhea
    c. intractable nausea
    d. projectile vomiting

49–21. Which active metabolite of sulfasalazine inhibits prostaglandin synthase?

    a. sulfazine-a
    b. sulfazine-b
    c. 2-aminosalicylic acid
    d. 5-aminosalicylic acid

49–22. Which of the following is NOT a manifestation of Crohn disease?

    a. genetic predisposition and association with certain HLA alleles
    b. disease confined to superficial layers of the colon
    c. disease involving bowel mucosa and deeper layers
    d. small and large bowel involvement

49–23. What is the most likely course for ulcerative colitis that is quiescent at the beginning of gestation?

    a. minimal activation of disease during pregnancy
    b. active disease during pregnancy in 33%

    c. active disease during pregnancy in 67%
    d. active disease during pregnancy in nearly 100%

49–24. What is a common long-term complication in a woman who has had a colectomy with mucosal proctectomy and ileal pouch-anal anastomosis?

    a. pouchitis
    b. large bowel obstruction
    c. proctitis
    d. fistula formation

49–25. What is the most common cause of bowel obstruction in pregnancy?

    a. infection
    b. adhesions
    c. cancer
    d. mechanical compression from the uterus

49–26. What is the most common symptom associated with bowel obstruction?

    a. nausea
    b. vomiting
    c. abdominal pain
    d. diarrhea

49–27. What is the cause of pseudo-obstruction of the colon (Ogilvie syndrome)?

    a. pelvic adhesions
    b. impacted stool
    c. adynamic colonic ileus
    d. medications used postpartum

49–28. Which of the following is NOT in the differential diagnosis of appendicitis in pregnancy?

    a. Crohn disease
    b. placental abruption
    c. pyelonephritis
    d. pneumonia

49–29. Which of the following complications is associated with ruptured appendix and peritonitis?

    a. fetal growth restriction
    b. oligohydramnios
    c. chorioamnionitis
    d. preterm birth

50

Hepatic, Biliary Tract, and Pancreatic Disorders

50–1. Pregnancy-induced liver disorders that resolve spontaneously following delivery include all of the following EXCEPT

    a. acute viral hepatitis
    b. intrahepatic cholestasis
    c. acute fatty liver
    d. severe preeclampsia

50–2. Which of the following findings would be expected in women with hyperemesis gravidarum?

    a. hematocrit <30 vol%
    b. creatinine 0.7 mg/dL
    c. ALT 86 IU/L
    d. K^+ 5.8 mEq/L

50–3. Which of the following gene mutations is associated with progressive familial intrahepatic cholestasis?

    a. LAP 1
    b. CBS 2
    c. Cox 9
    d. MDR 3 (multidrug resistance 3)

50–4. What is the suspected pathogenesis of intrahepatic cholestasis, as compared with controls?

    a. decreased human placental lactogen
    b. decreased human chorionic gonadotropin
    c. decreased progesterone
    d. unknown

50–5. What is the major histological lesion of intrahepatic cholestasis?

    a. centrilobular bile staining
    b. mesenchymal proliferation
    c. periportal necrosis
    d. centrilobular necrosis

50–6. Which of the following is appropriate in the management of intrahepatic cholestasis?

    a. azathioprine
    b. antihistamines
    c. ampicillin
    d. vitamin A

50–7. Which of the following is NOT an adverse pregnancy outcome associated with intrahepatic cholestasis?

    a. abruptio placenta
    b. preterm birth
    c. stillbirth
    d. meconium-stained amnionic fluid

50–8. What is the prominent histologic abnormality associated with acute fatty liver of pregnancy?

    a. intranuclear fat
    b. microvesicular fat
    c. massive hepatocellular necrosis
    d. all of the above

50–9. What is the etiology of acute fatty liver of pregnancy?

    a. autosomal recessive
    b. mitochondrial inheritance
    c. X-linked recessive
    d. polygenic

50–10. What is the major symptom in pregnancy complicated by acute fatty liver?

    a. malaise
    b. anorexia
    c. epigastric pain
    d. vomiting

50–11. Which of the following laboratory abnormalities would support a diagnosis of acute fatty liver?

	Fibrinogen	Platelets	Creatinine	AST
a.	140	100	1.4	1000
b.	400	190	1.4	100
c.	140	190	0.8	100
d.	400	100	0.8	1000

50–12. What is the etiology of diabetes insipidus in pregnancies complicated by acute fatty liver?

   a. excessive levels of oxytocin
   b. elevated vasopressinase concentrations
   c. fatty deposits in supraoptic nuclei
   d. decreased blood flow to posterior pituitary

50–13. Which of the following is due to a deoxyribonucleic acid virus?

   a. hepatitis A
   b. hepatitis B
   c. hepatitis C
   d. delta hepatitis

50–14. What is the most common complication of hepatitis B and C?

   a. intrahepatic cholestasis
   b. chronic hepatitis
   c. preeclampsia
   d. acute fatty liver

50–15. What is the incubation period for hepatitis A?

   a. 4 days
   b. 4 weeks
   c. 10 to 12 weeks
   d. >20 weeks

50–16. Which of the following hepatitis panels is associated with acute hepatitis A and chronic hepatitis B?

	HBsAg	IgM Anti-HAV	IgM Anti-HBc
a.	−	+	−
b.	+	+	+
c.	+	+	−
d.	+	−	+

50–17. Which of the following is recommended for a pregnant woman exposed to hepatitis A?

   a. immune globulin
   b. hepatitis A vaccine
   c. hepatitis B immunoglobulin (HBIG)
   d. HBIG plus gamma-globulin

50–18. What is the frequency of chronic hepatitis B following acute disease?

   a. <1%
   b. 5 to 10%
   c. 20 to 25%
   d. 40 to 50%

50–19. What percentage of hepatitis B-infected infants develop chronic infection?

   a. <1
   b. 15
   c. 35
   d. 85

50–20. What is the first virological marker for hepatitis B?

   a. HBeAg
   b. HBcAg
   c. HBsAg
   d. HB dane Ag

50–21. What is the significance of the e antigen of hepatitis B virus?

   a. indicates viral shedding in the feces
   b. associated with infectivity
   c. reflects number of circulating virus particles
   d. indicates chronic infection

50–22. How should infants delivered to chronic hepatitis B carriers be treated?

   a. isolated from their mothers
   b. treated with HBIG
   c. vaccinated with recombinant vaccine
   d. given HBIG and recombinant vaccine

50–23. When is the antibody first detected in the majority of patients with hepatitis C?

   a. at 3 weeks
   b. at 9 weeks
   c. at 15 weeks
   d. at 1 year

50–24. What is the incidence of persistent hepatitis C infection that progresses to cirrhosis within 20 years?

   a. 1 to 5%
   b. 10 to 15%
   c. 20 to 30%
   d. 50 to 60%

50–25. Which of the following adverse pregnancy outcomes is associated with hepatitis C?

   a. preterm birth
   b. abruptio placentae
   c. vertical transmission of hepatitis C
   d. fetal growth restriction

50–26. Which of the following agents may be effective or beneficial in producing remission in one half of chronic hepatitis B carriers?

    a. corticosteroids
    b. azathioprine
    c. interferon-α
    d. interleukin-2

50–27. Which of the hepatitis viruses are waterborne?

    a. A
    b. B
    c. C
    d. E

50–28. Which of the following is NOT a coexisting condition for fatty liver hepatitis?

    a. alcohol
    b. obesity
    c. type II diabetes
    d. hyperlipidemia

50–29. What is the most common cause of cirrhosis in young women?

    a. alcohol
    b. hepatitis
    c. illicit drug use
    d. prescribed drugs

50–30. What is the normal portal vein pressure?

    a. <5 mm Hg
    b. 10 to 15 mm Hg
    c. 30 to 40 mm Hg
    d. 60 to 80 mm Hg

50–31. What is the portal vein pressure associated with esophageal varices?

    a. >10 mm Hg
    b. >20 mm Hg
    c. >30 mm Hg
    d. >40 mm Hg

50–32. Which agent has been shown to substantially lower the likelihood of recurrence of bleeding from esophageal varices after treatment of an acute episode?

    a. β-blockers
    b. calcium channel blockers
    c. antihistamines
    d. proton pump inhibitors

50–33. What is the treatment of choice for acetaminophen overdosage?

    a. N-acetylcysteine
    b. glutathione
    c. induce emesis with charcoal
    d. aggressive fluids containing sodium bicarbonate

50–34. What is the most common pregnancy complication in women with liver transplants?

    a. anemia
    b. hypertension
    c. preterm delivery
    d. psychosis

50–35. What is the major component of gallstones?

    a. cholesterol
    b. calcium
    c. bile acids
    d. struvite

50–36. Which of the following is relatively contraindicated in pregnancy for the management of gallstones?

    a. laparoscopic cholecystectomy
    b. endoscopic retrograde cholangiopancreatography
    c. laparotomy at 12 weeks gestation
    d. none of the above

50–37. Which of the following is NOT a cause of pancreatitis in pregnancy?

    a. trauma
    b. hypotriglyceridemia
    c. alcoholism
    d. gallstones

50–38. Which of the following predispose to pancreatitis?

    a. acute fatty liver
    b. familial hypertriglyceridemia
    c. mutation of cystic fibrosis transmembrane conductance regulator gene
    d. all of the above

50–39. Which of the following portends a poor prognosis in women with pancreatitis?

    a. twin gestation
    b. hypercalcemia
    c. shock
    d. hypervolemia

50–40. Which laboratory finding confirms the diagnosis of pancreatitis?

    a. leukocytosis
    b. serum amylase three times normal
    c. low serum lipase
    d. hypocalcemia

Hematological Disorders

51–1. How does the Centers for Disease Control and Prevention define anemia in terms of hemoglobin concentration during the third trimester of pregnancy?

  a. <9 g/dL
  b. <10 g/dL
  c. <11 g/dL
  d. <12 g/dL

51–2. Which of the following may increase in pregnancies complicated by anemia in the second trimester?

  a. pregnancy-induced hypertension
  b. gestational diabetes
  c. preterm birth
  d. urinary tract infection

51–3. What are the most common causes of anemia during pregnancy?

  a. iron deficiency; acute blood loss
  b. iron deficiency; sickle-cell disease
  c. folate deficiency; acute blood loss
  d. folate deficiency; sickle-cell disease

51–4. What are the total iron requirements for the mother and fetus during a normal pregnancy?

  a. 100 mg
  b. 300 mg
  c. 1000 mg
  d. 3000 mg

51–5. What are the classical morphological features of iron-deficiency anemia?

  a. hyperchromia, macrocytosis
  b. hypochromia, microcytosis
  c. macrocytosis, teardrop cells
  d. spherocytosis, red cell fragments

51–6. Which of the following has the most influence on iron stores in the newborn?

  a. maternal iron status
  b. timing of cord clamping

  c. maternal vitamin C intake
  d. blood loss at time of delivery

51–7. Which of the following excludes iron deficiency as a cause of anemia?

  a. elevated serum iron-binding capacity
  b. normal serum ferritin
  c. bone marrow normoblastic hyperplasia
  d. positive sickle-cell preparation

51–8. How much elemental iron per day is needed for the treatment of iron-deficiency anemia during pregnancy?

  a. 50 mg
  b. 100 mg
  c. 200 mg
  d. 400 mg

51–9. Which of the following is NOT associated with anemia?

  a. inflammatory bowel disease
  b. chronic renal disease
  c. essential hypertension
  d. systemic lupus erythematosus

51–10. In women with chronic renal disease, which of the following characterizes the degree of red cell mass expansion during pregnancy?

  a. same as women with normal renal function
  b. increased compared with normal pregnancy
  c. decreased by the corresponding degree of renal impairment compared with normal pregnancy
  d. does not occur because of low levels of ferritin

51–11. What is the cause of anemia in women with acute antepartum pyelonephritis?

  a. decreased erythropoietin production
  b. increased red cell destruction due to endotoxemia
  c. dilution secondary to intravenous hydration
  d. decreased iron stores

51–12. What is a worrisome side effect of recombinant erythropoietin to treat chronic anemia?

    a. hypertension
    b. expanded red cell mass
    c. placenta previa
    d. allergic reaction

51–13. What is the earliest morphological evidence of folic acid deficiency?

    a. hypersegmentation of neutrophils
    b. microcytosis
    c. crenated erythrocytes
    d. nucleated red blood cells

51–14. What is the treatment for pregnancy-induced megaloblastic anemia?

    a. nutritious diet only
    b. 1000 μg vitamin B_{12} every month
    c. 200 mg/day iron (supplemental)
    d. folic acid 1 mg/day, nutritious diet, and iron

51–15. In which of the following circumstances is folic acid 4 mg/day indicated?

    a. multifetal pregnancy
    b. Crohn disease
    c. iron-deficiency anemia
    d. previous infant with neural-tube defect

51–16. Serum vitamin B_{12} levels are decreased in pregnancy secondary to which of the following?

    a. increased fibrinogen
    b. decreased fibrinogen
    c. increased transcobalamins
    d. decreased transcobalamins

51–17. What is the treatment for pregnant women who have undergone a total gastrectomy?

    a. 1 μg vitamin B_{12} daily
    b. 1000 μg vitamin B_{12} monthly
    c. 1 mg folic acid daily
    d. 4 mg folic acid daily

51–18. What is the most common cause of autoimmune hemolytic anemia?

    a. drug-induced cold autoantibodies
    b. chronic inflammatory disease
    c. warm, active autoantibodies
    d. connective tissue disease

51–19. Which of the following may induce cold-agglutinin disease?

    a. *Chlamydia trachomatis*
    b. *Neisseria gonorrhoeae*

    c. *Streptococcus agalactiae*
    d. *Mycoplasma pneumoniae*

51–20. What is effective therapy for autoimmune hemolytic anemia?

    a. corticosteroids (e.g., prednisone 1 mg/kg/day)
    b. supplemental iron 200 mg/day
    c. folate 1 mg/day
    d. corticosteroids plus vitamin B_{12}

51–21. Which of the following drugs may induce antierythrocyte antibodies?

    a. ibuprofen
    b. erythromycin
    c. rifampin
    d. acetaminophen

51–22. Which of the following is a hemopoietic stem-cell disorder characterized by formation of defective platelets, granulocytes, and erythrocytes?

    a. pregnancy-induced hemolytic anemia
    b. paroxysmal nocturnal hemoglobinuria
    c. autoimmune hemolytic anemia
    d. Diamond-Blackfan syndrome

51–23. Which of the following is the mutated gene responsible for paroxysmal nocturnal hemoglobinuria?

    a. PNH-1
    b. PIG-A
    c. URE-3
    d. XPN-F

51–24. What is the treatment for paroxysmal nocturnal hemoglobinuria?

    a. iron
    b. corticosteroids
    c. heparin
    d. bone marrow transplantation

51–25. How are most cases of spherocytosis inherited?

    a. autosomal recessive
    b. autosomal dominant
    c. X-linked recessive
    d. X-linked dominant

51–26. Autosomal recessive spherocytosis can be caused by a deficiency of which of the following?

    a. spectrin
    b. protein S
    c. ankyrin
    d. protein C

51–27. Which of the following treatments reduces hemolysis, anemia, and jaundice in women with hereditary spherocytosis?

    a. corticosteroids
    b. folic acid supplementation
    c. bone marrow transplantation
    d. splenectomy

51–28. How is glucose-6-phosphate dehydrogenase deficiency inherited?

    a. autosomal recessive
    b. autosomal dominant
    c. X-linked recessive
    d. X-linked dominant

51–29. What is the most common cause of aplastic anemia?

    a. drug-induced
    b. infection
    c. immunological disorder
    d. idiopathic

51–30. What is the major risk to a pregnant woman with aplastic anemia?

    a. hemorrhage and infection
    b. preterm labor and fetal growth restriction
    c. pregnancy-induced hypertension and fetal growth restriction
    d. anemia and infection

51–31. Hemoglobin S is caused by a substitution of which of the following?

    a. valine for glutamic acid at position 6
    b. glutamic acid for valine at position 6
    c. lysine for glutamic acid at position 6
    d. glutamic acid for leucine at position 6

51–32. What is the theoretical incidence of sickle-cell anemia among blacks?

    a. 1 in 12
    b. 1 in 144
    c. 1 in 576
    d. 1 in 2000

51–33. Which of the following is NOT associated with hemoglobin SC disease in pregnancy?

    a. severe bone pain
    b. pulmonary infarction
    c. placental abruption
    d. adult chest syndrome

51–34. Approximately how many blacks have the gene for hemoglobin C?

    a. 1 in 12
    b. 1 in 40
    c. 1 in 100
    d. 1 in 200

51–35. What is the approximate perinatal mortality in pregnancies complicated by sickle-cell anemia and hemoglobin SC disease?

    a. 10 in 1000
    b. 50 in 1000
    c. 75 in 1000
    d. 100 in 1000

51–36. Which of the following is NOT considered effective in the management of pain from intravascular sickling?

    a. intravenous hydration
    b. morphine
    c. prophylactic red cell transfusions
    d. therapeutic red cell transfusions

51–37. Prophylactic red cell transfusions in pregnant women with sickle-cell anemia is most likely to decrease which of the following?

    a. perinatal mortality
    b. maternal morbidity
    c. fetal growth retardation
    d. preterm delivery

51–38. In patients with sickle-cell disease, what is the incidence of isoimmunization per unit of blood transfused?

    a. 1%
    b. 3%
    c. 10%
    d. 30%

51–39. Which of the following is increased in pregnancies complicated by sickle-cell trait?

    a. perinatal mortality
    b. abortion (spontaneous)
    c. low birthweight
    d. urinary tract infection

51–40. Hemoglobin C results from substitution of glutamic acid by what amino acid at position 6 of the β-chain?

    a. valine
    b. leucine
    c. lysine
    d. phenylalanine

51–41. Which of the following adverse pregnancy outcomes is increased in women with hemoglobin C trait?

  a. preterm deliveries
  b. fetal growth retardation
  c. perinatal mortality
  d. none of the above

51–42. Which of the following peripheral blood smears would be expected in a patient with hemoglobin E?

  a. hypochromia; microcytosis; erythrocyte targeting
  b. hypochromia; macrocytosis; erythrocyte targeting
  c. hypochromia; microcytosis; hypersegmented neutrophils
  d. hypochromia; macrocytosis; hypersegmented neutrophils

51–43. Which chromosome contains the gene for α-globin chain synthesis?

  a. 6
  b. 11
  c. 16
  d. 21

51–44. Which of the following patterns characterizes hemoglobin Bart?

  a. $- -, a\,a$
  b. $-a, - a$
  c. β4
  d. γ4

51–45. Which of the following ethnic groups is most likely to have hemoglobin Bart?

  a. whites of Mediterranean descent
  b. Asians
  c. Africans
  d. Greeks

51–46. Which of the following characterizes β-thalassemias?

  a. impaired production of β-globin chains
  b. increased destruction of erythrocytes containing hemoglobin F
  c. increased production of α-globin chains
  d. decreased production of hemoglobin F

51–47. A fetus with hemoglobin Bart can be identified at 12 to 13 weeks by which of the following sonographic methods?

  a. abdominal circumference (AC)
  b. AC/BPD ratio

  c. cardiothoracic ratio
  d. AC/femur length ratio

51–48. Which chromosome contains the gene for β-globin chain synthesis?

  a. 6
  b. 11
  c. 16
  d. 21

51–49. Which of the following is elevated with β-thalassemias?

  a. hemoglobin A
  b. hemoglobin A_2
  c. hemoglobin F
  d. hemoglobin H

51–50. Which of the following characterizes β-thalassemia?

  a. increased β-chain production; decreased α-chain production
  b. increased β-chain production; increased α-chain production
  c. decreased β-chain production; decreased α-chain production
  d. decreased β-chain production; increased α-chain production

51–51. Which of the following helps to differentiate polycythemia vera (PCV) from secondary polycythemia?

  a. low values of erythropoietin in PCV
  b. low values of erythropoietin in secondary polycythemia
  c. peripheral smear with nucleated red cells
  d. peripheral smear with hypersegmented neutrophils in PCV

51–52. Which of the following causes of thrombocytopenia result from a lack of platelet membrane glycoprotein?

  a. May-Hegglin anomaly
  b. Bernand-Soulier syndrome
  c. hemolytic uremic syndrome
  d. drug-induced thrombocytopenia

51–53. What is the mechanism of action of corticosteroids in the therapy of immunological thrombocytopenia purpura?

  a. suppress phagocytic activity in the spleen
  b. increase platelet membrane stability
  c. cause short-term reticuloendothelial blockade and diminish platelet sequestration
  d. increase platelet production

51–54. What is the fetal or neonatal risk of maternal immune thrombocytopenia purpura?

   a. increased abortion rate
   b. thrombocytopenia
   c. necrotizing enterocolitis
   d. no risk

51–55. Which of the following findings in women with immune thrombocytopenia purpura correlate closely with fetal platelet counts?

   a. maternal platelet count
   b. circulating antiplatelet antibodies
   c. indirect platelet antiglobulin
   d. no correlation with maternal status

51–56. What is the risk of severe neonatal thrombocytopenia in women with chronic immunological thrombocytopenia?

   a. 3%
   b. 7%
   c. 13%
   d. 25%

51–57. The platelet count in women with essential thrombocytosis is greater than which of the following?

   a. 200,000
   b. 400,000
   c. 800,000
   d. 1,000,000

51–58. Which of the following is used to treat thrombocytosis complicating pregnancy?

   a. hydroxyurea
   b. coumadin
   c. heparin
   d. γ-interferon

51–59. Which of the following is NOT part of the pentad of thrombotic thrombocytopenic purpura?

   a. fever
   b. neurological abnormalities
   c. hemolytic anemia
   d. liver abnormalities

51–60. What is the pathogenesis of thrombotic microangiopathies?

   a. unknown
   b. microthrombi of hyaline material and platelets producing fluctuating ischemia
   c. microthrombi (multiple) of erythrocyte clumps causing multiple infarctions
   d. intravascular neutrophil aggregation stimulating cytokine production leading to end-organ failure

51–61. What is the most common presenting symptom in women with thrombotic thrombocytopenic syndrome?

   a. fever
   b. fatigue
   c. hemorrhage
   d. neurological abnormalities

51–62. What is the most common laboratory finding in women with thrombotic thrombocytopenic syndrome?

   a. mild anemia
   b. erythrocyte fragmentation
   c. decreased leukocytes
   d. fibrin-split products

51–63. What is the treatment for thrombotic thrombocytopenic syndromes?

   a. heparin
   b. aspirin and dipyridamole
   c. glucocorticoids
   d. exchange transfusion with donor plasma and plasmapheresis

51–64. Moderate hemophilia is defined as plasma factor levels of which percentage?

   a. <0.1
   b. <1
   c. 2 to 5
   d. 6 to 30

51–65. Which factor is deficient in individuals with hemophilia A?

   a. von Willebrand factor
   b. antithrombin III
   c. factor VIII:C
   d. factor IX

51–66. Which of the following stimulates factor VIII:C release?

   a. prednisone
   b. γ-globulin
   c. desmopressin
   d. plasmapheresis

51–67. What is the most commonly inherited bleeding disorder?

   a. von Willebrand disease
   b. antithrombin III deficiency
   c. factor VIII:C deficiency
   d. factor IX deficiency

51–68. What is the site of synthesis of von Willebrand factor?

    a. liver
    b. endothelium and megakaryocytes
    c. megakaryocytes only
    d. kidney

51–69. Control of the synthesis of von Willebrand factor is on autosomal genes on which chromosome?

    a. 3
    b. 6
    c. 9
    d. 12

51–70. On which chromosome is the gene that codes for factor VII?

    a. 6
    b. 11
    c. 13
    d. 21

51–71. You are called to evaluate a 23 y/o G1P1, one day postpartum, because the lab called a panic value of hemoglobin 7.2 mg/dL. The patient is feeling well, has no chest pain or dizziness, is not complaining of vaginal bleeding, and has been to the nursery by herself to see her baby. Her antepartum hematocrit was 34%. Her vital signs are normal. Your best plan of management includes which of the following?

    a. blood transfusion with packed RBCs
    b. blood transfusion with whole blood
    c. iron therapy for 1 month
    d. iron therapy for 3 months

51–72. A 17 y/o G2 P0 African American presents for prenatal care at 19 weeks. She gives no past history of any medical complications. Sickle prep is positive, and electrophoresis confirms sickle cell–hemoglobin C disease. Your counseling is likely to include all of the following EXCEPT:

    a. the need for supplemental folic acid
    b. genetic counseling and testing for the father of the baby
    c. her risk of perinatal mortality being greater than that of sickle-cell (SS) disease
    d. the risk of maternal mortality being about 2%

51–73. The thrombophilia most commonly diagnosed in patients presenting with deep vein thrombosis, pulmonary embolism, early-onset preeclampsia, and placental infarction/abruption is which of the following?

    a. antithrombin III deficiency
    b. protein S deficiency
    c. protein C deficiency
    d. resistance to activated protein C

52

Diabetes

52–1. What is the likely etiology of insulin resistance in childhood?

    a. maternal hyperglycemia
    b. fetal hypoinsulinemia
    c. decreased fetal fat cells
    d. maternal ketonuria

52–2. Which of the following is the pathophysiology of type 2 diabetes?

    a. absence of the islet cells
    b. destruction of the islet cells
    c. insulin resistance in target tissues
    d. develops ketoacidosis if untreated

52–3. Which of the following is the most common medical complication in pregnancy?

    a. hypertension
    b. diabetes
    c. deep venous thrombosis
    d. asthma

52–4. What is the overall percentage of pregnancies complicated by diabetes?

    a. <1
    b. 3 to 4
    c. 6 to 8
    d. >10

52–5. How is overt diabetes diagnosed during pregnancy?

    a. random plasma glucose >200 mg/dL
    b. polydipsia, polyuria, unexplained weight loss with glucose >200 mg/dL
    c. fasting glucose >125 mg/dL
    d. all of the above

52–6. What is the most common etiology of glycosuria in pregnancy?

    a. false positive from lactose
    b. gestational diabetes
    c. augmented glomerular filtration of glucose
    d. insulin resistance

52–7. Which of the following is NOT a risk factor for gestational diabetes?

    a. age <25 years
    b. prior macrosomic infant
    c. prior stillborn infant
    d. sister with diabetes

52–8. Screening for diabetes is recommended for all EXCEPT which of the following?

    a. age >30 years
    b. obesity
    c. Hispanic ethnicity
    d. prior postterm pregnancy

52–9. What lower-limit level for the 50-g glucose screen would improve its sensitivity to >90% for detection of gestational diabetes?

    a. 130 mg/dL
    b. 135 mg/dL
    c. 140 mg/dL
    d. 145 mg/dL

52–10. How is gestational diabetes diagnosed?

    a. 1-hr value after a 50-g glucose load exceeds 140 mg/dL

    b. elevated fasting value after a 100-g glucose load
    c. elevated 1-hr value after a 100-g glucose load
    d. two abnormal values after a 100-g glucose load

52–11. Which sequence correctly identifies the plasma glucose threshold values for the 100-g oral glucose tolerance test according to the 2001 ACOG criteria for the diagnosis of gestational diabetes?

    a. Fasting: 95; 1 hr: 190; 2 hr: 155; 3 hr: 140
    b. Fasting: 105; 1 hr: 180; 2 hr: 155; 3 hr: 145
    c. Fasting: 95; 1 hr: 190; 2 hr: 165; 3 hr: 140
    d. Fasting: 95; 1 hr: 180; 2 hr: 155; 3 hr: 140

52–12. What percentage of women with gestational diabetes will later develop overt diabetes?

    a. none
    b. 10
    c. 25
    d. 50

52–13. Which class of gestational diabetics is NOT at increased risk for unexplained stillbirth?

    a. A_1
    b. A_2
    c. B
    d. C

52–14. How is macrosomia defined?

    a. >3750 g
    b. >4000 g
    c. >4250 g
    d. >4500 g

52–15. In diabetes, which fetal organ is unaffected by fetal macrosomia?

    a. heart
    b. kidney
    c. liver
    d. brain

52–16. Which of the following factors is increased in large-for-gestational age infants?

    a. insulin-like growth factor I and II
    b. leptin
    c. C peptide insulin
    d. all of the above

52–17. What is the daily caloric recommendation for a nonobese woman with gestational diabetes?

    a. 20 kcal/kg
    b. 30 kcal/kg
    c. 40 kcal/kg
    d. 50 kcal/kg

52–18. What are the benefits of postprandial glucose surveillance?

    a. better glucose control
    b. less neonatal hypoglycemia
    c. less macrosomia
    d. all of the above

52–19. In the study by Philipson (1989), what was the recurrence rate for gestational diabetes in subsequent pregnancies?

    a. 33%
    b. 50%
    c. 67%
    d. 90%

52–20. Using White's classification for diabetes in pregnancy (1978), related which of the following is characteristic of class C?

    a. retinopathy
    b. age of onset before 10
    c. age of onset over 20
    d. age of onset 10 to 20

52–21. What is the prevalence of preeclampsia or eclampsia in type 1 diabetic pregnancies as compared with normal pregnancies?

    a. not increased
    b. increased twofold
    c. increased threefold
    d. increased fourfold

52–22. Which factor increases a diabetic's risk for spontaneous abortion?

    a. $HgA_1C = 6.3\%$
    b. poor general glycemic control
    c. preprandial glucose 115 mg/dL
    d. postprandial glucose 125 mg/dL

52–23. With overt diabetes, what fetal malformation is most strongly associated with diabetes?

    a. congenital heart defects
    b. neural-tube defects
    c. caudal regression
    d. renal agenesis

52–24. In general, what is true of "unexplained" fetal demise in overt diabetics?

    a. usually occurs before 30 weeks gestation
    b. fetus usually small for gestational age
    c. oligohydramnios is usually present
    d. suspected due to chronic metabolic aberrations

52–25. For which diabetic complication may pregnancy have a detrimental effect?

    a. proliferative retinopathy
    b. nephropathy
    c. hypertension
    d. neuropathy

52–26. What is the incidence of ketoacidosis in diabetic pregnancies?

    a. <0.5%
    b. 1.0%
    c. 3.0%
    d. 5.0%

52–27. The incidence of antepartum pyelonephritis in pregnancy is increased to what degree with overt diabetics (Cousins, 1987)?

    a. no change
    b. twofold
    c. fourfold
    d. eightfold

52–28. Which of the following is true concerning preconceptional glycemic control in overtly diabetic women?

    a. may reduce congenital anomalies
    b. may reduce spontaneous abortions
    c. does not reduce the congenital anomaly rate to that of those who do not have diabetes
    d. all of the above

52–29. What is the most attractive method of contraception for overtly diabetic patients who do not desire future pregnancy?

    a. abstinence
    b. oral contraceptives
    c. intrauterine device
    d. puerperal sterilization

53

Thyroid and Other Endocrine Disorders

53–1. The autoimmune component of endocrinopathies may be initiated by which of the following?

   a. environmental factors
   b. genetic predisposition
   c. viral infection
   d. all of the above

53–2. What is the incidence of hyperthyroidism and hypothyroidism in prenatal patients undergoing screening?

   a. 1 to 3%
   b. 3 to 5%
   c. 5 to 7%
   d. 9 to 11%

53–3. The thyroid undergoes which of the following structural changes during pregnancy?

   a. enlarges
   b. decreases in size
   c. remains the same size
   d. becomes nodular

53–4. Which of the following levels increases markedly during pregnancy?

   a. thyroid-binding globulin (TBG)
   b. thyrotropin-releasing hormone (TRH)
   c. thyrotropin
   d. none of the above

53–5. Which of the following is most useful in screening for thyroid disorders?

   a. thyroid-binding globulin (TBG)
   b. thyroid-releasing hormone (TRH)
   c. thyrotropin (TSH)
   d. none of the above

53–6. Which autoantibody is strongly associated with thyroid failure as well as with Down syndrome and miscarriage in pregnancy?

   a. thyroid antinuclear antibodies
   b. thyroid peroxidase antibodies
   c. thyroid-stimulating blocking antibodies
   d. thyroid-stimulating immunoglobulins

53–7. What is the incidence of symptomatic thyrotoxicosis during pregnancy?

   a. 1 in 20
   b. 1 in 100
   c. 1 in 1000
   d. 1 in 10,000

53–8. Thyrotoxicosis in pregnancy may be associated with elevated levels of all of the following EXCEPT

   a. autoantibodies
   b. thyroxine (T_4)
   c. thyrotropin (TSH)
   d. triiodothyronine (T_3)

53–9. What is the primary treatment approach for thyrotoxicosis during pregnancy?

   a. medical
   b. surgical
   c. combination of medical and surgical
   d. no treatment necessary

53–10. Use of which of the following medications early in pregnancy is associated with congenital-esophageal atresia and *aplasia cutis*?

   a. propylthiouracil
   b. methimazole
   c. verapamil
   d. captopril

53–11. Which of the following is a rare but potentially serious maternal complication of thioamide therapy?

   a. agranulocytosis
   b. gastrointestinal bleeding
   c. polycythemia
   d. seizures

53–12. Following initiation of one of the thioamide drugs for hyperthyroidism, what is the median time to normalization of the free thyroxine index?

    a. 1 to 2 weeks
    b. 3 to 4 weeks
    c. 7 to 8 weeks
    d. 12 to 14 weeks

53–13. Which of the following complications is NOT increased with untreated maternal thyrotoxicosis?

    a. adverse perinatal outcome
    b. deep vein thrombosis
    c. heart failure
    d. preeclampsia

53–14. Which of the following fetal complications is NOT increased with uncontrolled maternal thyrotoxicosis?

    a. growth restriction
    b. preterm delivery
    c. postterm pregnancy
    d. stillbirth

53–15. Drugs useful in the treatment of thyrotoxic storm include all of the following EXCEPT

    a. dexamethasone
    b. magnesium sulfate
    c. propylthiouracil
    d. potassium iodide

53–16. Treatment of maternal hyperthyroidism with propylthyiouracil rarely can lead to what neonatal abnormality?

    a. hearing loss
    b. hypocalcemia
    c. goiter
    d. seizures

53–17. Which of the following is NOT associated with elevated serum levels of thyroxine?

    a. gestational trophoblastic disease
    b. Graves disease
    c. hyperemesis gravidarum
    d. subclinical hyperthyroidism

53–18. Which of the following complications is NOT increased in pregnant women with hypothyroidism?

    a. cardiac dysfunction
    b. macrosomia
    c. abruptio placenta
    d. preeclampsia

53–19. Serum levels of which marker are monitored to assess thyroxine therapy for maternal hypothyroidism?

    a. thyroid-stimulating hormone or thyrotropin (TSH)
    b. thyrotropin-releasing hormone (TRH)
    c. total T_4 plus total T_3
    d. thyroid antibodies

53–20. Untreated maternal subclinical hypothyroidism increases the risk of which of the following?

    a. abnormal psychomotor development in child
    b. placental abruption
    c. preterm delivery
    d. all of the above

53–21. Which of the following is the current recommendation regarding prenatal screening for subclinical hypothyroidism?

    a. screen all women preconceptually
    b. screen all pregnant women at initial prenatal visit
    c. screen women with a history of a child with unexplained neuropsychomotor delay
    d. screening not recommended pending further studies

53–22. Endemic cretinism is seen in countries with high incidences of which dietary problem?

    a. low protein intake
    b. iodide deficiency
    c. elevated lithium levels in water supply
    d. manganese deficiency

53–23. What is the frequency of congenital hypothyroidism?

    a. 1 in 40 to 70 infants
    b. 1 in 400 to 700 infants
    c. 1 in 4000 to 7000 infants
    d. 1 in 40,000 to 70,000 infants

53–24. What is the most common etiology of congenital hypothyroidism?

    a. idiopathic
    b. thyroid agenesis
    c. therapeutic radioiodine
    d. transient hypothyroidism

53–25. What percentage of women will have transient autoimmune thyroid dysfunction during the first year postpartum?

    a. 1 to 2
    b. 5 to 10
    c. 15 to 20
    d. 25 to 30

53–26. What medical condition most strongly predisposes a woman to postpartum thyroid dysfunction?

  a. diabetes type I
  b. lupus erythematosus
  c. psoriasis
  d. renal insufficiency

53–27. Transient postpartum thyroiditis is associated with which of the following nonspecific symptoms?

  a. depression
  b. fatigue
  c. palpitations
  d. all of the above

53–28. What percentage of women with postpartum thyroiditis will develop permanent hypothyroidism?

  a. 10
  b. 30
  c. 60
  d. 90

53–29. What is the most common histological diagnosis of thyroid nodules biopsied during pregnancy?

  a. carcinoma
  b. cystic degeneration
  c. granulomatous disease
  d. nodular hyperplasia

53–30. What is the physiological role of calcitonin?

  a. increases serum calcium levels
  b. decreases serum calcium levels
  c. maintains steady calcium levels
  d. has no effect on calcium levels

53–31. What happens to parathyroid hormone levels during pregnancy?

  a. increase
  b. decrease
  c. remain unchanged
  d. unclear

53–32. What happens to ionized calcium levels in pregnancy?

  a. increase
  b. decrease
  c. remain unchanged
  d. vary widely

53–33. Which of the following is NOT a complication of hyperparathyroidism in pregnancy?

  a. generalized weakness
  b. hyperemesis
  c. pancreatitis
  d. thyrotoxicosis

53–34. Which of the following is generally NOT used for the treatment of hypercalcemic crisis in pregnancy?

  a. calcium gluconate
  b. furosemide
  c. intravenous normal saline
  d. mithramycin

53–35. What is the preferred treatment of hypoparathyroidism during pregnancy?

  a. calcitrol (1,25-dihdyroxyvitamin D)
  b. vitamin K
  c. phosphorus
  d. calcitonin

53–36. What is the most common etiology of pregnancy-associated osteoporosis?

  a. bed rest
  b. corticosteroids
  c. heparin therapy
  d. idiopathic

53–37. Which of the following hormone levels increase during pregnancy?

  a. cortisol
  b. renin
  c. aldosterone
  d. all of the above

53–38. What percentage of pheochromocytomas are bilateral?

  a. 1
  b. 10
  c. 20
  d. 40

53–39. Urine levels of which of the following is NOT used for the diagnosis of pheochromocytomas?

  a. cortisol
  b. vanillylmandelic acid
  c. metanephrines
  d. free catecholamines

53–40. Which of the following is most useful for the treatment of pheochromocytoma?

  a. α-adrenergic blockade
  b. benzodiazepines

c. calcium channel blockers

d. corticosteroids

53–41. What is the most common etiology of Cushing syndrome in the general population?

a. iatrogenic corticosteroid treatment

b. adrenal adenomas

c. adrenal carcinomas

d. pituitary adenomas

53–42. Maternal complications of Cushing syndrome include all of the following EXCEPT

a. heart failure

b. hypertension

c. gestational diabetes

d. liver failure

53–43. What is the most common cause of Addison disease today?

a. tuberculosis

b. histoplasmosis

c. nonspecific granulomatous disease

d. idiopathic autoimmune adrenalitis

53–44. Primary aldosteronism presents with which of the following?

a. hypotension

b. hypokalemia

c. hypercalcemia

d. tetany

53–45. Enlargement of the pituitary in pregnancy is due primarily to what process?

a. generalized pituitary edema

b. lactotrophic cellular hyperplasia

c. thyrotrophic cellular hypertrophy

d. increased vascular supply

53–46. Bromocriptine has proven efficacy for which of the following conditions during pregnancy?

a. Graves disease

b. Addison disease

c. primary aldosteronism

d. pituitary prolactinoma

53–47. Bromocriptine increases which of the following fetal effects?

a. stillbirth

b. growth restriction

c. microcephaly

d. no adverse effects

53–48. What is the specific drug used to treat diabetes insipidus during pregnancy?

a. angiotensin

b. desmopressin

c. oxytocin

d. renin

53–49. Transient diabetes insipidus is most likely encountered in pregnant women with which of the following complications?

a. acute fatty liver

b. preeclampsia

c. prolactin-secreting macroadenoma

d. hemorrhage

53–50. What syndrome is caused by pituitary ischemia and necrosis secondary to obstetrical blood loss?

a. Kalman syndrome

b. Hing syndrome

c. Morris syndrome

d. Sheehan syndrome

53–51. A pregnant patient with a history of Graves disease presents with new-onset, severe headaches. Subsequent evaluation reveals a visual-field defect. A large sellar mass is seen on computed tomography imaging. Serum prolactin level is 48 pg/mL. What is the most likely diagnosis?

a. craniopharyngioma

b. lymphocytic hypophysitis

c. prolactinoma

d. Sheehan syndrome

Connective Tissue Disorders

54–1. On which chromosome is the human leukocyte antigen (HLA) complex located?

  a. 6p
  b. 11p
  c. 14q
  d. 17q

54–2. Genes located in the "HLA" complex encode cell-surface antigens. What is "HLA" an acronym for?

  a. human leukocyte antigen
  b. histological locator antigens
  c. heredity locus assemblage
  d. heterogenous lipoprotein aggregate

54–3. What percentage of systemic lupus erythematosus (SLE) cases occur in women?

  a. 30
  b. 50
  c. 70
  d. 90

54–4. What is the 20-year survival rate of patients with lupus?

  a. 20%
  b. 50%
  c. 70%
  d. 90%

54–5. What is the frequency of SLE in women with one affected family member?

  a. <1%
  b. 3%
  c. 10%
  d. 25%

54–6. At least how many women with SLE have renal involvement?

  a. 10%
  b. 25%
  c. 50%
  d. 90%

54–7. Which is the best screening test for SLE?

  a. anti-Sm (Smith) antibodies
  b. cardiolipin antibodies
  c. antiplatelet antibodies
  d. antinuclear antibodies

54–8. Which of the following autoantibodies is most specific for SLE?

  a. anti-ribonucleic acid (RNA)
  b. anti-nuclear
  c. anti-double-stranded deoxyribonucleic acid (dsDNA)
  d. anti-ribonucleoprotein

54–9. How many of the 11 criteria of the American Rheumatism Association must be present serially or simultaneously to make the diagnosis of SLE?

  a. 2
  b. 4
  c. 8
  d. 10

54–10. Which of the following is most common among the clinical manifestations of SLE?

  a. arthralgias
  b. seizures
  c. gastrointestinal lesions
  d. venous thrombosis

54–11. Which of the following drugs is NOT known to induce a lupus-like syndrome?

  a. hydralazine
  b. methyldopa
  c. phenytoin
  d. verapamil

54–12. What is the rate of major morbidity seen in pregnant patients with SLE?

  a. 1%
  b. 3%
  c. 5%
  d. 7%

54–13. What is the most common complication in pregnant women with lupus nephritis?

    a. renal failure
    b. hypertension
    c. abruption
    d. fetal demise

54–14. Which of the following is the usual first-line therapy for severe manifestations of SLE in pregnancy?

    a. corticosteroids
    b. nonsteroidal anti-inflammatory drugs
    c. azathioprine
    d. cyclophosphamide

54–15. In the management of SLE, azathioprine should be reserved for which of the following?

    a. arthritis
    b. steroid-resistant disease
    c. serositis
    d. thrombocytopenia

54–16. Which of the following forms of reversible contraception is probably the most advantageous and safest for women with SLE?

    a. combination oral contraceptives
    b. intrauterine devices
    c. progesterone-only implants or injections
    d. vaginal spermicides

54–17. What is the incidence of neonatal lupus?

    a. <1%
    b. 5 to 10%
    c. 40 to 50%
    d. 80 to 90%

54–18. Which of the following maternal antibodies is/are associated with congenital heart block in the newborn?

    a. anti-SS-A and anti-SS-B
    b. anti-dsDNA
    c. ANA
    d. anti-RNA

54–19. What is the incidence of congenital heart block in the presence of the associated antibodies?

    a. 3%
    b. 33%
    c. 66%
    d. 99%

54–20. On average, how long does congenital heart block secondary to maternal lupus last?

    a. 6 days
    b. 6 weeks

    c. 6 months
    d. permanent lesion requiring pacemaker

54–21. What percentage of infants with congenital heart block secondary to lupus will die within the first 3 years of life?

    a. 5
    b. 15
    c. 33
    d. 50

54–22. Antibodies of which class are antiphospholipid antibodies?

    a. IgG
    b. IgM
    c. IgA
    d. all of the above

54–23. Which of the following is associated with antiphospholipid antibody syndrome?

    a. arterial thromboses
    b. fetal losses
    c. venous thromboses
    d. all of the above

54–24. Which of the following may be directly bound by antiphospholipid antibodies, causing venous, arterial, or decidual thrombosis in antiphospholipid antibody syndrome?

    a. annexin V
    b. β_2-glycoprotein I
    c. protein S
    d. all of the above

54–25. Approximately what percentage of women with SLE will have the lupus anticoagulant?

    a. 5
    b. 10
    c. 33
    d. 75

54–26. What percentage of women with anticardiolipin antibodies will have the lupus anticoagulant?

    a. 5
    b. 20
    c. 50
    d. 90

54–27. Approximately what percentage of normal pregnant women will have nonspecific antiphospholipid antibodies in low titers?

    a. <1
    b. 5
    c. 15
    d. 25

54–28. Which clotting test is most specific for identifying the lupus anticoagulant?

    a. platelet neutralization procedure
    b. bleeding time
    c. prothrombin time
    d. partial thromboplastin time

54–29. What is the most commonly used test for identifying anticardiolipin antibodies?

    a. polymerase chain reaction (PCR)
    b. prothrombin time
    c. enzyme-linked immunosorbent assay (ELISA)
    d. monoclonal antibody assay

54–30. Which of the following treatment protocols appears to result in the best pregnancy outcome for women with antiphospholipid antibodies and a history of fetal loss?

    a. corticosteroids plus low-dose aspirin
    b. corticosteroids plus heparin
    c. heparin plus low-dose aspirin
    d. aspirin alone

54–31. Which of the following characterizes rheumatoid arthritis?

    a. association with cigarette smoking
    b. genetic predisposition
    c. joint deformation
    d. all of the above

54–32. What is the cornerstone of symptomatic therapy for rheumatoid arthritis?

    a. NSAIDs
    b. corticosteroids
    c. sulfasalazine
    d. cyclosporine

54–33. What is the most likely course of rheumatoid arthritis in pregnancy?

    a. stable during and postpartum
    b. mild flare during and postpartum
    c. serious flare during, remission postpartum
    d. marked improvement during, flare postpartum

54–34. Which of the following proteins or hormones is likely to be responsible for the improvement in rheumatoid arthritis during pregnancy?

    a. cortisol
    b. estrogen
    c. pregnancy associated α_2-glycoprotein
    d. human placental lactogen

54–35. What adverse perinatal outcome is associated with rheumatoid arthritis?

    a. stillbirth
    b. fetal growth restriction
    c. preterm birth
    d. none of the above

54–36. What percentage of women with systemic sclerosis (scleroderma) will have antinuclear antibodies?

    a. 5
    b. 20
    c. 50
    d. 95

54–37. The manifestations of systemic sclerosis (scleroderma) are caused by overproduction of which of the following?

    a. collagen
    b. desmoplastin
    c. elastin
    d. epithelial growth factor

54–38. What is the 10-year survival rate of systemic sclerosis (scleroderma) when there is renal or pulmonary involvement?

    a. <90%
    b. <75%
    c. <50%
    d. <10%

54–39. Which of the following is NOT a characteristic of the CREST syndrome?

    a. calcinosis
    b. Raynaud phenomenon
    c. seizures
    d. telangectasia

54–40. What is the treatment for systemic sclerosis (scleroderma)?

    a. aspirin
    b. cortisol
    c. sulfasalazine
    d. tailored to specific end-organ dysfunction

54–41. Which of the following vasculitis syndromes is associated with hepatitis B antigenemia?

    a. polyarteritis nodosa
    b. Wegener granulomatosis
    c. Grant cell arteritis
    d. dermatomyositis

54–42. What percentage of adults developing dermatomyositis will have an associated malignant tumor?

    a. 5
    b. 15
    c. 25
    d. 50

54–43. Which of the following is inherited as an autosomal dominant trait?

    a. polymyositis
    b. polyarteritis nodosa
    c. Marfan syndrome
    d. dermatomyositis

54–44. Which of the following is characterized by hyperelasticity of the skin?

    a. dermatomyositis
    b. polyarteritis nodosa
    c. Marfan syndrome
    d. Ehlers-Danlos syndrome

54–45. Which of the following obstetrical complications is increased in Ehlers-Danlos syndrome?

    a. preterm ruptured fetal membranes
    b. eclampsia
    c. gestational diabetes
    d. twinning

55

Neurological and Psychiatric Disorders

55–1. Which of the following is true regarding the evaluation of neurological symptoms during pregnancy?

    a. postpone until puerperium
    b. avoid magnetic resonance imaging (MRI)
    c. avoid computed tomographic (CT) scanning
    d. comparable to that of a nonpregnant patient

55–2. Which of the following is true of cranial CT scanning during pregnancy?

    a. safe during pregnancy
    b. should be replaced by MRI
    c. unsafe amounts of radiation exposure to the fetus
    d. inferior to MRI for diagnosis of hemorrhagic lesions

55–3. Which of the following may be used safely during pregnancy?

    a. MRI
    b. CT scanning
    c. cerebral angiography
    d. all of the above

55–4. What percentage of women will, at some time, suffer from migraine headache?

    a. 6
    b. 12
    c. 18
    d. 24

55–5. Risk of stroke in migraine sufferers is increased by which of the following?

    a. obesity
    b. smoking
    c. ergotamine use
    d. none of the above

55–6. What is the usual course of migraine headaches during pregnancy?

    a. slight improvement
    b. dramatic improvement
    c. slight worsening
    d. dramatic worsening

55–7. Which of the following drugs should NOT be used for the treatment of migraine headaches during pregnancy?

   a. meperidine
   b. propranolol
   c. ergonovine
   d. amitriptyline

55–8. Which of the following may be used for the successful treatment of migraine headaches during pregnancy?

   a. atenolol
   b. acupuncture
   c. sumatriptan
   d. all of the above

55–9. Typically, which of the following is true of new-onset migraine headaches during pregnancy?

   a. associated with an aura
   b. develop in the third trimester
   c. associated with fetal growth restriction
   d. should receive thorough evaluation post-partum

55–10. How often is pregnancy complicated by maternal epilepsy?

   a. 1 in 200
   b. 1 in 500
   c. 1 in 1000
   d. 1 in 2000

55–11. Your patient is brought to the emergency room awake and alert by members of her family. They describe jerking muscle movements of her right arm and right leg. She did not lose consciousness. This neuromuscular activity is best described by which of the following seizure categories?

   a. absence
   b. petit mal
   c. generalized
   d. simple motor

55–12. Seizure frequency during pregnancy in epileptic women most commonly follows which pattern of change?

   a. decreases
   b. does not change
   c. slightly increases
   d. markedly increases

55–13. Neonates born to epileptic mothers not taking medication are at increased for which of the following?

   a. perinatal death
   b. seizure disorder
   c. fetal growth restriction
   d. congenital malformation

55–14. Epileptic pregnant women are at increased risk for which of the following?

   a. cesarean delivery
   b. placental abruption
   c. first-trimester abortion
   d. none of the above

55–15. Optimal initial management of epileptic drugs during pregnancy should include which of the following?

   a. attempt switch to newer anticonvulsants
   b. attempt switch to anticonvulsant mono-therapy
   c. add anticonvulsants to ensure seizure control
   d. avoid medication changes if seizures are well-controlled

55–16. Which of the following should be supplemented during pregnancy, particularly if a woman is taking anticonvulsants?

   a. zinc
   b. cobalt
   c. folic acid
   d. pyridoxine

55–17. Parenteral administration of which of the following vitamins may be needed for newborns whose mothers take anticonvulsants?

   a. A
   b. D
   c. E
   d. K

55–18. Which of the following is the most reasonable approach to monitoring of pregnancy when the mother is epileptic in the absence of other complications?

   a. hospitalization in the third trimester
   b. regular nonstress testing in the third trimester
   c. anticonvulsant levels drawn every 2 to 4 weeks
   d. targeted midtrimester ultrasonographic examination

55–19. Which of the following is most strongly associated with peripartum stroke?

   a. hypertension
   b. chorioamnionitis
   c. sickle-cell disease
   d. placental abruption

55–20. Which of the following time periods has the highest risk of pregnancy-associated stroke?

   a. labor
   b. puerperium
   c. third trimester
   d. second trimester

55–21. Evaluation of a patient suspected of having suffered a stroke does NOT include which of the following?

   a. echocardiography
   b. serum lipid profile
   c. serum antiphospholipid antibody screen
   d. peripheral venous Doppler ultrasonography

55–22. Approximately what percentage of ischemic strokes in women of reproductive age is caused by antiphospholipid antibodies?

   a. 5
   b. 10
   c. 30
   d. 50

55–23. In patients who suffer ischemic stroke without a persistent cause during pregnancy, what is the magnitude of risk of recurrent stroke in future pregnancies?

   a. low
   b. proportionate with parity
   c. proportionate with maternal age
   d. proportionate with socioeconomic level

55–24. What is the most common source of cerebral emboli?

   a. cardiac arrhythmia
   b. mitral valve prolapse
   c. infective endocarditis
   d. peripheral deep venous thrombosis

55–25. Cerebral venous thrombosis is NOT associated with which of the following?

   a. sepsis
   b. preeclampsia
   c. thrombophilias
   d. hemorrhage with shock

55–26. What is the most common cause of subarachnoid hemorrhage during pregnancy?

   a. preeclampsia
   b. cocaine abuse
   c. aneurysm rupture
   d. arteriovenous malformation (AVM) rupture

55–27. What is the cardinal symptom of aneurysm rupture?

   a. seizure
   b. vertigo
   c. epistaxis
   d. headache

55–28. Which of the following statements is true regarding arteriovenous malformations (AVMs) and pregnancy?

   a. bleeding risk is increased by pregnancy
   b. bleeding risk is increased by advanced maternal age
   c. route of delivery is based on obstetrical indications
   d. pregnancy delivery or termination should promptly follow bleeding from an AVM

55–29. Which of the following is true of multiple sclerosis demographics?

   a. symptoms begin in the third and fourth decades
   b. men are affected more commonly than women
   c. disproportionately affects those of African descent
   d. no increased incidence in offspring of affected individuals

55–30. All of the following are common presenting symptoms of multiple sclerosis EXCEPT

   a. diplopia
   b. hyperreflexia
   c. bladder dysfunction
   d. simple motor seizure

55–31. Which of the following is used to treat multiple sclerosis?

   a. mitomycin
   b. lamivudine
   c. natalizumab
   d. all of the above

55–32. Multiple sclerosis is commonly associated with which of the following pregnancy outcomes?

   a. cesarean delivery
   b. perinatal mortality
   c. fetal growth restriction
   d. none of the above

55–33. Myasthenia gravis results from the IgG-mediated destruction which of the following?

   a. actin filaments
   b. myosin heavy chain
   c. calcium ATPase pumps
   d. acetylcholine receptors

55–34. All of the following may be used in the successful treatment of myasthenia gravis EXCEPT

    a. azathioprine
    b. thymectomy
    c. mitoxantrone
    d. pyridostigmine

55–35. Which of the following antimicrobials should be used with caution in pregnant women with myasthenia gravis?

    a. penicillins
    b. quinolones
    c. sulfonamides
    d. aminoglycosides

55–36. With maternal disease, what percentage of newborns will develop neonatal myasthenia gravis?

    a. <5
    b. 10 to 20
    c. 30 to 40
    d. 50 to 60

55–37. Which of the following is true regarding the incidence of Guillain-Barré syndrome?

    a. increases during pregnancy
    b. increases during puerperium
    c. majority of cases follow viral vaccination
    d. majority of cases follow surgical procedures

55–38. What percentage of patients with Guillain-Barré syndrome will have full recovery?

    a. 50
    b. 66
    c. 85
    d. 99

55–39. Your pregnant patient presents with abrupt onset of unilateral facial paralysis and pain. You counsel her that this condition is associated with an increased risk for which of the following?

    a. preeclampsia
    b. gestational diabetes
    c. congenital malformation
    d. none of the above

55–40. Which of the following is an indicator of poor prognosis for Bell palsy during pregnancy?

    a. bilateral disease
    b. recurrence in subsequent pregnancy
    c. electromyographic evidence of denervation extends beyond 10 days
    d. all of the above

55–41. Your pregnant patient complains of bilateral numbness along the medial aspect of her forearm, wrists, and hands that worsens during sleep. Most cases of this condition eventually require which of the following treatments?

    a. wrist splinting
    b. oral corticosteroids
    c. corticosteroid injections
    d. surgical ligament release

55–42. Which of the following is NOT a complication of pregnancy in patients with spinal cord injury?

    a. constipation
    b. urinary tract infection
    c. low-birthweight neonate
    d. hypotonic labor

55–43. Which of the following is NOT typically associated with autonomic hyperreflexia?

    a. headache
    b. hypertension
    c. facial flushing
    d. loss of consciousness

55–44. Which of the following is used to decrease the frequency of autonomic hyperreflexia during labor?

    a. nifedipine
    b. propranolol
    c. general anesthesia
    d. epidural anesthesia

55–45. Your pregnant patient with a body mass index of 30 presents during the first trimester with new-onset headache, loss of central visual acuity, and neck stiffness. She is afebrile; BP 120/60; respirations 14/min; pulse 80 bpm. Her head MRI was unremarkable. Spinal tap revealed elevated cerebrospinal fluid (CSF) pressure but normal CSF composition. The next most appropriate treatment includes which of the following?

    a. oral acetazolamide
    b. lumboperitoneal shunting of CSF
    c. prompt pregnancy termination using D&C
    d. all of the above

55–46. The most common potential long-term sequela of benign intracranial hypertension is which of the following?

    a. seizure
    b. loss of vision
    c. intracranial tumor
    d. facial muscle paralysis

55–47. Management of pregnancy in women with benign intracranial hypertension includes which of
the following?

   a. serial visual-field testing
   b. mandatory cesarean delivery
   c. avoidance of epidural anesthesia
   d. prompt pregnancy termination or delivery

55–48. Chorea gravidarum is more commonly associated
with which of the following conditions?

   a. hyperthyroidism
   b. hydrocephalus
   c. systemic lupus erythematosus
   d. benign intracranial hypertension

55–49. During which of the following time periods do
women most frequently suffer depression?

   a. first trimester
   b. second trimester
   c. third trimester
   d. puerperium

55–50. All of the following may be risk factors for pregnancy-related depression EXCEPT

   a. cigarette smoking
   b. young maternal age
   c. high serum estrogen levels
   d. family history of alcoholism

55–51. In what percentage of suicides are major mood
disorders a predisposing factor?

   a. 10
   b. 25
   c. 50
   d. 66

55–52. Evaluation of a patient with schizophrenia typically reveals all EXCEPT which of the following?

   a. other affected family members
   b. brain atrophy found on imaging
   c. abnormal EEG reading
   d. symptom onset in patient's 30s

55–53. Treatment of postpartum blues primarily involves which of the following?

   a. reassurance
   b. psychological consultation
   c. serotonin-reuptake inhibitors
   d. Child Protective Service consultation

55–54. What percentage of women after delivery will
develop postpartum blues?

   a. 10
   b. 30

   c. 50
   d. 70

55–55. What percentage of women after delivery will
develop postpartum depression?

   a. 10
   b. 25
   c. 33
   d. 50

55–56. Treatment of postpartum depression primarily
should involve which of the following?

   a. reassurance
   b. serotonin-reuptake inhibitors
   c. electroconvulsive therapy
   d. Child Protective Services consultation

55–57. Recurrence rates of depression after recovery
from postpartum depression approximate which
of the following?

   a. 2 to 30%
   b. 30 to 50%
   c. 50 to 85%
   d. 80 to 95%

55–58. What is the recurrence risk of postpartum depression?

   a. 5%
   b. 20%
   c. 70%
   d. 90%

55–59. All EXCEPT which of the following are adverse
neonatal outcomes attributable to psychiatric
diagnoses?

   a. infanticide
   b. low birthweight
   c. insecure maternal attachment
   d. breast feeding–related sertraline toxicity

55–60. What is currently considered the primary treatment for postpartum depression?

   a. tricyclic antidepressants
   b. electroconvulsant therapy
   c. monoamine oxidase inhibitors
   d. selective serotonin reuptake inhibitors

55–61. Counseling your patient regarding electroconvulsive therapy and pregnancy should include
which of the following?

   a. should not be used in pregnancy
   b. carries significant fetal risk
   c. carries a 10% complication risk
   d. carries a 25% preterm labor risk

56

Dermatological Disorders

56–1. Hyperpigmentation of pregnancy is related to which of the following?

   a. cortisol
   b. aldosterone
   c. melanocyte-stimulating hormone
   d. unknown cause

56–2. What percentage of pregnant women demonstrate some skin darkening?

   a. 10
   b. 25
   c. 50
   d. 90

56–3. Which of the following terms describe the non-palpable brown to blue-gray patches of skin containing spindle-shaped melanocytes often seen in pregnancy?

   a. pruritic papules of pregnancy
   b. linea nigra
   c. acquired dermal melanocytes
   d. chloasma

56–4. Severe or persistent chloasma can be treated postpartum with which of the following?

   a. hydrocortisone
   b. oral contraceptive pills
   c. tretinoin ointment
   d. ultraviolet light

56–5. Chloasma is a pigmentation of which of the following?

   a. areolae
   b. linea alba
   c. face
   d. inner thighs

56–6. Chloasma is seen in what percentage of pregnant women?

   a. 10
   b. 25

   c. 50
   d. 75

56–7. Which of the following is the most common behavior of nevi during pregnancy?

   a. decrease size
   b. increase size
   c. malignant transformation
   d. no size change

56–8. Which of the following best describes telogen effluvium?

   a. caused by high levels of melanocyte-stimulating hormone
   b. self-limited and usually resolves in 6 to 12 months
   c. associated with oral contraceptives
   d. all of the above

56–9. Which of the following hormones most likely causes spider angiomas during pregnancy?

   a. estrogen
   b. progesterone
   c. cortisol
   d. chorionic gonadotropin

56–10. Which ethnic group is most likely to have spider angiomas?

   a. African Americans
   b. Caucasians
   c. Hispanics
   d. Asians

56–11. Which of the following conditions results from a mild form of cholestatic jaundice?

   a. pruritis gravidarum
   b. capillary hemangiomas
   c. palmar erythema
   d. pruritic urticarial papules and plaques of pregnancy (PUPPP)

56–12. Cholestasis of pregnancy is caused by the dermal deposition of which of the following?

   a. bile acids
   b. bile salts
   c. bilirubin
   d. biliverdin

56–13. Lesions of PUPPP usually appear first in which of the following locations?

   a. abdomen
   b. buttocks
   c. extremities
   d. face

56–14. What is the likely pathophysiology of PUPPP?

   a. allergic
   b. autoimmune
   c. infectious
   d. uncertain

56–15. What effect does PUPPP have on perinatal morbidity?

   a. decreased
   b. increased in primigravidas
   c. increased in all gravidas
   d. no effect

56–16. Which of the following dermatological conditions is characterized by bite-like papules on the forearm and trunk?

   a. prurigo
   b. herpes gestationis
   c. pruritic urticarial papules and plaques of pregnancy
   d. chloasma

56–17. Which of the following is characteristic of prurigo of pregnancy?

   a. adversely affects perinatal outcome
   b. develops early in pregnancy
   c. involves the lower legs and feet
   d. treated with antihistamines and topical steroids

56–18. Herpes gestationis is occasionally associated with which of the following?

   a. chorioangioma
   b. trophoblastic disease
   c. preeclampsia
   d. herpes zoster

56–19. Herpes gestationis typically shows which of the following behaviors in subsequent pregnancies?

   a. always recurs
   b. milder course
   c. never recurs
   d. presents later in gestation

56–20. What is the pathophysiology of herpes gestationis?

   a. allergic
   b. autoimmune
   c. infectious
   d. unknown

56–21. Of the following, which is most strongly associated with Graves disease?

   a. pruritus gravidarum
   b. pruritic urticarial papules and plaques of pregnancy
   c. herpes gestationis
   d. impetigo herpetiformis

56–22. Herpes gestationis usually responds to which of the following therapies?

   a. antihistamines
   b. high-dose oral steroids
   c. topical steroids
   d. ultraviolet light therapy

56–23. What is the hallmark lesion of impetigo herpetiformis?

   a. sterile pustules with margins of erythematous patches
   b. infected pustules surrounded by erythema
   c. erythematous, scaly, dry lesions
   d. infected apocrine gland plugging

56–24. Which of the following is accompanied by constitutional symptoms?

   a. hidradentis suppurativa
   b. impetigo herpetiformis
   c. melanosis gravidarum
   d. pruritus gravidarum

56–25. Which of the following is thought to pose no teratogenic risk to the fetus?

   a. isotretinoin
   b. etretinate
   c. oral tretinoin
   d. benzoyl peroxide

57

Neoplastic Diseases

57–1. What is the approximate incidence of cancer in pregnancy?

   a. 1 in 100
   b. 1 in 1,000
   c. 1 in 10,000
   d. 1 in 100,000

57–2. What is the most common malignancy diagnosed in pregnancy?

   a. breast
   b. cervix
   c. lymphoma
   d. melanoma

57–3. What is the earliest gestational age at which the ovaries may be removed safely because placental progesterone production is adequate to maintain the pregnancy?

   a. 4 weeks
   b. 6 weeks
   c. 8 weeks
   d. 12 weeks

57–4. What is the optimal timing of therapeutic surgeries for non-ovarian cancers in pregnancy?

   a. second trimester
   b. third trimester
   c. postpartum
   d. as indicated, regardless of gestational age

57–5. What are the characteristic adverse fetal effects of high-dose radiation in pregnancy?

   a. leukemia and cardiac defects
   b. radiation nephritis and anal atresia
   c. microcephaly and mental retardation
   d. fetal cardiac defects and hydrocephalus

57–6. Which of the following radiation-dose thresholds poses a negligible risk for major fetal malformations?

   a. <5 cGy
   b. <10 cGy
   c. <15 cGy
   d. <20 cGy

57–7. During what gestational period are antineoplastic drugs most harmful to the fetus?

   a. first trimester
   b. second trimester
   c. late third trimester
   d. postpartum if breast feeding

57–8. Embryonic exposure to cytotoxic drugs causes major malformations in what percentage of cases?

   a. 0 to 5
   b. 10 to 20
   c. 30 to 40
   d. 50 to 60

57–9. How often is childhood malignancy seen in the offspring of women treated with chemotherapy during pregnancy?

   a. 1 in 2
   b. 1 in 10
   c. 1 in 50
   d. <1 in 100

57–10. What is the major potential reproductive sequela subsequent to multi-drug therapy for Hodgkin lymphoma?

   a. ovarian fibrosis
   b. incompetent cervix
   c. recurrent abortion
   d. preterm delivery

57–11. Low birthweight has been associated with in utero exposure to which chemotherapeutic agent?

   a. 5-fluuoruracil
   b. chlorambucil
   c. doxorubicin
   d. methotrexate

57–12. Which of the following are risk factors for the diagnosis of breast cancer during pregnancy?

    a. BRCA1 and BRCA2 genes
    b. breast feeding after previous pregnancy
    c. chemotherapy in past for other malignancy
    d. prior induced abortion

57–13. According to post-1990 data, how often are axillary lymph nodes positive for cancer in pregnant women with breast cancer?

    a. 10%
    b. 30%
    c. 60%
    d. 90%

57–14. Stage for stage, what influence does pregnancy have on the course of breast cancer?

    a. decreases survival
    b. increases survival
    c. no influence
    d. unknown

57–15. Pregnant women with breast cancer are more likely to present with what stage disease?

    a. stage 0
    b. stage 1
    c. stage 2
    d. stages 3 and 4

57–16. What is the false-negative rate of mammography performed during pregnancy?

    a. 5%
    b. 15%
    c. 25%
    d. 35%

57–17. A 27-year-old G1P0 at 32 weeks gestation has a breast mass with features worrisome for malignancy. Ultrasound and mammography are inconclusive. Which of the following would be the most appropriate approach?

    a. await delivery at term and evaluate further postpartum
    b. deliver preterm when fetal lungs mature and evaluate further postpartum
    c. perform core biopsy now
    d. repeat ultrasound and mammogram in 4 weeks

57–18. Metastatic work-up for breast cancer during pregnancy may include all of the following EXCEPT

    a. chest x-ray
    b. radionuclide liver scan
    c. MRI
    d. ultrasonography

57–19. Which of the following is NOT a recommended therapy for breast cancer during pregnancy?

    a. mastectomy with lymph node dissection
    b. adjuvant chemotherapy
    c. radiotherapy
    d. wide local excision

57–20. What apparent effect do future pregnancy and lactation have on the course of previously treated breast cancer?

    a. do not affect prognosis
    b. improve long-term survival
    c. increase local recurrence rate
    d. worsen long-term prognosis

57–21. What is the recommended delay for future pregnancy following treatment of breast cancer?

    a. 6 months to 1 year
    b. 2 to 3 years
    c. 5 to 6 years
    d. 7 to 8 years

57–22. What is NOT a common presenting finding of Hodgkin disease in pregnancy?

    a. fever
    b. peripheral adenopathy
    c. seizures
    d. weight loss

57–23. What is the name of the staging system commonly used for Hodgkin disease and other lymphomas?

    a. Ann Arbor
    b. Detroit
    c. Green Bay
    d. Mayo

57–24. Staging of Hodgkin disease does NOT include which of the following?

    a. abdominal imaging
    b. bone marrow biopsy
    c. chest x-ray
    d. intravenous pyelogram

57–25. Pregnant women with Hodgkin disease have a greatly increased risk of which of the following, particularly if undergoing chemotherapy or radiation therapy?

    a. infection
    b. gestational diabetes
    c. renal insufficiency
    d. pregnancy wastage

57–26. Approximately what percentage of women treated for Hodgkin disease with chemotherapy will resume normal menses?

　　a. 5
　　b. 25
　　c. 50
　　d. 95

57–27. What percentage of women with Hodgkin disease will develop a second different cancer within 15 years?

　　a. 5
　　b. 20
　　c. 40
　　d. 60

57–28. What is the incidence of lymphoma in a woman with human immunodeficiency virus (HIV)?

　　a. equal to that of the general population
　　b. 1%
　　c. 5 to 10%
　　d. 15 to 20%

57–29. What is the reported incidence of leukemia in pregnancy?

　　a. 1 per 1000
　　b. 1 per 10,000
　　c. 1 per 100,000
　　d. 1 per 1,000,000

57–30. What percentage of pregnant women with acute leukemia will have a remission with chemotherapy?

　　a. 10
　　b. 25
　　c. 40
　　d. 75

57–31. Which is NOT increased in the presence of maternal leukemia?

　　a. eclampsia
　　b. hemorrhage
　　c. preterm delivery
　　d. stillbirth

57–32. What is the most important prognostic feature of stage 1 melanoma, measured by both the Clark classification and Breslow scale?

　　a. cellular atypia
　　b. color-tone irregularity
　　c. lateral spread
　　d. thickness

57–33. Which of the following is true of melanoma in pregnant women?

　　a. Disease diagnosis tends to occur at a later stage than in nonpregnant women.
　　b. Future pregnancies increase future recurrence risk.
　　c. Stage for stage, prognosis is worse than for nonpregnant women.
　　d. Therapeutic abortion improves survival.

57–34. How long should pregnancy be avoided following treatment for melanoma?

　　a. 1 to 2 years
　　b. 3 to 5 years
　　c. 8 to 10 years
　　d. should not become pregnant

57–35. A 32-year-old at 14 weeks gestation has abnormal cervical cytology and unsatisfactory colposcopy during initial evaluation. What is the most appropriate plan?

　　a. cervical cone biopsy
　　b. endocervical curettage
　　c. loop excision
　　d. repeat colposcopy in 6 to 12 weeks

57–36. What is the complication rate of colposcopy with biopsies during pregnancy?

　　a. <1%
　　b. 10%
　　c. 20%
　　d. 50%

57–37. Which of the following is NOT a complication of conization and loop excision during pregnancy?

　　a. cervical stenosis
　　b. incomplete excision of the neoplasia
　　c. hemorrhage
　　d. preterm delivery

57–38. Which of the following is true regarding the natural history of cervical intraepithelial neoplasia during pregnancy?

　　a. 10% progress to invasive cancer
　　b. 70% progress to invasive cancer
　　c. 10% regress postpartum
　　d. 70% regress postpartum

57–39. In general, how does pregnancy affect the survival rate for invasive carcinoma of the cervix?

　　a. increases
　　b. decreases
　　c. no effect
　　d. varies with route of delivery

57–40. A microinvasive cervical cancer is diagnosed by conization at 12 weeks gestation. Frank invasion has been ruled out. Which of the following would NOT be part of a reasonable follow-up strategy?

    a. pregnancy termination followed by radical hysterectomy
    b. periodic colposcopic surveillance
    c. vaginal delivery unless obstetrical indications for cesarean delivery
    d. definitive treatment deferred until postpartum

57–41. Which is the most common cancer involving the ovary associated with pregnancy?

    a. epithelial
    b. germ cell
    c. stromal
    d. metastatic from distant primary

57–42. Where are 80% of colorectal cancers located when diagnosed during pregnancy?

    a. appendix
    b. descending colon
    c. transverse colon
    d. rectum

57–43. What is the most common presenting symptom in a pregnant woman with renal cell carcinoma?

    a. hematuria
    b. pain
    c. fever
    d. abdominal mass

57–44. What is the most common site of genital tract cancer diagnosed in pregnancy?

    a. cervix
    b. endometrium
    c. ovary
    d. vulva/vagina

58

Infections

58–1. The early stages of neonatal infection may be associated with all of the following clinical signs EXCEPT

    a. jaundice
    b. respiratory depression
    c. hypothermia
    d. jitteriness

58–2. The most common pathogens of ascending infection leading to neonatal sepsis and stillbirth do NOT include which of the following?

    a. *Escherichia coli*
    b. *Ureaplasma urealyticum*
    c. *Bacteroides fragilis*
    d. Group B streptococcus

58–3. Varicella-zoster infection is typically most severe in which of the following?

    a. adolescents
    b. children
    c. nonpregnant adults
    d. pregnant women

58–4. Your susceptible patient with an uncomplicated pregnancy states that she was exposed to varicella-zoster 24 hours ago. The correct statement regarding varicella-zoster immunoglobulin (VZIG) administration in this patient would be which of the following?

    a. She may be tested for immunity before VZIG administration.
    b. She should receive VZIG no later than 72 hr after exposure.
    c. VZIG, in most cases, should be reserved for immunocompromised pregnant patients.
    d. She should receive VZIG immediately.

58–5. In which group of patients should VARIVAX vaccine be withheld?

a. children who have no history of varicella infection
b. breast-feeding women who have no history of varicella infection
c. pregnant women who have no history of varicella infection
d. adolescents who have no history of varicella infection

58–6. Your pregnant patient develops a varicella-zoster infection at 22 weeks gestation. You counsel her that the risk of congenital varicella infection is which of the following?

a. highest after 20 weeks gestation
b. highest between 13 and 20 weeks gestation
c. the same regardless of gestational age
d. highest prior to 13 weeks gestation

58–7. Which of the following is NOT part of the varicella embryopathy?

a. chorioretinitis
b. multicystic kidneys
c. limb atrophy
d. cerebral cortical atrophy

58–8. When should varicella-zoster immunoglobulin be administered to the newborn in the presence of maternal chicken pox?

a. delivery within 21 days of maternal disease
b. delivery within 10 days of maternal disease
c. delivery within 5 days of maternal disease
d. maternal disease occurs at 7 days of newborn age

58–9. Your patient with an uncomplicated pregnancy presents for a scheduled prenatal visit in November. Her EDC is April 30th. Which of the following would be the most appropriate use of the influenza vaccine in this patient?

a. She should receive the inactivated-virus vaccine injection.
b. The inactivated-virus vaccine should be withheld due to teratogenicity concerns.
c. She should receive the intranasal viral vaccine.
d. The influenza vaccine should be reserved for patients with chronic underlying disease.

58–10. Which of the following agents has specific activity against influenza A?

a. acyclovir
b. ganciclovir
c. adenosine arabinoside
d. amantadine

58–11. Which of the following adult psychiatric diseases may be related to fetal exposure to influenza A?

a. schizophrenia
b. bipolar disorder
c. depression
d. acute psychosis

58–12. Your patient has just received the MMR vaccine. Conception should be avoided for how many weeks following this vaccination?

a. 4
b. 6
c. 8
d. 12

58–13. You are providing prepregnancy counseling to your patient. She was born abroad and did not receive childhood immunizations. You counsel her that mumps during pregnancy may be associated with which of the following?

a. no increased risk of abortion
b. no increased risk of congenital malformations
c. an increased risk cardiac malformations
d. an increased risk of deafness

58–14. What associated pregnancy complications are increased in women with measles?

a. preeclampsia
b. abortion
c. fetal anomalies
d. abruptio placentae

58–15. Which of the following is most likely to produce a cough and lower respiratory tract infection (i.e., pneumonia)?

a. rhinovirus
b. coronavirus
c. adenovirus
d. echovirus

58–16. The classical hantaviral syndrome presents clinically as which entity?

a. pulmonary edema
b. encephalitis
c. gastroenteritis
d. hepatitis

58–17. Which of the following is associated with coxsackie viremia in the fetus?

a. pancreatitis
b. cholecystitis
c. cystitis
d. encephalomyelitis

58–18. Which of the following tests is used to confirm the diagnosis of erythema infectiosum?

    a. antistreptolysis titer
    b. parvovirus IgM titer
    d. rubella IgM titer
    d. coxsackie IgM titer

58–19. A classic clinical sign of fifth disease includes which of the following?

    a. punctuate skin ulcers
    b. herpetiform vesicles
    c. erythroderma
    d. skin desquamation

58–20. Which of the following adverse fetal effects has been reported to be caused by maternal parvovirus infection?

    a. microcephaly
    b. hydrocephaly
    c. hydrops
    d. cardiac defects

58–21. A boy with fifth disease poses what risk to his social contacts?

    a. Casual contacts have an approximately 20% risk of infection.
    b. His mother's risk of infection is equal to his teacher's.
    c. His teacher has an approximately 50% risk of infection.
    d. His teacher has an approximately 20% risk of infection.

58–22. In addition to a maculopapular rash, maternal rubella infection commonly presents with which of the following?

    a. pneumonitis
    b. arthritis
    c. esophagitis
    d. encephalitis

58–23. Congenital rubella syndrome is most commonly acquired during which weeks of gestation?

    a. 8 to 10
    b. 12 to 14
    c. 16 to 18
    d. 36 to 38

58–24. Congenital rubella syndrome may include all of the following EXCEPT

    a. limb atrophy
    b. eye defects
    c. heart defects
    d. deafness

58–25. Maternal cytomegaloviral infection commonly presents with which of the following?

    a. gastroenteritis
    b. maculopapular dermatitis
    c. vertigo
    d. no symptoms

58–26. Which of the following is an associated fetal risk with cytomegalovirus infection?

    a. diabetes
    b. cataracts
    c. spastic paralysis
    d. deafness

58–27. Which of the following techniques is best for the diagnosis of fetal cytomegalovirus infection?

    a. amniocentesis or cordocentesis
    b. chorionic villus sampling
    c. ultrasonography
    d. magnetic resonance imaging

58–28. Which of the following management options should be recommended to women with documented maternal cytomegaloviral infection?

    a. antepartum ganciclovir administration
    b. no specific management
    c. fetal ultrasonography and amniocentesis
    d. CMV immunoglobulin administered to neonates delivered within 10 days of maternal infection

58–29. You counsel your pregnant patient that the most effective prevention of maternal CMV infection involves which of the following?

    a. prepregnancy inactivated-virus vaccine administration
    b. good hygiene and hand washing
    c. CMV immunoglobulin given within 72 hr of viral exposure
    d. ganciclovir administered within 72 hr of viral exposure

58–30. Pregnancy-related group A streptococcal infections commonly present as which of the following maternal complications?

    a. pneumonia
    b. meningitis
    c. pyelonephritis
    d. postpartum endometritis

58–31. What percent of pregnant women are colonized with *Streptococcus agalactiae*?

    a. <1
    b. 5 to 10
    c. 15 to 20
    d. 40 to 50

58–32. Pregnancy-related group B streptococcal infections can commonly present as which of the following maternal complications?

   a. pyelonephritis
   b. pneumonia
   c. postpartum endometritis
   d. septic arthritis

58–33. Which of the following is a characteristic of early-onset group B streptococcus neonatal sepsis?

   a. onset at 1 to 2 weeks of age
   b. respiratory distress
   c. nearly always fatal
   d. cardiac arrhythmia

58–34. Late-onset group B streptococcal infection in the neonate classically manifests as which of the following?

   a. jejunal perforation
   b. meningitis
   c. respiratory distress
   d. osteochondritis

58–35. Current prevention strategies for group B streptococcus infections from the American College of Obstetricians and Gynecologists and the Centers for Disease Control and Prevention include which of the following?

   a. vaginal culture screening at 32 to 35 weeks
   b. antepartum antimicrobial prophylaxis given to women with positive GBS cultures
   c. antepartum vaginal lavage with chlorhexidine for women with positive GBS cultures
   d. intrapartum antimicrobial prophylaxis given to women with GBS bacteriuria

58–36. Antimicrobial prophylaxis for group B streptococcus may include all of the following EXCEPT

   a. penicillin G
   b. trimethoprim-sulfamethoxazole
   c. cefazolin
   d. clindamycin

58–37. Preventive counseling of your pregnant patient for listeriosis should include avoidance of which of the following?

   a. small children
   b. processed meats
   c. rodents
   d. cat feces

58–38. Which of the following is associated with fetal listerial infection?

   a. osteochondritis
   b. neuronal destruction
   c. microabscess formation
   d. myocarditis

58–39. Fetal infection with *Listeria monocytogenes* may lead to which of the following?

   a. stillbirth
   b. limb atrophy
   c. cardiac defects
   d. cataract formation

58–40. What is the treatment of choice for listeriosis during the third trimester?

   a. metronidazole plus ampicillin
   b. clindamycin plus gentamicin
   c. ciprofloxacin plus metronidazole
   d. ampicillin plus gentamicin

58–41. Treatment of uncomplicated salmonellosis in pregnancy should include which of the following?

   a. ampicillin plus gentamicin
   b. intravenous hydration
   c. anti-salmonella vaccination after recovery
   d. azithromycin

58–42. What is one of the antimicrobial agents used in pregnancy for the treatment of *Salmonella typhi*?

   a. ampicillin
   b. erythromycin
   c. azithromycin
   d. clindamycin

58–43. Adults with shigellosis commonly manifest which of the following symptoms?

   a. nonproductive cough
   b. jaundice
   c. polyarthralgia
   d. diarrhea

58–44. Adults with Lyme disease commonly manifest symptoms of which of the following?

   a. hepatitis
   b. pneumonia
   c. carditis
   d. gastroenteritis

58–45. What is the treatment choice for Lyme disease in pregnancy?

   a. amoxicillin
   b. clindamycin
   c. gentamicin
   d. ciprofloxacin

58–46. Maternal Lyme disease during pregnancy has been associated with an increased incidence of which of the following?

　　a. abortion
　　b. placental abruption
　　c. maternal meningitis
　　d. fetal cardiac defects

58–47. Your pregnant patient is traveling to a Lyme disease endemic area. Which of the following is true regarding prevention strategies against maternal infection?

　　a. Chemoprophylaxis for tick bites typically lowers maternal infection rates.
　　b. Removal of attached ticks typically does not reduce maternal infection rates.
　　c. A vaccine is currently available against Lyme disease.
　　d. Immunoglobulin administered within 72 hr of a tick bite typically reduces maternal infection rates.

58–48. Maternal toxoplasmosis infection commonly presents with which of the following?

　　a. maculopapular rash
　　b. mild gastroenteritis
　　c. pneumonia
　　d. no symptoms

58–49. Which of the following may be associated with congenital toxoplasmosis infection?

　　a. polyhydramnios
　　b. cardiomegaly
　　c. microcephaly
　　d. polycystic kidneys

58–50. The classical triad of findings with congenital toxoplasmosis infection include all of the following EXCEPT

　　a. intracranial calcifications
　　b. hydrocephaly
　　c. chorioretinitis
　　d. limb atrophy

58–51. Which of the following is used as part of the treatment for fetal toxoplasmosis infection?

　　a. spectinomycin
　　b. erythromycin
　　c. sulfasalazine
　　d. spiramycin

58–52. Your otherwise healthy pregnant patient is concerned about her risk for toxoplasmosis because of her cat. An appropriate management strategy for this patient includes which of the following?

　　a. antimicrobial prophylaxis following exposure to cat feces
　　b. screen for toxoplasmosis IgG antibodies
　　c. avoid feeding her cat raw meat
　　d. receive toxoplasmosis immunoglobulin within 96 hr following exposure to cat feces

58–53. Which of the following is associated with malarial infections in pregnancy?

　　a. fetal hydrops
　　b. preterm labor
　　c. congenital blindness
　　d. congenital cardiac defects

58–54. Preventive strategies for the effects of malaria in pregnancy include which of the following?

　　a. chemoprophylaxis for pregnant travelers on arrival to malaria-endemic areas
　　b. chemoprophylaxis for pregnant travelers initiated before arrival to endemic areas
　　c. inactivated malarial vaccine administered prior to travel to endemic areas
　　d. no preventive method available

58–55. The transmitting vector of the West Nile virus to humans is which of the following?

　　a. rodent
　　b. cat
　　c. mosquito
　　d. bird

58–56. Adults infected with the West Nile virus most commonly present with which of the following?

　　a. no symptoms
　　b. coma
　　c. mental status changes
　　d. jaundice

58–57. Patients in the third phase of Severe Acute Respiratory Syndrome (SARS) may develop which of the following conditions?

　　a. pulmonary edema
　　b. asthma
　　c. congestive heart failure
　　d. ARDS

58–58. Treatment of SARS includes which of the following?

　　a. acyclovir plus corticosteroids
　　b. clarithromycin plus amoxicillin/clavulanate
　　c. acyclovir plus ventilatory support
　　d. ventilatory support alone

58–59. Pregnancy-related methicillin-resistant *Staphylo-coccus aureus* infections commonly present as which of the following?

   a. mastitis
   b. sinusitis
   c. epiglottitis
   d. septic arthritis

58–60. Recommendations regarding the smallpox vaccine include which of the following?

   a. Vaccination should be withheld in pregnancy, even following smallpox exposure.
   b. Vaccination should not be withheld in pregnancy following smallpox exposure.

   c. Vaccination during pregnancy should be an indication for pregnancy termination.
   d. Vaccination may be administered routinely in pregnancy.

58–61. Treatment recommendations regarding anthrax exposure during pregnancy include which of the following?

   a. clarithromycin
   b. ciprofloxacin
   c. ciprofloxacin plus anthrax vaccination
   d. clarithromycin plus anthrax vaccination

59

Sexually Transmitted Diseases

59–1. Which of the following is true concerning syphilis in reproductive-age women?

   a. rates peaked in 1950
   b. rates peaked in 1975
   c. rates peaked in 1990
   d. rates continue to rise

59–2. Increased rates of maternal syphilis are linked to which of the following?

   a. substance abuse
   b. inadequate prenatal care
   c. human immunodeficiency virus (HIV) infection
   d. all of the above

59–3. Antepartum syphilis is NOT associated with which of the following?

   a. fetal death
   b. preterm labor
   c. neonatal infection
   d. placental abruption

59–4. At what gestational age does the fetus first manifest clinical disease if infected by syphilis?

   a. 6 weeks
   b. 8 to 10 weeks
   c. 12 weeks
   d. 18 weeks or more

59–5. What is the gross appearance of the placenta in syphilitic infection?

   a. congested and small
   b. congested and large
   c. pale and small
   d. pale and large

59–6. Which of the following is NOT a specific treponemal test?

   a. RPR
   b. FTA-ABS
   c. MHA-TP
   d. TP-PA

59–7. Which of the following is the most specific test for syphilis?

   a. fluorescent treponemal antibody absorption test (FTA-ABS)
   b. Gram stain of lesion exudate
   c. rapid plasma reagin test (RPR)
   d. venereal disease research laboratory test (VDRL)

59–8. What is the best test for diagnosis of neonatal syphilis?

   a. cord blood VDRL
   b. motile spirochetes in amnionic fluid
   c. amnionic fluid polymerase chain reaction
   d. sonographic evidence of an enlarged placenta

59–9. Which of the following is NOT typical of congenital syphilis?

   a. ascites
   b. cerebral calcifications
   c. lymphadenopathy
   d. rhinitis

59–10. What is the treatment of choice for syphilis in pregnancy?

   a. tetracycline
   b. doxycycline
   c. erythromycin
   d. penicillin

59–11. Penicillin G cures what percentage of maternal and neonatal syphilis infections?

   a. 70
   b. 80
   c. 90
   d. 98

59–12. Syphilis of more than 1-year duration should be treated with which of the following?

   a. penicillin V, 250 mg po qid × 10 days
   b. benzathine penicillin G, 2.4 million units IM × 1 dose
   c. benzathine penicillin G, 2.4 million units IM weekly × 3 doses
   d. aqueous penicillin G, 4 million units every 4 hr for 10 days

59–13. What is the best treatment of syphilis in pregnant women who are allergic to penicillin?

   a. ceftriaxone
   b. erythromycin
   c. tetracycline
   d. penicillin desensitization

59–14. Which of the following antibiotics may be curative of syphilis in the mother but may not prevent congenital syphilis?

   a. penicillin
   b. erythromycin
   c. tetracycline
   d. ceftriaxone

59–15. Which of the following is commonly observed with the Jarisch-Herxheimer reaction in pregnancy?

   a. hypotension
   b. uterine quiescence
   c. fetal heart rate decelerations
   d. maternal rash

59–16. In pregnant women with latent syphilis of more than 1-year duration, which of the following is NOT a criterion for recommending lumbar puncture?

   a. neurological symptoms
   b. treatment failures
   c. concomitant human immunodeficiency virus (HIV) infection
   d. serological titer of 1 to 4

59–17. Which of the following treatment protocols is appropriate for the asymptomatic infant whose mother was treated with erythromycin for syphilis?

   a. penicillin G, IV or IM for 10 days
   b. erythromycin, 500 mg po for 4 doses
   c. treat only if stigmata are present
   d. no treatment necessary

59–18. Which of the following is a risk factor for gonorrhea?

   a. married
   b. age >35 years
   c. high socioeconomic status
   d. lack of prenatal care

59–19. Pregnant women with gonorrhea frequently have concurrent infection with which of the following?

   a. *Chlamydia trachomatis*
   b. herpes simplex virus
   c. *Trichomonas vaginalis*
   d. *Haemophilus ducreyi*

59–20. What is the treatment of choice for uncomplicated gonorrhea in pregnancy?

   a. ceftriaxone
   b. penicillin
   c. erythromycin
   d. azithromycin

59–21. Which of the following is used to treat gonorrhea in pregnant women allergic to β-lactam drugs?

    a. ciprofloxacin
    b. cefixime
    c. doxycycline
    d. spectinomycin

59–22. Which of the following is NOT a manifestation or sign of disseminated gonococcal infection in adults?

    a. blindness
    b. pustular skin lesions
    c. arthralgias
    d. endocarditis

59–23. Which of the following is an obligate intracellular bacterium?

    a. *Treponema pallidum*
    b. *Borrelia burgdorferi*
    c. *Chlamydia trachomatis*
    d. *Escherichia coli*

59–24. Which of the following is the most common bacterial sexually transmitted disease in women?

    a. gonorrhea
    b. herpes simplex virus infection
    c. chancroid
    d. chlamydial infection

59–25. Which of the following is the most common presentation of chlamydial infection in pregnancy?

    a. asymptomatic infection
    b. complaint of vaginal discharge
    c. septic abortion
    d. fetal growth restriction

59–26. Vertical transmission of chlamydia is associated with which of the following neonatal infections?

    a. sepsis
    b. conjunctivitis
    c. urinary tract infection
    d. dermatitis

59–27. What percentage of infants born through an infected cervix will develop chlamydial conjunctivitis?

    a. 1 to 5
    b. 10 to 20
    c. 30 to 50
    d. 90 to 100

59–28. Infants who develop *C. trachomatis* pneumonitis are LEAST likely to demonstrate which of the following clinical features?

    a. chronic cough
    b. fever
    c. poor weight gain
    d. pulmonary infiltrates

59–29. Of the following, which is the best treatment for chlamydial cervicitis in pregnancy?

    a. erythromycin estolate, 250 mg po qid × 4 days
    b. tetracycline, 500 mg po qid × 7 days
    c. erythromycin base, 500 mg po qid × 7 days
    d. ciprofloxacin, 500 mg po bid × 14 days

59–30. What is the cure rate for chlamydial infections in pregnancy treated with azithromycin?

    a. 22%
    b. 44%
    c. 66%
    d. 88%

59–31. Lymphogranuloma venereum is most difficult to differentiate from which of the following?

    a. chancroid
    b. granuloma inguinale
    c. herpesvirus vulvitis
    d. syphilis

59–32. Nongenital herpesvirus infections are generally caused by which of the following?

    a. HSV 1
    b. HSV 2
    c. HSV 6
    d. HSV 11

59–33. Serological screening of couples during pregnancy for HSV 2 has been shown to prevent which of the following?

    a. HSV transmission
    b. neonatal infection
    c. sexual relations during pregnancy
    d. none of the above

59–34. What is the average incubation time for primary herpesvirus infection?

    a. 3 to 6 days
    b. 14 to 21 days
    c. 28 to 40 days
    d. 100 to 120 days

59–35. How long does it take for all signs and symptoms of primary herpesvirus infection to resolve?

    a. 3 to 5 days
    b. 7 to 10 days
    c. 14 to 28 days
    d. 35 to 50 days

59–36. Which of the following is the "gold standard" for the diagnosis of genital herpesvirus infection in adults?

   a. tissue culture
   b. enzyme-linked immunosorbent assay (ELISA) tests or serology
   c. deoxyribonucleic acid (DNA) probes
   d. cervical smear cytological examination

59–37. What proportion of women overall will have a positive herpes culture result during labor?

   a. <0.03
   b. 0.3
   c. 3
   d. 13

59–38. Acquisition of neonatal herpesvirus infection occurs most frequently in which of the following settings?

   a. antepartum
   b. across intact fetal membranes
   c. peripartum
   d. postnatally

59–39. What is the risk of neonatal herpesvirus infection with primary maternal infection during labor?

   a. <1%
   b. 5%
   c. 20%
   d. 50%

59–40. What is the risk of neonatal herpesvirus infection with recurrent maternal infection during labor?

   a. 5%
   b. 15%
   c. 25%
   d. 50%

59–41. What is the mortality rate of disseminated neonatal herpesvirus infection?

   a. 10%
   b. 30%
   c. 50%
   d. 70%

59–42. In disseminated neonatal herpesvirus infection, serious nervous system damage is seen in at least what percentage of survivors?

   a. 5 to 10
   b. 20 to 50

   c. 70 to 80
   d. 100

59–43. How often is HIV infection responsible for death in persons between the ages of 25 and 44 years?

   a. tenth leading cause
   b. fifth leading cause
   c. third leading cause
   d. most common cause

59–44. What type of virus is the human immunodeficiency virus (HIV)?

   a. ribonucleic acid (RNA) virus
   b. deoxyribonucleic acid (DNA) virus
   c. RNA retrovirus
   d. DNA retrovirus

59–45. What is the most common mode of transmission of HIV-1?

   a. fecal–orally
   b. parenterally
   c. sexually
   d. perinatally

59–46. What is the median time interval from asymptomatic viremia to the acquired immunodeficiency syndrome in HIV infection?

   a. 2 years
   b. 5 years
   c. 10 years
   d. 20 years

59–47. What CD4+ count is definitive for a diagnosis of acquired immune deficiency syndrome (AIDS)?

   a. <50 mm^3
   b. <100 mm^3
   c. <200 mm^3
   d. <500 mm^3

59–48. What is the screening test for HIV?

   a. viral p24 antigen assay
   b. HIV antibody enzyme immunoassay (EIA)
   c. HIV antibody Western blot
   d. HIV antibody immunofluorescence assay (IFA)

59–49. Rapid tests can detect HIV antibodies in what length of time?

   a. 1 to 6 min
   b. 10 to 60 min
   c. 1 to 2 hr
   d. 4 to 5 hr

59–50. Prenatal testing rates are higher with which approach to the patient?

    a. risk factor assessment approach
    b. age assessment approach
    c. opt-in approach
    d. opt-out approach

59–51. Combination antiretroviral therapy is indicated when the maternal HIV RNA exceeds which of the following?

    a. 50 copies/mL
    b. 100 copies/mL
    c. 500 copies/mL
    d. 1000 copies/mL

59–52. What is the rate of perinatal transmission of the HIV virus in untreated women?

    a. 5 to 10%
    b. 15 to 40%
    c. 50 to 60%
    d. 80 to 90%

59–53. Which of the following increases the risk of perinatal HIV transmission?

    a. high maternal plasma HIV RNA level
    b. premature delivery
    c. prolonged rupture of membranes
    d. all of the above

59–54. At what CD4+ count minimum level is primary prophylaxis for *Pneumocystis carinii* pneumonia recommended?

    a. $<200/\mu L$
    b. $<100/\mu L$
    c. $<75/\mu L$
    d. $<50/\mu L$

59–55. What is the rate of perinatal transmission in women given HAART (highly active antiretroviral therapy)?

    a. $<2\%$
    b. 8%
    c. 15%
    d. 25%

59–56. The U.S. Public Health Service perinatal guidelines state that zidovudine treatment alone is acceptable for all of the following scenarios EXCEPT

    a. maternal HIV RNA level is 600 copies/mL
    b. maternal HIV RNA level is 1500 copies/mL
    c. treatment of newborn with no maternal intrapartum treatment
    d. no prior treatment, in active labor at 34 weeks

59–57. How is the HIV transmission risk affected by breast feeding?

    a. increased
    b. decreased
    c. unaffected
    d. unknown

59–58. What is the etiology of mucocutaneous external genital warts?

    a. *Treponema pallidum*
    b. human papillomavirus
    c. parvovirus
    d. *Hemophilus ducreyi*

59–59. What is a useful modality for treatment of condylomata accuminata during pregnancy?

    a. podophyllin resin
    b. interferon
    c. trichloracetic acid
    d. 5-fluorouracil

59–60. Of the following viral types, which are associated with laryngeal papillomatosis?

    a. HPV 6/11
    b. HPV 16/18
    c. HPV 31/35
    d. HPV 51/52

59–61. What is the etiology of soft chancres?

    a. *Treponema pallidum*
    b. *Haemophilus ducreyi*
    c. *Trichomonas vaginalis*
    d. *Calymmatobacterium granulomatis*

59–62. Which of the following is a recommended treatment for chancroid in pregnancy?

    a. ceftriaxone, 125 mg IM once
    b. erythromycin, 250 mg bid for 3 days
    c. azithromycin, 1 g po once
    d. metronidazole, 2 g po once

59–63. How sensitive is a vaginal secretion wet mount for the detection of trichomoniasis?

    a. 20%
    b. 40%
    c. 60%
    d. 100%

59–64. Which drug is an alternative to metronidazole for the treatment of trichomoniasis?

    a. ampicillin
    b. ciprofolxacin
    c. spectinomycin
    d. none is available

ANSWERS

CHAPTER 1

1–1. **b** (*p. 4*) Vital Statistics

1–2. **b** (*p. 4*) Vital Statistics

1–3. **a** (*p. 5*) Definitions

1–4. **b** (*p. 5*) Definitions

1–5. **b** (*p. 5*) Definitions

1–6. **d** (*p. 5*) Definitions

1–7. **a** (*p. 5*) Definitions

1–8. **c** (*p. 5*) Definitions

1–9. **d** (*p. 5*) Definitions

1–10. **d** (*p. 5*) Definitions

1–11. **b** (*p. 5*) Definitions

1–12. **b** (*p. 5*) Definitions

1–13. **c** (*p. 6*) Pregnancy in the US

1–14. **b** (*p. 6*) Pregnancy in the US

1–15. **b** (*p. 6*) Pregnancy in the US

1–16. **b** (*p. 6*) Pregnancy in the US

1–17. **d** (*p. 6*) Pregnancy in the US

1–18. **c** (*p. 6*) Pregnancy in the US

1–19. **a** (*p. 6*) Pregnancy in the US

1–20. **d** (*p. 7*) Infant Deaths

1–21. **a** (*p. 7*) Maternal Deaths

1–22. **d** (*p. 7*) Maternal Deaths

1–23. **a** (*p. 7*) Maternal Deaths

1–24. **c** (*p. 7*) Maternal Deaths

1–25. **b** (*p. 8*) Maternal Deaths

1–26. **c** (*p. 8*) Rising Cesarean Delivery

1–27. **d** (*p. 8*) Rising Cesarean Delivery

1–28. **c** (*p. 8*) Women in Obstetrics

1–29. **d** (*p. 9*) Medical Liability

1–30. **d** (*p. 10*) Uninsured People

1–31. **a** (*p. 10*) Birth Control

CHAPTER 2

2–1. **b** (*p. 16*) Labia Majora

2–2. **a** (*p. 17*) Clitoris

2–3. **b** (*p. 17*) Clitoris

2–4. **c** (*p. 17*) Labia Minora

2–5. **c** (*p. 17*) Clitoris

2–6. **b** (*p. 17*) Vestibule

2–7. **d** (*p. 17*) Vestibule

2–8. **d** (*p. 17*) Vaginal Opening and Hymen

2–9. **c** (*p. 18*) Vaginal Opening and Hymen

2–10. **c** (*p. 18*) Vagina

2–11. **b** (*p. 18*) Vagina

2–12. **d** (*p. 18*) Vagina

2–13. **d** (*p. 19*) Vagina

2–14. **a** (*p. 19*) Vagina

2–15. **b** (*p. 19*) Vagina

2–16. **c** (*p. 20*) Perineum

2–17. **d** (*p. 21*) Size and Shape

2–18. **a** (*p. 22*) Size and Shape

2–19. **c** (*pp. 16, 17, 22, 23*) External Generative Organs

2–20. **b** (*p. 23*) Myometrium

2–21. **a** (*p. 22*) Pregnancy-Induced Werine Changes

2–22. **a** (*p. 24*) Ligaments

2–23. **d** (*p. 24*) Ligaments

2–24. **c** (*p. 24*) Ligaments

2–25. **b** (*p. 24*) Blood Vessels

2–26. **b** (*p. 25*) Blood Vessels

2–27. **a** (*p. 25*) Blood Vessels

2–28. **a** (*p. 26*) Blood Vessels

2–29. **c** (*p. 26*) Lymphatics

2–30. **b** (*p. 27*) Innervation

2–31. **d** (*p. 27*) Oviducts

2–32. **a** (*p. 28*) Embryological Development of the Uterus and Oviducts

2–33. **a** (*p. 29*) Ovaries

2–34. **b** (*p. 30*) Histology

2–35. **b** (*p. 31*) Histology

2–36. **a** (*p. 31*) Embryological Remnants

2–37. **a** (*p. 31*) Embryological Remnants

2–38. **d** (*p. 31*) The Bony Pelvis

2–39. **b** (*p. 34*) Relaxation of the Pelvic Joints

2–40. **a** (*p. 31*) Pelvic Anatomy

2–41. **d** (*p. 34*) Pelvic Inlet

2–42. **b** (*p. 34*) Pelvic Inlet

2–43. **b** (*p. 34*) Pelvic Inlet

2–44. **c** (*p. 34*) Midpelvis

2–45. **a** (*p. 35*) Fig. 2-24

2–46. **b** (*p. 35*) Fig. 2-24

2–47. **c** (*p. 35*) Fig. 2-24

2–48. **a** (*p. 35*) Pelvic Shapes

2–49. **d** (*p. 36*) Pelvic Inlet Measurements

2–50. **b** (*p. 37*) Engagement

2–51. **c** (*p. 37*) Pelvic Outlet Measurements

CHAPTER 3

3–1. **c** (*p. 40*) Follicular Ovarian Phase

3–2. **c** (*p. 40*) Follicular Ovarian Phase

3–3. **c** (*p. 41*) Follicular Ovarian Phase

3–4. **a** (*p. 42*) Follicular Ovarian Phase

3–5. **b** (*p. 42*) Follicular Ovarian Phase

3–6. **d** (*p. 42*) Follicular Ovarian Phase

3–7. **a** (*p. 42*) Ovulation

3–8. **c** (*p. 43*) Luteal Phase of Ovary

3–9. **c** (*p. 43*) Estrogen and Progesterone Action

3–10. **c** (*p. 43*) Estrogen and Progesterone Action

3–11. **a** (*p. 43*) Estrogen and Progesterone Action

3–12. **b** (*p. 44*) Proliferative Phase of the Endometrium

3–13. **d** (*p. 46*) Secretory Phase of the Endometrium

3–14. **b** (*p. 47*) Menstruation

3–15. **c** (*p. 48*) Prostaglandins and Menstruation

3–16. **b** (*p. 49*) Decidual Structure

3–17. **b** (*p. 51*) Decidual Histology

3–18. **a** (*p. 51*) Decidual Prolactin Production

3–19. **d** (*p. 51*) Decidual Prolactin Production

3–20. **a** (*p. 52*) Ovum Fertilization and Zygote Cleavage

3–21. **b** (*p. 52*) Ovum Fertilization and Zygote Cleavage

3–22. **b** (*p. 52*) Ovum Fertilization and Zygote Cleavage

3–23. **d** (*p. 52*) Ovum Fertilization and Zygote Cleavage

3–24. **b** (*p. 52*) Implantation of the Blastocyst

3–25. **c** (*p. 52*) Implantation of the Blastocyst

3–26. **a** (*p. 52*) Implantation of the Blastocyst

3–27. **d** (*p. 54*) Trophoblast Differentiation

3–28. **c** (*p. 56*) Chorionic Villi

3–29. **d** (*p. 57*) Development of the Chorion and Decidua

3–30. **c** (*p. 58*) Development of the Chorion and Decidua

3–31. **c** (*p. 59*) Trophoblast Invasion of the Endometrium

3–32. **b** (*p. 61*) Placental Growth

3–33. **b** (*p. 61*) Placental Growth

3–34. **c** (*p. 61*) Placental Maturation

3–35. **a** (*p. 63*) Fetal Circulation

3–36. **d** (*p. 64*) Maternal Circulation

3–37. **d** (*p. 64*) Breaks in the Placental 'Barrier'

3–38. **d** (*p. 66*) Uterine Large Granular Lymphocytes (LGLs)

3–39. **c** (*p. 66*) HLA-G Expression in Human Trophoblasts

3–40. **b** (*p. 66*) Amnion Structure

3–41. **d** (*p. 67*) Amnion Epithelial Cells

3–42. **c** (*p. 68*) Amnionic Fluid

3–43. **b** (*p. 69*) Cord Development

3–44. **b** (*p. 69*) Cord and Structure

3–45. **a** (*p. 69*) Cord and Structure

3–46. **d** (*p. 71*) Chemical Characteristics

3–47. **b** (*p. 71*) Chemical Characteristics

3–48. **c** (*p. 71*) Biosynthesis

3–49. **b** (*p. 71*) Free Subunits

3–50. **b** (*p. 71*) Concentrations of hCG in Plasma and Urine

3–51. **b** (*p. 72*) Elevated or Depressed hCG Levels in Maternal Plasma or Urine

3–52. **d** (*p. 72*) Biological Functions

3–53. **a** (*p. 72*) Biological Functions

3–54. **d** (*p. 73*) Chemical Characteristics

3–55. **c** (*p. 73*) Gene Structure and Expression

3–56. **d** (*p. 73*) Serum Concentration

3–57. **d** (*p. 74*) Metabolic Actions

3–58. **c** (*p. 74*) Relaxin

3–59. **c** (*p. 74*) Growth Hormone-Variant (hGH-V)

3–60. **b** (*p. 75*) Gonadotropin-Releasing Hormone (GnRH)

3–61. **a** (*p. 76*) Inhibin and Activin

3–62. **b** (*p. 76*) Placental Progesterone Production

3–63. **c** (*p. 77*) Source of Cholesterol for Placental Progesterone Biosynthesis

3–64. **c** (*p. 77*) Source of Cholesterol for Placental Progesterone Biosynthesis

3–65. **d** (*p. 77*) Placental Estrogen Biosynthesis

3–66. **d** (*p. 77*) Placental Estrogen Biosynthesis

3–67. **b** (*p. 78*) Plasma C19-Steroids as Estrogen Precursors

3–68. **c** (*p. 78*) Fetal Adrenal Glands

3–69. **a** (*p. 79*) Fetal Adrenal Morphology

3–70. **a** (*p. 80*) Fetal Adrenal Steroid Production

3–71. **c** (*p. 81*) Fetal Anencephaly

3–72. **d** (*p. 81*) Deficiency in Fetal LDL Cholesterol Biosynthesis

3–73. **b** (*p. 81*) Fetal-Placental Sulfatase Deficiency

CHAPTER 4

4–1. **c** (*p. 92*) Determination of Gestational Age

4–2. **d** (*p. 92*) Determination of Gestational Age

4–3. **b** (*p. 92*) Determination of Gestational Age

4–4. **d** (*p. 92*) Determination of Gestational Age

4–5. **c** (*p. 93*) Embryo

4–6. **a** (*p. 93*) Embryo

4–7. **b** (*p. 93*) Embryo

4–8. **c** (*p. 93*) 12 Gestational Weeks

4–9. **b** (*p. 93*) 12 Gestational Weeks

4–10. **c** (*p. 93*) 12 Gestational Weeks

4–11. **c** (*p. 94*) 24 Gestational Weeks

4–12. **b** (*p. 94*) 24 Gestational Weeks

4–13. **c** (*p. 94*) 28 Gestational Weeks

4–14. **d** (*p. 94*) 28 Gestational Weeks

4–15. **d** (*p. 94*) 28 Gestational Weeks

4–16. **c** (*p. 94*) 32 Gestational Weeks

4–17. **b** (*p. 95*) 36 Gestational Weeks

4–18. **c** (*p. 95*) 40 Gestational Weeks

4–19. **c** (*p. 95*) Fetal Head

4–20. **d** (*p. 96*) Fetal Head

4–21. **b** (*p. 97*) Fetal Head

4–22. **a** (*p. 97*) Fetal Head

4–23. **b** (*p. 97*) Fetal Head

4–24. **d** (*p. 97*) Fetal Head

4–25. **c** (*p. 97*) The Intervillous Space: Maternal Blood

4–26. **a** (*p. 97*) The Intervillous Space: Maternal Blood

4–27. **c** (*p. 98*) Chorionic Villus

4–28. **a** (*p. 99*) Mechanisms of Transfer

4–29. **a** (*p. 99*) Mechanisms of Transfer

4–30. **c** (*p. 99*) Mechanisms of Transfer

4–31. **b** (*p. 99*) Transfer of Oxygen and Carbon Dioxide

4–32. **c** (*p. 99*) Transfer of Oxygen and Carbon Dioxide

4–33. **c** (*p. 100*) Glucose Transport

4–34. **a** (*p. 100*) Glucose Transport

4–35. **b** (*p. 101*) Amino Acids

4–36. **d** (*p. 101*) Proteins

4–37. **a** (*p. 101*) Placental Sequestration of Heavy Metals

4–38. **a** (*p. 101*) Calcium and Phosphorus

4–39. **b** (*p. 102*) Amnionic Fluid

4–40. **d** (*p. 102*) Amnionic Fluid

4–41. **c** (*p. 102*) Fetal Circulation

4–42. **b** (*p. 103*) Fetal Circulation

4–43. **b** (*p. 103*) Fetal Circulation

4–44. **d** (*p. 103*) Hemopoiesis

4–45. **d** (*p. 104*) Hemopoiesis

4–46. **a** (*p. 104*) Erythropoiesis

4–47. **d** (*p. 104*) Fetal Blood Volume

4–48. **c** (*p. 105*) Fetal Hemoglobin

4–49. **c** (*p. 105*) Fetal Hemoglobin

4–50. **a** (*p. 105*) Fetal Coagulation Factors

4–51. **d** (*p. 105*) Fetal Coagulation Factors

4–52. **d** (*p. 106*) Immunoglobulin G

4–53. **c** (*p. 106*) Immunoglobulin A

4–54. **b** (*p. 106*) Nervous System and Sensory Organs

4–55. **b** (*p. 106*) Nervous System and Sensory Organs

4–56. **c** (*p. 106*) Nervous System and Sensory Organs

4–57. **d** (*p. 107*) Meconium

4–58. **a** (*p. 107*) Liver

4–59. **b** (*p. 108*) Pancreas

4–60. **b** (*p. 108*) Urinary System

4–61. **c** (*p. 108*) Urinary System

4–62. **a** (*p. 109*) Surfactant

4–63. **d** (*p. 109*) Surfactant Composition

4–64. **a** (*p. 109*) Surfactant Synthesis

4–65. **c** (*p. 110*) Surfactant Synthesis

4–66. **a** (*p. 110*) Respiration

4–67. **d** (*p. 111*) Anterior Pituitary

4–68. **b** (*p. 111*) Thyroid Gland

4–69. **a** (*p. 111*) Thyroid Gland

4–70. **d** (*p. 112*) Gonadal Gender

4–71. **c** (*p. 113*) Gonadal Gender

4–72. **c** (*p. 114*) Fetal Testicular Contributions to Male Sexual Differentiation

4–73. **c** (*p. 114*) Fetal Testosterone Secretion

4–74. **a** (*p. 114*) Genital Ambiguity of the Newborn

4–75. **d** (*p. 114*) Category 1. Female Pseudohermaphroditism

4–76. **c** (*p. 115*) Category 2. Male Pseudohermaphroditism

4–77. **d** (*p. 115*) Androgen Insensitivity Syndrome

4–78. **b** (*p. 115*) Androgen Insensitivity Syndrome

4–79. **c** (*p. 115*) Androgen Insensitivity Syndrome

4–80. **a** (*p. 116*) Category 3. Dysgenetic Gonads

CHAPTER 5

5–1. **d** (*p. 122*) Uterus

5–2. **b** (*p. 122*) Uterus

5–3. **b** (*p. 122*) Uterine Size, Shape, and Position

5–4. **a** (*p. 123*) Contractility

5–5. **c** (*p. 123*) Contractility

5–6. **d** (*p. 123*) Contractility

5–7. **a** (*p. 123*) Cervix

5–8. **a** (*p. 124*) Ovaries

5–9. **d** (*p. 124*) Relaxin

5–10. **b** (*p. 125*) Pregnancy Luteoma

5–11. **d** (*p. 125*) Theca-Lutein Cysts

5–12. **a** (*p. 125*) Theca-Lutein Cysts

5–13. **a** (*p. 125*) Vagina and Perineum

5–14. **b** (*p. 126*) Pigmentation

5–15. **d** (*p. 126*) Skin

5–16. **b** (*p. 126*) Breasts

5–17. **c** (*p. 126*) Weight Gain

5–18. **c** (*p. 127*) Water Metabolism

5–19. **c** (*p. 127*) Protein Metabolism

5–20. **b** (*p. 127*) Carbohydrate Metabolism

5–21. **b** (*p. 128*) Fat Metabolism

5–22. **a** (*p. 129*) Electrolyte and Mineral Metabolism

5–23. **c** (*p. 129*) Blood Volume

5–24. **c** (*p. 129*) Blood Volume

5–25. **c** (*p. 129*) Hemoglobin Concentration and Hematocrit

5–26. **a** (*p. 130*) Iron Stores

5–27. **c** (*p. 130*) Iron Requirements

5–28. **b** (*p. 130*) Iron Requirements

5–29. **c** (*p. 130*) Iron Requirements

5–30. **b** (*p. 130*) Blood Loss

5–31. **c** (*p. 130*) Blood Loss

5–32. **d** (*p. 130*) Immunological and Leukocyte Function

5–33. **c** (*p. 131*) Coagulation

5–34. **d** (*p. 131*) Coagulation

5–35. **d** (*p. 132*) Regulatory Proteins

5–36. **a** (*p. 132*) Regulatory Proteins

5–37. **a** (*p. 132*) Cardiovascular System

5–38. **c** (*p. 132*) Heart

5–39. **b** (*p. 132*) Heart

5–40. **d** (*p. 133*) Heart

5–41. **c** (*p. 133*) Heart

5–42. **a** (*p. 133*) Cardiac Output

5–43. **d** (*p. 134*) Hemodynamic Function in Late Pregnancy

5–44. **a** (*p. 134*) Circulation and Blood Pressure

5–45. **c** (*p. 135*) Renin, Angiotensin II, and Plasma Volume

5–46. **d** (*p. 135*) Prostaglandins

5–47. **c** (*p. 136*) Respiratory Tract

5–48. **d** (*p. 136*) Pulmonary Function

5–49. **d** (*p. 137*) Acid-Base Equilibrium

5–50. **d** (*p. 137*) Kidney

5–51. **b** (*p. 137*) Urinalysis

5–52. **b** (*p. 139*) Ureters

5–53. **d** (*p. 139*) Bladder

5–54. **b** (*p. 139*) Bladder

5–55. **d** (*p. 140*) Gastrointestinal Tract

5–56. **c** (*p. 140*) Liver

5–57. **a** (*p. 140*) Gallbladder

5–58. **a** (*p. 141*) Pituitary Gland

5–59. **b** (*p. 141*) Growth Hormone

5–60. **d** (*p. 141*) Prolactin

5–61. b (*p. 141*) Prolactin

5–62. a (*p. 142*) Thyroid Gland

5–63. d (*p. 142*) Parathyroid Hormone and Calcium

5–64. a (*p. 143*) Calcitonin and Calcium

5–65. a (*p. 143*) Vitamin D and Calcium

5–66. b (*p. 143*) Cortisol

5–67. b (*p. 143*) Aldosterone

5–68. a (*p. 144*) Androstenedione and Testosterone

5–69. d (*p. 144*) Musculoskeletal System

5–70. c (*p. 145*) Central Nervous System

CHAPTER 6

6–1. c (*p. 152*) Phases of Parturition

6–2. d (*p. 152*) Phase 0 of Parturition: Uterine Quiescence

6–3. c (*p. 153*) Phase 1 of Parturition: Preparation for Labor

6–4. c (*p. 153*) Myometrial Changes

6–5. d (*p. 154*) Uterine Contractions Characteristic of Labor

6–6. c (*p. 155*) Uterine Contractions Characteristic of Labor

6–7. a (*p. 156*) Formation of Distinct Lower and Upper Uterine Segments

6–8. c (*p. 156*) Ancillary Forces in Labor

6–9. b (*p. 156*) Ancillary Forces in Labor

6–10. d (*p. 157*) Cervical Changes Induced During the First Stage of Labor

6–11. a (*p. 157*) Cervical Changes Induced During the First Stage of Labor

6–12. a (*p. 160*) Changes in the Pelvic Floor During Labor

6–13. c (*p. 160*) Changes in the Pelvic Floor During Labor

6–14. b (*p. 161*) Placental Extrusion

6–15. d (*p. 161*) Phase 3 of Parturition: The Pueperium

6–16. c (*p. 162*) Physiological and Biochemical Processes Regulating Parturition

6–17. b (*p. 162*) Regulation of Myometrial Contraction and Relaxation

6–18. b (*p. 162*) Regulation of Myometrial Contraction and Relaxation

6–19. d (*p. 162*) Regulation of Myometrial Contraction and Relaxation

6–20. c (*p. 163*) Myometrial Gap Junction

6–21. a (*p. 163*) A Fail-Safe System that Maintains Uterine Quiescence

6–22. b (*p. 165*) Progesterone and Estrogen Contributions to Phase 0 of Parturition

6–23. b (*p. 165*) Steroid Hormone Regulation of Myometrial . . .

6–24. b (*p. 166*) Relaxin

6–25. b (*p. 166*) Relaxin

6–26. b (*p. 166*) Corticotropin-Releasing Hormone (CRH)

6–27. a (*p. 166*) Parathyroid Hormone-Related Protein

6–28. b (*p. 166*) Prostaglandins

6–29. d (*p. 167*) Accelerated Uterotonin Degradation . . .

6–30. c (*p. 168*) Functional Progesterone Withdrawal . . .

6–31. c (*p. 169*) Oxytocin Receptors

6–32. d (*p. 172*) Fetal Contributions to Initiation . . .

6–33. c (*p. 172*) Oxytocin and Phase 2 of Parturition

6–34. **a** (*p. 172*) Oxytocin and Phase 2 of Parturition

6–35. **d** (*p. 175*) Platelet-Activating Factor (PAF)

6–36. **d** (*p. 175*) Endothelin-1

6–37. **a** (*p. 175*) Amnion

6–38. **c** (*p. 176*) Decidua Parietalis

6–39. **d** (*p. 177*) Preterm Premature Rupture of the Membranes

6–40. **c** (*p. 179*) Infection and Preterm Labor

6–41. **a** (*p. 180*) Origins of Cytokines in Intrauterine Infection

6–42. **d** (*p. 180*) Origins of Cytokines in Intrauterine Infection

6–43. **c** (*p. 180*) Intrauterine Inflammatory Response to Infection

CHAPTER 7

7–1. **d** (*pp. 190, 191*) Benefits of Preconceptual Counseling

7–2. **b** (*p. 190*) Prenatal Counseling

7–3. **d** (*p. 190*) Unplanned Pregnancy

7–4. **d** (*p. 191*) Diabetes Mellitus

7–5. **d** (*p. 198*) Screening Tests

7–6. **b** (*p. 198*) Screening Tests

7–7. **a** (*p. 191*) Epilepsy

7–8. **c** (*p. 191*) Epilepsy

7–9. **c** (*p. 192*) Epilepsy

7–10. **a** (*p. 192*) Genetic Diseases

7–11. **c** (*p. 192*) Neural-Tube Defects (NTDs)

7–12. **c** (*p. 192*) Neural-Tube Defects (NTDs)

7–13. **d** (*p. 192*) Neural-Tube Defects (NTDs)

7–14. **c** (*p. 192*) Phenylketonuria (PKU)

7–15. **d** (*p. 192*) Tay-Sachs Disease

7–16. **d** (*p. 192*) Thalassemias

7–17. **d** (*p. 193*) Thalassemias

7–18. **c** (*p. 194*) Teenage Pregnancy

7–19. **d** (*p. 194*) Pregnancy after Age 35

7–20. **a** (*p. 195*) Pregnancy after Age 35

7–21. **b** (*p. 195*) Pregnancy after Age 35

7–22. **b** (*p. 195*) Pregnancy after Age 35

7–23. **b** (*p. 195*) Recreational Drugs & Smoking

7–24. **c** (*p. 195*) Environmental Exposures

7–25. **c** (*p. 196*) Diet

7–26. **d** (*p. 196*) Diet

7–27. **d** (*p. 196*) Diet

7–28. **c** (*p. 197*) Domestic Abuse

7–29. **b** (*p. 197*) Immunizations

CHAPTER 8

8–1. **d** (*p. 202*) Overview of Prenatal Care

8–2. **a** (*p. 202*) Overview of Prenatal Care

8–3. **a** (*p. 202*) Inadequate Prenatal Care

8–4. **b** (*p. 202*) Inadequate Prenatal Care

8–5. **c** (*p. 202*) Inadequate Prenatal Care

8–6. **b** (*p. 204*) Effectiveness of Prenatal Care

8–7. **b** (*p. 204*) Effectiveness of Prenatal Care

8–8. **d** (*p. 204*) Organization of Prenatal Care

8–9. **b** (*p. 204*) Changes in Cervical Mucus

8–10. **b** (*p. 205*) Discoloration of the Vaginal Mucosa

8–11. **c** (*p. 205*) Changes in the Uterus

8–12. **a** (*p. 205*) Fetal Heart Action

8–13. **c** (*p. 206*) Fetal Heart Action

8–14. **c** (*p. 206*) Perception of Fetal Movement

8–15. **b** (*p. 206*) Chorionic Gonadotropin

8–16. **b** (*p. 206*) Chorionic Gonadotropin

8–17. **b** (*p. 206*) Measurement of hCG

8–18. **b** (*p. 207*) Measurement of hCG

8–19. **b** (*p. 207*) Home Pregnancy Tests

8–20. **c** (*p. 207*) Ultrasonic Recognition of Pregnancy

8–21. **a** (*p. 207*) Ultrasonic Recognition of Pregnancy

8–22. **d** (*p. 207*) Definitions

8–23. **c** (*p. 207*) Definitions

8–24. **b** (*p. 207*) Definitions

8–25. **d** (*p. 207*) Definitions

8–26. **c** (*p. 208*) Definitions

8–27. **d** (*p. 208*) Normal Pregnancy Duration

8–28. **a** (*p. 208*) Normal Pregnancy Duration

8–29. **d** (*p. 208*) Normal Pregnancy Duration

8–30. **a** (*p. 209*) Normal Pregnancy Duration

8–31. **b** (*p. 209*) Cigarette Smoking

8–32. **d** (*p. 209*) Cigarette Smoking

8–33. **d** (*p. 210*) Alcohol and Illicit Drugs During Pregnancy

8–34. **b** (*p. 210*) Domestic Violence Screening

8–35. **d** (*p. 210*) Domestic Violence Screening

8–36. **b** (*p. 208*) Table 8-3

8–37. **c** (*p. 211*) Subsequent Prenatal Visits

8–38. **c** (*p. 212*) Fundal Height

8–39. **d** (*p. 212*) Fetal Heart Sounds

8–40. **c** (*p. 212*) Gestational Diabetes

8–41. **d** (*pp. 210, 212, 213*) Laboratory Tests/ Subsequent Laboratory Tests/Ancillary Prenatal Tests

8–42. **d** (*p. 213*) Group B Streptococcal (GBS) Infection

8–43. **b** (*p. 213*) Special Screening for Genetic Diseases

8–44. **c** (*p. 213*) Nutrition

8–45. **d** (*p. 213*) Recommendations for Weight Gain

8–46. **a** (*p. 213*) Recommendations for Weight Gain

8–47. **d** (*p. 215*) Recommended Daily Allowances

8–48. **b** (*p. 215*) Calories

8–49. **c** (*p. 216*) Minerals

8–50. **d** (*p. 216*) Iron

8–51. **a** (*p. 216*) Iron

8–52. **a** (*p. 216*) Calcium

8–53. **c** (*p. 216*) Calcium

8–54. **d** (*p. 216*) Zinc

8–55. **b** (*p. 216*) Zinc

8–56. **a** (*p. 217*) Iodine

8–57. **c** (*p. 217*) Iodine

8–58. **d** (*p. 217*) Copper

8–59. **a** (*p. 217*) Selenium

8–60. **d** (*p. 218*) Folic Acid

8–61. **c** (*p. 218*) Folic Acid

8–62. **a** (*p. 218*) Folic Acid

8–63. **b** (*p. 218*) Folic Acid

8–64. **c** (*p. 218*) Vitamin A

8–65. **b** (*p. 218*) Vitamin B12

8–66. **c** (*p. 218*) Vitamin B12

8–67. **d** (*p. 218*) Vitamin C

8–68. **c** (*p. 219*) Exercise

8–69. **b** (*p. 219*) Employment

8–70. **d** (*p. 219*) Employment

8–71. **d** (*p. 220*) Travel

8–72. **d** (*p. 220*) Travel

8–73. **b** (*p. 220*) Travel

8–74. **a** (*p. 221*) Coitus

8–75. **b** (*p. 222*) Table 8-9

8–76. **b** (*p. 223*) Table 8-9

8–77. **a** (*p. 222*) Table 8-9

8–78. **b** (*p. 222*) Table 8-9

8–79. **a** (*p. 222*) Table 8-9

8–80. **d** (*p. 222*) Table 8-9

8–81. **d** (*p. 221*) Biological Warfare and Vaccines

8–82. **d** (*p. 224*) Caffeine

8–83. **d** (*p. 224*) Medications

8–84. **d** (*p. 224*) Nausea and Vomiting

8–85. **a** (*p. 224*) Nausea and Vomiting

8–86. **d** (*pp. 224, 225*) Backache/Varicosities/ Heartburn

8–87. **c** (*p. 225*) Pica

8–88. **c** (*p. 225*) Fatigue

8–89. **d** (*pp. 225, 226*) Bacterial Vaginosis/ Trichomoniasis/Candidiasis

CHAPTER 9

9–1. **d** (*p. 232*) Abortion

9–2. **a** (*p. 232*) Pathology

9–3. **a** (*p. 232*) Etiology

9–4. **d** (*p. 232*) Etiology

9–5. **c** (*p. 233*) Aneuploid Abortion

9–6. **d** (*p. 233*) Euploid Abortion

9–7. **b** (*pp. 232, 233, 234, 235*) Etiology/Infections/ Diabetes Mellitus/ Autoimmune Factors

9–8. **a** (*p. 234*) Caffeine/Nutrition

9–9. **a** (*p. 235*) Environmental Toxins

9–10. **d** (*p. 236*) Acquired Uterine Defects

9–11. **b** (*p. 235*) Autoimmune Factors

9–12. **a** (*p. 235*) Autoimmune Factors

9–13. **a** (*p. 235*) Autoimmune Factors

9–14. **c** (*p. 236*) Acquired Uterine Defects

9–15. **c** (*p. 236*) Acquired Uterine Defects

9–16. **d** (*p. 236*) Acquired Uterine Defects

9–17. **a** (*p. 237*) Etiology

9–18. **b** (*p. 236*) Incomplete Cervix

9–19. **d** (*p. 237*) Treatment

9–20. **d** (*p. 237*) Cerclage Procedures

9–21. **c** (*p. 237*) Preoperative Evaluation

9–22. **b** (*p. 238*) Complications

9–23. **c** (*p. 239*) Threatened Abortion

9–24. **d** (*p. 239*) Threatened Abortion

9–25. **d** (*p. 240*) Threatened Abortion

9–26. **a** (*p. 240*) Complete and Incomplete Abortion

9–27. **b** (*p. 240*) Threatened Abortion

9–28. **a** (*p. 240*) Inevitable Abortion

9–29. **d** (*p. 240*) Missed Abortion

9–30. **c** (*pp. 242, 245*) Surgical Techniques for Abortion/Early Abortion

9–31. **d** (*pp. 243, 245, 247*) Surgical Techniques for Abortion/ Complications/Impact on Future Pregnancy

9–32. **a** (*p. 247*) Impact on Future Pregnancy

9–33. **b** (*p. 243*) Surgical Techniques for Abortion

9–34. **c** (*p. 244*) Hygroscopic Dilators

9–35. **b** (*pp. 243, 244*) Hygroscopic Dilators/ Prostaglandins/Technique for Dilatation and Curettage

9–36. **a** (*p. 244*) Technique for D and C

9–37. **b** (*p. 245*) Early Abortion

9–38. **a** (*p. 246*) Early Abortion

9–39. **b** (*p. 246*) Second-Trimester Abortion

9–40. **a** (*p. 247*) Prostaglandin E$_2$

9–41. **a** (*p. 247*) Resumption of Ovulation After Abortion

CHAPTER 10

10–1. **a** (*p. 254*) Epidemiology

10–2. **a** (*p. 255*) Mortality

10–3. **d** (*p. 254*) Risk Factors

10–4. **b** (*p. 254*) Risk Factors

10–5. **d** (*p. 254*) Failed Contraception

10–6. **b** (*p. 254*) Epidemiology

10–7. **b** (*p. 256*) Tubal Pregnancy

10–8. **d** (*pp. 256, 257*) Tubal Rupture/Interstitial Pregnancy

10–9. **a** (*p. 257*) Heterotypic Ectopic Pregnancy

10–10. **d** (*p. 258*) Clinical Features of Ectopic Pregnancy

10–11. **c** (*p. 258*) Pain

10–12. **d** (*p. 259*) Chorionic Gonadotropin Assays

10–13. **c** (*p. 259*) Serum Progesterone Levels

10–14. **d** (*p. 259*) Abdominal Sonography

10–15. **c** (*p. 259*) Vaginal Sonography

10–16. **c** (*p. 259*) Multimodality Diagnosis

10–17. **b** (*p. 260*) Multimodality Diagnosis

10–18. **d** (*p. 260*) Multimodality Diagnosis

10–19. **d** (*p. 260*) Multimodality Diagnosis

10–20. **d** (*p. 261*) Salpingostomy

10–21. **d** (*p. 261*) Surgical Management

10–22. **d** (*p. 262*) Persistent Trophoblast

10–23. **d** (*p. 262*) Persistent Trophoblast

10–24. **c** (*p. 262*) Systemic Methotrexate

10–25. **d** (*p. 262*) Systemic Methotrexate

10–26. **b** (*p. 263*) Patient Selection

10–27. **d** (*p. 263*) Patient Selection

10–28. **c** (*p. 263*) Dose and Administration

10–29. **a** (*p. 263*) Monitoring Toxicity

10–30. a (*p. 264*) Monitoring Efficacy of Therapy

10–31. c (*p. 265*) Abdominal Pregnancy

10–32. a (*p. 265*) Laboratory Tests

10–33. c (*p. 265*) Sonography

10–34. b (*p. 266*) Management

10–35. b (*p. 267*) Cervical Pregnancy

10–36. d (*p. 268*) Medical Management

CHAPTER 11

11–1. c (*p. 274*) Complete Hydatiform Mole

11–2. d (*p. 275*) Partial Hydatiform Mole

11–3. a (*p. 276*) Partial Hydatiform Mole

11–4. c (*p. 274*) Table 11-2

11–5. c (*p. 276*) Theca-lutein Cysts

11–6. d (*p. 276*) Theca-lutein Cysts

11–7. a (*pp. 276–7*) Age

11–8. c (*p. 277*) Thyrotoxicosis

11–9. a (*p. 277*) Hyperemesis

11–10. d (*p. 277*) Clinical Course

11–11. b (*p. 277*) Diagnostic Features

11–12. b (*p. 278*) Vacuum Aspiration

11–13. a (*p. 278*) Follow Up Evacuation

11–14. d (*p. 279*) Gestational Trophoblastic Neoplasia

11–15. b (*p. 279*) Pathology

11–16. a (*p. 279*) Choriocarcinoma

11–17. b (*p. 279*) Choriocarcinoma

11–18. c (*p. 279*) Gestational Trophoblastic Neoplasic

11–19. c (*p. 281*) Clinical Course

11–20. a (*p. 281*) Diagnosis

11–21. b (*p. 282*) Prognostic Scoring System

11–22. d (*p. 282*) Treatment

11–23. b (*p. 282*) High-Risk Trophoblastic Neoplasic

11–24. d (*p. 282*) Prognosis

11–25. c (*p. 283*) Pregnancy after Gestational Trophoblastic Disease

CHAPTER 12

12–1. b (*p. 286*) Genetics

12–2. b (*p. 286*) Genetics

12–3. c (*p. 286*) Etiology of Birth Defects

12–4. d (*p. 286*) Etiology of Birth Defects

12–5. c (*p. 286*) Standard Nomenclature

12–6. c (*p. 286*) Standard Nomenclature

12–7. a (*p. 289*) Monosomy

12–8. a (*p. 289*) Polyploidy

12–9. d (*p. 289*) Paternal Effects

12–10. a (*p. 289*) Paternal Effects

12–11. d (*p. 289*) Paternal Effects

12–12. a (*p. 290*) Trisomy 21

12–13. a (*p. 290*) Recurrence Risk

12–14. c (*p. 288*) Table 12-4

12–15. a (*p. 288*) Table 12-4

12–16. c (*p. 288*) Table 12-5

12–17. b (*p. 290*) Trisomy 18

12–18. d (*p. 290*) Trisomy 18

12–19. c (*p. 291*) Trisomy 13

12–20. c (*p. 291*) XXX and XXY

12–21. d (*p. 291*) 47 XYY

12–22. d (*p. 291*) 45, X

12–23. b (*p. 292*) Chromosomal Deletions

12–24. b (*p. 292*) Deletion 4p

12–25. c (*p. 292*) Shprintzen and DiGeorge Phenotypes

12–26. a (*p. 293*) Robertsonian Translocation

12–27. a (*p. 294*) Robertsonian Translocation

12–28. a (*p. 294*) Robertsonian Translocation

12–29. b (*p. 294*) Chromosomal Inversion

12–30. a (*p. 295*) Chromosomal Mosaicism

12–31. b (*p. 296*) Autosomal Dominant/Penetrance

12–32. d (*p. 296*) Anticipation

12–33. d (*p. 296*) Table 12-6

12–34. c (*p. 296*) Table 12-6

12–35. c (*p. 296*) Table 12-6

12–36. d (*p. 297*) Phenylketonuria

12–37. c (*p. 297*) Consanguinity

12–38. d (*p. 297*) Consanguinity

12–39. a (*p. 298*) X-linked and Y-linked Genes

12–40. a (*p. 298*) Fragile X Syndrome

12–41. c (*p. 298*) Fragile X Syndrome

12–42. d (*p. 298*) Fragile X Syndrome

12–43. d (*p. 298*) Fragile X Syndrome

12–44. a (*p. 299*) Myotonic Dystrophy

12–45. c (*p. 299*) Myotonic Dystrophy

12–46. b (*p. 299*) Imprinting

12–47. c (*p. 299*) Imprinting

12–48. c (*p. 300*) Uniparental Disomy

12–49. d (*p. 300*) Mitochondrial Inheritance

12–50. d (*p. 302*) Examples of Multifactorial or Polygenic Defects

12–51. d (*p. 302*) Neural-Tube Defects

12–52. c (*pp. 302, 303*) Neural-Tube Defects/Cardiac Defects

12–53. c (*p. 304*) Molecular Genetics

12–54. b (*p. 305*) Organization of the Genome

12–55. a (*p. 305*) Coding DNA: Genes

12–56. d (*p. 305*) Coding DNA: Genes

12–57. c (*p. 307*) Fluorescence In Situ Hybrid (FISH)

12–58. b (*p. 308*) Southern Blotting

12–59. c (*p. 308*) Polymerase Chain Reaction (PCR)

12–60. c (*p. 310*) DNA Chips

CHAPTER 13

13–1. b (*p. 314*) Prenatal Diagnosis and Fetal Therapy

13–2. c (*pp. 330, 331, 333, 334*) Percutaneous Umbilical Cord Blood Sampling/ Fetal Tissue Biopsy/Fetal Surgery/Stem Cell Transplantation

13–3. a (*p. 314*) Fetal Aneuploidy

13–4. b (*p. 314*) Fetal Aneuploidy

13–5. b (*p. 314*) Fetal Aneuploidy

13–6. b (*p. 314*) Fetal Aneuploidy

13–7. b (*p. 314*) Fetal Aneuploidy

13–8. c (*p. 314*) Table 13-1

13–9. c (*p. 314*) Fetal Aneuploidy

13–10. a (*p. 315*) Fetal Aneuploidy

13–11. c (*p. 316*) Isolated Structural Anomalies

13–12. d (*p. 316*) Isolated Structural Anomalies

13–13. b (*p. 316*) Congenital Heart Defects

13–14. d (*p. 316*) Congenital Heart Defects

13–15. c (*p. 316*) Congenital Heart Defects

13–16. d (*p. 317*) Neural-Tube Defects

13–17. c (*p. 317*) Neural-Tube Defects

13–18. d (*p. 317*) Neural-Tube Defects

13–19. d (*p. 318*) Ethic Groups at High Risk

13–20. d (*p. 318*) Jewish Ancestry

13–21. c (*p. 319*) Alpha-Fetoprotein (AFP)

13–22. d (*p. 319*) Alpha-Fetoprotein (AFP)

13–23. c (*p. 319*) Alpha-Fetoprotein (AFP)

13–24. d (*p. 319*) Figure 13-2

13–25. d (*p. 319*) Maternal Serum AFP Screening

13–26. a (*p. 320*) Maternal Serum AFP Screening

13–27. d (*p. 320*) Maternal Serum AFP Screening

13–28. d (*p. 321*) Table 13-7

13–29. a (*p. 320*) Maternal Serum AFP Screening

13–30. c (*p. 321*) Ultrasonographic Examination

13–31. d (*p. 321*) Ultrasonographic Examination

13–32. d (*p. 322*) Amniocentesis

13–33. d (*p. 322*) Amniocentesis

13–34. d (*p. 322*) Unexplained Elevated Abnormal Maternal Serum AFP Levels

13–35. b (*p. 323*) Multiple-Marker Screening

13–36. c (*p. 323*) Multiple-Marker Screening

13–37. c (*p. 323*) Multiple-Marker Screening

13–38. c (*p. 324*) First-Trimester Down Syndrome Screening

13–39. c (*p. 325*) Cystic Fibrosis

13–40. b (*p. 325*) Carrier Screening

13–41. d (*p. 325*) Fragile X Syndrome

13–42. d (*p. 326*) Carrier Screening

13–43. b (*p. 326*) Incidental Findings of a Major Structural Defect

13–44. b (*p. 326*) Incidental Findings of a Major Structural Defect

13–45. a (*p. 327*) Nasal Bone

13–46. d (*p. 328*) Second-Trimester Amniocentesis

13–47. d (*p. 328*) Early Amniocentesis

13–48. a (*p. 329*) Chorionic Villus Sampling

13–49. b (*p. 329*) Chorionic Villus Sampling

13–50. b (*p. 329*) Chorionic Villus Sampling

13–51. d (*p. 330*) Percutaneous Umbilical Cord Blood Sampling (PUBS)

13–52. d (*p. 331*) Fetal Tissue Biopsy

13–53. a (*p. 331*) Preimplantation Genetic Diagnosis

13–54. b (*p. 332*) Fetal Medical Therapy

13–55. c (*pp. 332, 333*) Fetal Medical Therapy/Fetal Surgery

13–56. d (*p. 332*) Fetal Surgery

13–57. b (*p. 332*) Urinary Shunts

13–58. c (*p. 333*) Thoracic Shunts

13–59. d (*p. 333*) Congenital Diaphragmatic Hernia

13–60. c (*p. 333*) Congenital Cystic Adenomatoid . . .

13–61. d (*p. 334*) Neural-Tube Defects

CHAPTER 14

14–1. b (*p. 342*) Teratology, Drugs, and Other Medications

14–2. c (*p. 342*) Teratology, Drugs, and Other Medications

14–3. a (*p. 342*) Teratology, Drugs, and Other Medications

14–4. a (*p. 342*) Teratology, Drugs, and Other Medications

14–5. b (*p. 342*) Teratology

14–6. c (*p. 343*) The Defect Must Be Completely Characterized

14–7. c (*p. 343*) Exposure Must Occur During a Critical Developmental Period

14–8. c (*p. 343*) Exposure Must Occur During a Critical Developmental Period

14–9. b (*p. 343*) Exposure Must Occur During a Critical Developmental Period

14–10. c (*p. 343*) Exposure Must Occur During a Critical Developmental Period

14–11. a (*p. 343*) Figure 14-1

14–12. d (*pp. 342, 343, 344*) Evaluation of Potential Teratogens

14–13. c (*p. 344*) Epidemiological Findings Must Be Consistent

14–14. d (*p. 345*) Disruption of Folic Acid Metabolism

14–15. a (*p. 345*) Disruption of Folic Acid Metabolism

14–16. c (*p. 345*) Oxidative Intermediates

14–17. b (*p. 345*) Homeobox Genes

14–18. c (*p. 346*) Paternal Exposures

14–19. a (*p. 342*) Table 14-1

14–20. a (*pp. 346, 347*) Alcohol

14–21. d (*p. 347*) Dose Effect

14–22. b (*p. 347*) Dose Effect

14–23. a (*p. 348*) Anticonvulsant Medications

14–24. c (*pp. 348, 349*) Anticonvulsant Medications

14–25. a (*p. 348*) Table 14-4

14–26. c (*p. 349*) Warfarin Compounds

14–27. b (*p. 349*) Angiotensin-Converting Enzyme (ACE) Inhibitors

14–28. b (*p. 350*) Vitamin A

14–29. a (*p. 351*) Isoretinoin

14–30. c (*p. 351*) Isoretinoin

14–31. b (*p. 351*) Etretinate

14–32. a (*p. 351*) Etretinate

14–33. b (*p. 352*) Hormones

14–34. a (*p. 352*) Danazol

14–35. c (*p. 352*) Diethylstilbestrol

14–36. c (*p. 352*) Diethylstilbestrol

14–37. b (*p. 353*) Cyclophosphamide

14–38. c (*p. 353*) Methotrexate and Aminopterin

14–39. b (*p. 353*) Tetracyclines

14–40. d (*p. 353*) Sulfonamides

14–41. a (*p. 353*) Sulfonamides

14–42. d (*p. 353*) Griseofulvin

14–43. d (*p. 353*) Antivirals

14–44. d (*p. 354*) Antimalarials

14–45. b (*p. 354*) Tobacco

14–46. b (*p. 354*) Tobacco

14–47. d (*p. 354*) Cocaine

14–48. c (*p. 354*) Cocaine

14–49. d (*p. 354*) Cocaine

14–50. b (*p. 355*) Thalidomide

14–51. d (*p. 355*) Thalidomide

14–52. d (*p. 355*) Methyl Mercury

14–53. d (*p. 355*) Salicylates and Acetaminophen

14–54. b (*p. 356*) Other Nonsteroidal Anti-Inflammatory Drugs (NSAIDs)

14–55. a (*p. 356*) Narcotic Analgesics

14–56. d (*p. 356*) Migraine Headache Medications

14–57. c (*p. 356*) General Anesthesia

14–58. b (*p. 356*) Anticoagulants

14–59. c (*p. 357*) Anticoagulants

14–60. d (*p. 357*) Antihypertensives

14–61. c (*p. 357*) Calcium-Channel Blockers

14–62. c (*p. 358*) Diuretics

14–63. a (*p. 358*) Diuretics

14–64. b (*p. 358*) Antibacterial Agents

14–65. a (*p. 358*) Antibacterial Agents

14–66. a (*pp. 358, 359*) Antibacterial Agents

14–67. b (*p. 359*) Antibacterial Agents

14–68. d (*p. 359*) Antiviral Agents

14–69. b (*p. 359*) Antiviral Agents

14–70. a (*p. 360*) Antiparasitic Agents

14–71. b (*p. 360*) Antiparasitic Agents

14–72. d (*p. 360*) Asthma Medications

14–73. a (*p. 361*) Cardiac Medications

14–74. d (*p. 361*) Herbal Remedies

14–75. b (*p. 362*) Table 14-5

14–76. c (*p. 361*) Herbal Remedies

14–77. c (*p. 361*) Hormones

14–78. c (*p. 363*) Psychotropic Drugs

14–79. d (*p. 363*) Antidepressant Drugs

14–80. d (*p. 364*) Recreational Drugs

14–81. a (*p. 364*) Recreational Drugs

CHAPTER 15

15–1. a (*p. 374*) Antepartum Assessment

15–2. d (*p. 374*) Antepartum Assessment

15–3. b (*p. 374*) Antepartum Assessment

15–4. b (*p. 374*) Fetal Movements

15–5. c (*p. 374*) Fetal Movements

15–6. a (*p. 374*) Fetal Movements

15–7. a (*p. 374*) Fetal Movements

15–8. a (*p. 374*) Fetal Movements

15–9. b (*p. 374*) Fetal Movements

15–10. b (*p. 375*) Fetal Movements

15–11. d (*p. 375*) Clinical Application

15–12. d (*p. 375*) Fetal Movements

15–13. c (*p. 376*) Fetal Breathing

15–14. c (*p. 376*) Fetal Breathing

15–15. **d** (*p. 376*) Fetal Breathing

15–16. **d** (*p. 376*) Fetal Breathing

15–17. **c** (*p. 377*) Contraction Stress Test

15–18. **b** (*p. 377*) Contraction Stress Test

15–19. **a** (*p. 377*) Fetal Heart Rate Accelerations

15–20. **b** (*p. 377*) Fetal Heart Rate Accelerations

15–21. **b** (*p. 378*) Normal Nonstress Tests

15–22. **d** (*p. 379*) Abnormal Nonstress Tests

15–23. **d** (*p. 379*) Interval Between Testing

15–24. **a** (*p. 380*) False-Normal Nonstress Tests

15–25. **b** (*p. 380*) Acoustic Stimulation Tests

15–26. **c** (*p. 381*) Biophysical Profile

15–27. **c** (*p. 381*) Biophysical Profile

15–28. **b** (*p. 382*) Modified Biophysical Profile

15–29. **d** (*p. 383*) Umbilical Artery Doppler Velocimetry

15–30. **c** (*p. 383*) Umbilical Artery Doppler Velocimetry

15–31. **d** (*p. 383*) Current Antenatal Testing Rec.

15–32. **a** (*p. 384*) Current Antenatal Testing Rec.

CHAPTER 16

16–1. **b** (*p. 390*) Technology

16–2. **a** (*p. 390*) Safety

16–3. **d** (*p. 390*) Clinical Applications

16–4. **b** (*p. 390*) Clinical Applications

16–5. **d** (*p. 390*) First Trimester

16–6. **c** (*p. 390*) First Trimester

16–7. **c** (*p. 391*) First Trimester

16–8. **c** (*p. 391*) Table 16-2

16–9. **b** (*p. 392*) Fetal Measurements

16–10. **a** (*p. 392*) Fetal Measurements

16–11. **d** (*p. 392*) Fetal Measurements

16–12. **b** (*p. 393*) Central Nervous System

16–13. **b** (*p. 393*) Neural-Tube Defects

16–14. **b** (*p. 394*) Neural-Tube Defects

16–15. **d** (*p. 394*) Neural-Tube Defects

16–16. **d** (*p. 394*) Neural-Tube Defects

16–17. **b** (*p. 395*) Ventriculomegaly

16–18. **a** (*p. 395*) Ventriculomegaly

16–19. **a** (*p. 395*) Cystic Hygroma

16–20. **c** (*p. 395*) Cystic Hygroma

16–21. **d** (*p. 395*) Cystic Hygroma

16–22. **b** (*p. 396*) Thorax

16–23. **b** (*p. 396*) Diaphragmatic Hernia

16–24. **d** (*p. 396*) Diaphragmatic Hernia

16–25. **b** (*p. 396*) Heart

16–26. **d** (*p. 396*) Heart

16–27. **b** (*p. 396*) Heart

16–28. **c** (*p. 396*) Heart

16–29. **d** (*p. 396*) Heart

16–30. **c** (*p. 396*) Heart

16–31. **a** (*p. 397*) Accuracy

16–32. **d** (*p. 397*) Gastrointestinal Tract

16–33. **c** (*p. 397*) Gastrointestinal Tract

16–34. **b** (*p. 397*) Gastroschisis

16–35. **c** (*p. 398*) Gastrointestinal Tract

16–36. **b** (*p. 399*) Gastrointestinal Atresia

16–37. **c** (*p. 399*) Gastrointestinal Atresia

16–38. **a** (*pp. 397-99*) Gastrointestinal Tract

16–39. **c** (*p. 399*) Kidneys and Urinary Tract

16–40. **a** (*p. 399*) Renal Agenesis

16–41. **d** (*pp. 399-400*) Kidneys and Urinary Tract

16–42. **d** (*p. 400*) Ureteropelvic Junction Obstruction

16–43. **b** (*p. 401*) Umbilical Artery

16–44. **c** (*p. 401*) Ductus Arteriosus

16–45. **a** (*p. 402*) Middle Cerebral Artery

CHAPTER 17

17–1. **c** (*p. 410*) Normal Labor & Delivery

17–2. **b** (*p. 410*) Fetal lie

17–3. **c** (*p. 410*) Fetal lie

17–4. **d** (*p. 410*) Fetal lie

17–5. **b** (*p. 410*) Fetal lie

17–6. **a** (*p. 410*) Cephalic Presentation

17–7. **b** (*p. 410*) Cephalic Presentation

17–8. **d** (*p. 411*) Cephalic Presentation

17–9. **a** (*p. 411*) Fetal Attitude or Posture

17–10. **a** (*p. 411*) Cephalic Presentation

17–11. **c** (*p. 411*) Varieties of Presentations and Positions

17–12. **a** (*p. 412*) First Maneuver

17–13. **c** (*p. 412*) Third Maneuver

17–14. **b** (*p. 412*) Second Maneuver

17–15. **d** (*p. 413*) Fourth Maneuver

17–16. **d** (*p. 415*) Labor with Occiput Presentations

17–17. **a** (*p. 415*) Labor with Occiput Presentations

17–18. **c** (*p. 415*) Occiput Anterior Presentations

17–19. **b** (*p. 415*) Occiput Anterior Presentations

17–20. **c** (*p. 415*) Asynclitism

17–21. **c** (*p. 416*) Asynclitism

17–22. **c** (*pp. 416, 417*) Descent

17–23. **a** (*p. 417*) Flexion

17–24. **b** (*p. 417*) Expulsion

17–25. **c** (*p. 417*) External rotation

17–26. **a** (*p. 417*) Extension

17–27. **c** (*p. 417*) Occiput Posterior Position

17–28. **d** (*pp. 417, 418*) Occiput Posterior Position

17–29. **b** (*p. 418*) Caput Succedaneum

17–30. **d** (*p. 419*) Molding

17–31. **c** (*p. 420*) Characteristics of Normal Labor

17–32. **d** (*p. 422*) First Stage of Labor

17–33. **a** (*p. 422*) First Stage of Labor

17–34. **d** (*p. 422*) Latent Phase

17–35. **c** (*p. 422*) Latent Phase

17–36. **c** (*p. 422*) Latent Phase

17–37. **d** (*p. 422*) Latent Phase

17–38. **b** (*p. 422*) Active Labor

17–39. **c** (*p. 423*) Active Labor

17–40. **b** (*p. 423*) Active Labor

17–41. **b** (*p. 423*) Active Labor

17–42. **b** (*p. 423*) Second Stage of Labor

17–43. **a** (*p. 423*) Second Stage of Labor

17–44. **b** (*p. 424*) Duration of Labor

17–45. **d** (*p. 425*) Admission Procedures

17–46. **b** (*p. 425*) Emergency Medical Treatment & Labor Act (EMTLA)

17–47. **d** (*p. 425*) Home Births

17–48. **a** (*p. 425*) Vaginal Examination

17–49. **a** (*p. 426*) Detection of Ruptured Membranes

17–50. **c** (*p. 426*) Detection of Ruptured Membranes

17–51. **b** (*p. 426*) Detection of Ruptured Membranes

17–52. **c** (*p. 426*) Cervical Effacement

17–53. **c** (*p. 426*) Station

17–54. **d** (*p. 426*) Station

17–55. **d** (*p. 426*) Station

17–56. **c** (*p. 427*) Monitoring Fetal Well-Being During Labor

17–57. **c** (*p. 427*) Monitoring Fetal Well-Being During Labor

17–58. **b** (*p. 427*) Monitoring Fetal Well-Being During Labor

17–59. **c** (*p. 427*) Monitoring Fetal Well-Being During Labor

17–60. **c** (*p. 427*) Maternal Vital Signs

17–61. **d** (*p. 428*) Maternal Position During Labor

17–62. **b** (*p. 429*) Delivery of the Head

17–63. **b** (*p. 429*) Delivery of the Head

17–64. **c** (*p. 429*) Ritgen Maneuver

17–65. **d** (*p. 431*) Nuchal Cord

17–66. **d** (*p. 431*) Timing of Cord Clamping

17–67. **d** (*pp. 431, 432*) Signs of Placental Separation

17–68. **d** (*p. 432*) Delivery of the Placenta

17–69. **d** (*p. 432*) Manual Removal of Placenta

17–70. **b** (*p. 433*) "Fourth Stage" of Labor

17–71. **a** (*p. 433*) Oxytotic Agents

17–72. **a** (*p. 434*) Oxytocin

17–73. **b** (*p. 434*) Cardiovascular Effects

17–74. **d** (*p. 434*) Water Intoxication

17–75. **b** (*p. 434*) Ergonovine and Methylergonovine

17–76. **d** (*p. 434*) Lacerations of the Birth Canal

17–77. **a** (*p. 434*) Lacuations of the Birth Canal

17–78. **c** (*p. 434*) Lacuations of the Birth Canal

17–79. **d** (*p. 436*) Table 17-4

17–80. **a** (*p. 435*) Purposes of Episiotomy

17–81. **d** (*p. 435*) Purposes of Episiotomy

17–82. **d** (*p. 436*) Midline versus Mediolateral Episiotomy

17–83. **d** (*p. 439*) Active Management of Labor

CHAPTER 18

18–1. **c** (*p. 444*) Internal Electronic Fetal Heart Rate Monitoring

18–2. **b** (*p. 446*) Fetal Heart Rate Patterns

18–3. **c** (*p. 447*) Rate

18–4. **b** (*p. 447*) Rate

18–5. **c** (*p. 447*) Rate

18–6. **a** (*p. 447*) Rate

18–7. **b** (*p. 447*) Bradycardia

18–8. **c** (*p. 447*) Tachycardia

18–9. **c** (*p. 447*) Beat-to-Beat Variability

18–10. **d** (*p. 448*) Beat-to-Beat Variability

18–11. **d** (*p. 448*) Beat-to-Beat Variability

18–12. **a** (*p. 449*) Beat-to-Beat Variability

18–13. **d** (*p. 450*) Cardiac Arrhythmia

18–14. **c** (*p. 450*) Cardiac Arrhythmia

18–15. **a** (*pp. 450, 451*) Cardiac Arrhythmia

18–16. **c** (*p. 451*) Sinusoidal Heart Rate

18–17. **d** (*p. 451*) Sinusoidal Heart Rate

18–18. **a** (*p. 451*) Sinusoidal Heart Rate

18–19. **b** (*p. 452*) Accelerations

18–20. **b** (*p. 452*) Early Deceleration

18–21. **a** (*p. 452*) Late Deceleration

18–22. **d** (*p. 452*) Early Deceleration

18–23. **d** (*p. 453*) Late Deceleration

18–24. **b** (*pp. 453, 454*) Variable Decelerations

18–25. **c** (*p. 453*) Variable Decelerations

18–26. **d** (*p. 455*) Variable Decelerations

18–27. **a** (*p. 456*) Prolonged Deceleration

18–28. **b** (*p. 456*) Fetal Heart Rate Patterns During Second-Stage Labor

18–29. **d** (*p. 457*) Complications of Electronic Fetal Monitoring

18–30. **d** (*p. 457*) Complications of Electronic Fetal Monitoring

18–31. **a** (*p. 458*) Scalp Stimulation

18–32. **a** (*p. 458*) Fetal Pulse Oximetry

18–33. **a** (*p. 458*) Fetal Pulse Oximetry

18–34. **b** (*p. 460*) Fetal Echocardiography

18–35. **d** (*pp. 455, 456, 461*) Diagnosis

18–36. **d** (*p. 461*) Meconium in the Amnionic Fluid

18–37. **b** (*p. 461*) Meconium in the Amnionic Fluid

18–38. **c** (*p. 462*) Management Options with "Fetal Distress"

18–39. **a** (*p. 462*) Amnioinfusion

18–40. **a** (*p. 463*) Table 18-3

18–41. **d** (*p. 465*) Table 18-5

18–42. **a** (*p. 466*) Patterns of Uterine Activity

18–43. **c** (*p. 466*) Patterns of Uterine Activity

18–44. **c** (*p. 466*) Patterns of Uterine Activity

18–45. **c** (*p. 467*) Origin & Propagation of Contractions

18–46. **a** (*p. 467*) Origin & Propagation of Contractions

18–47. **c** (*pp. 467, 468*) Origin & Propagation of Contractions

CHAPTER 19

19–1. **a** (*p. 474*) Obstetrical Anesthesia

19–2. **d** (*p. 474*) Table 19-1

19–3. **c** (*p. 474*) Obstetrical Anesthesia

19–4. **d** (*p. 475*) Nonpharmacological Methods of Pain Control

19–5. **c** (*p. 476*) Meperidine and Promethazine

19–6. **a** (*p. 476*) Meperidine and Promethazine

19–7. **b** (*p. 476*) Meperidine and Promethazine

19–8. **b** (*p. 476*) Butorphanol (Stadol)

19–9. **c** (*p. 476*) Butorphanol (Stadol)

19–10. **d** (*p. 476*) Efficacy and Safety of Parenteral Agents

19–11. **b** (*p. 476*) Narcotic Antagonists

19–12. **b** (*p. 477*) Uterine Innervation

19–13. **d** (*p. 477*) Lower Genital Tract Innervation

19–14. **d** (*p. 478*) Central Nervous System Toxicity

19–15. **b** (*p. 478*) Central Nervous System Toxicity

19–16. **c** (*p. 478*) Cardiovascular Toxicity

19–17. **c** (*p. 478*) Cardiovascular Toxicity

19–18. **c** (*p. 480*) Complications [under "Paracenical Block"]

19–19. **a** (*p. 481*) Spinal (Postdural Puncture) Headache

19–20. **c** (*p. 482*) Spinal (Postdural Puncture) Headache

19–21. **b** (*p. 482*) Table 19-5

19–22. **b** (*p. 483*) Continuous Lumbar Epidural Block

19–23. **b** (*p. 481*) Table 19-4

19–24. **d** (*p. 484*) Maternal Pyrexia

19–25. **a** (*pp. 485, 486*) Cesarean Delivery

19–26. **c** (*p. 487*) Epidural Opiate Analgesia

19–27. **c** (*p. 487*) Epidural Opiate Analgesia

19–28. **d** (*pp. 488, 489*) General Anesthesia

19–29. **b** (*p. 489*) Preoxygenation

19–30. **a** (*p. 489*) Thiopental

19–31. **a** (*p. 489*) Ketamine

19–32. **c** (*p. 489*) Intubation

19–33. **a** (*p. 490*) Gas Anesthetics

19–34. **d** (*p. 490*) Volatile Anesthetics

19–35. **c** (*p. 490*) Aspiration

19–36. **a** (*p. 490*) Pathophysiology

19–37. **d** (*p. 491*) Pathophysiology

CHAPTER 20

20–1. **c** (*p. 496*) Dystocia: Abnormal Labor

20–2. **d** (*p. 496*) Dystocia

20–3. **d** (*p. 496*) Overdiagnosis of Dystocia

20–4. **d** (*p. 496*) Overdiagnosis of Dystocia

20–5. **c** (*p. 497*) Overdiagnosis of Dystocia

20–6. **a** (*p. 498*) Types of Uterine Dysfunction

20–7. **b** (*p. 498*) Types of Uterine Dysfunction

20–8. **b** (*p. 499*) Table 20-2

20–9. **b** (*p. 500*) Table 20-3

20–10. **b** (*p. 500*) Table 20-3

20–11. **b** (*p. 499*) Table 20-2

20–12. **d** (*p. 499*) Figure 20-3

20–13. **b** (*p. 498*) Active-Phase Disorders

20–14. **b** (*p. 498*) Active-Phase Disorders

20–15. **c** (*p. 500*) Table 20-3

20–16. **d** (*p. 502*) Maternal Effects

20–17. **a** (*p. 502*) Maternal Effects

20–18. **c** (*p. 503*) Contracted Pelvic Inlet

20–19. **c** (*p. 503*) Contracted Pelvic Inlet

20–20. **c** (*p. 503*) Contracted Pelvic Inlet

20–21. **b** (*p. 503*) Contracted Pelvic Inlet

20–22. **d** (*p. 503*) Contracted Midpelvis

20–23. **b** (*p. 503*) Contracted Midpelvis

20–24. **d** (*pp. 503, 504*) Contracted Midpelvis

20–25. **c** (*p. 504*) X-ray Pelvimetry

20–26. **b** (*p. 504*) Computed Tomographic (CT) Scanning

20–27. b (*p. 504*) Computed Tomographic (CT) Scanning

20–28. a (*p. 506*) Estimation of Fetal Head Size

20–29. c (*p. 506*) Face Presentation

20–30. a (*p. 506*) Face Presentation

20–31. b (*p. 506*) Face Presentation

20–32. a (*p. 507*) Etiology

20–33. c (*p. 507*) Etiology

20–34. b (*p. 508*) Brow Presentation

20–35. a (*p. 508*) Brow Presentation

20–36. a (*p. 509*) Transverse Lie

20–37. c (*p. 509*) Transverse Lie

20–38. d (*p. 510*) Etiology

20–39. b (*pp. 510, 511*) Management

20–40. a (*p. 510*) Mechanism of Labor

20–41. c (*p. 511*) Incidence and Etiology

20–42. d (*p. 511*) Persistent Occiput Posterior Position

20–43. c (*p. 513*) Shoulder Dystocia

20–44. c (*p. 513*) Shoulder Dystocia

20–45. b (*p. 514*) Risk Factors

20–46. d (*pp. 514, 515*) Risk Factors

20–47. b (*p. 514*) Management

20–48. c (*p. 516*) Management

20–49. d (*p. 518*) Technique of Cephalocentesis

20–50. b (*pp. 518, 519*) Fetal Abdomen as a Cause of Dystocia

20–51. b (*p. 520*) Pelvic Floor Injury

20–52. c (*p. 520*) Pelvic Floor Injury

20–53. a (*p. 520*) Fetal Head Molding

CHAPTER 21

21–1. b (*p. 526*) Normal Amnionic Fluid Volume

21–2. a (*p. 526*) Measurement of Amnionic Fluid

21–3. c (*p. 526*) Measurement of Amnionic Fluid

21–4. d (*p. 527*) Incidence

21–5. d (*p. 527*) Causes of Hydramnios

21–6. c (*p. 529*) Pathogenesis

21–7. b (*p. 528*) Causes of Hydramnios

21–8. a (*p. 528*) Causes of Hydramnios

21–9. a (*pp. 527, 528*) Measurement of Amnionic Fluid/Pathogenesis

21–10. b (*p. 528*) Pathogenesis

21–11. c (*p. 529*) Symptoms

21–12. d (*p. 529*) Pregnancy Outcomes

21–13. c (*p. 529*) Pregnancy Outcomes

21–14. a (*p. 529*) Management

21–15. b (*p. 529*) Amniocentesis

21–16. d (*p. 530*) Indomethacin Therapy

21–17. c (*p. 530*) Indomethacin Therapy

21–18. b (*p. 530*) Oligohydramnios

21–19. b (*p. 530*) Oligohydramnios

21–20. c (*p. 530*) Early-Onset Oligohydramnios

21–21. a (*p. 530*) Early-Onset Oligohydramnios

21–22. d (*p. 530*) Oligohydramnios

21–23. c (*p. 531*) Prognosis

21–24. a (*p. 531*) Pulmonary Hypoplasia

21–25. c (*p. 532*) Oligohydramnios in Late Pregnancy

21–26. b (*p. 533*) Amnioinfusion

CHAPTER 22

22–1. d (*p. 536*) Induction and Augmentation of Labor

22–2. d (*p. 536*) Elective Induction of Labor

22–3. c (*p. 537*) Preinduction Cervical Ripening

22–4. a (*p. 537*) Indicated Labor Induction

22–5. d (*p. 537*) Contraindications

22–6. a (*p. 537*) Table 22-1

22–7. b (*p. 537*) Preinduction Cervical Ripening

22–8. a (*p. 537*) Prostaglandin E_2

22–9. d (*p. 537*) Administration

22–10. d (*p. 538*) Prostaglandin E_1

22–11. a (*p. 538*) Vaginal Administration

22–12. d (*p. 538*) Vaginal Administration

22–13. d (*p. 538*) Transcervical Catheter

22–14. d (*p. 539*) Membrane Stripping

22–15. d (*p. 540*) Labor Induction and Augmentation in Oxytocin

22–16. a (*p. 540*) Intravenous Oxytocin Administration

22–17. d (*p. 540*) Intravenous Oxytocin Administration

22–18. c (*p. 540*) Intravenous Oxytocin Administration

22–19. b (*p. 541*) Risks Versus Benefits

22–20. d (*p. 541*) Uterine Contraction Pressures

22–21. b (*p. 541*) Uterine Contraction Pressures

22–22. b (*p. 541*) Duration of Oxytocin Administration

CHAPTER 23

23–1. b (*p. 548*) Forcep Delivery & Vacuum Extraction

23–2. d (*p. 548*) Design of Forceps

23–3. a (*p. 548*) Design of Forceps

23–4. c (*p. 548*) Design of Forceps

23–5. b (*p. 548*) Classification of Forceps Deliveries

23–6. d (*p. 548*) Classification of Forceps Deliveries

23–7. d (*p. 548*) Incidence of Forceps Delivery

23–8. a (*p. 549*) Table 23-1

23–9. b (*p. 549*) Table 23-1

23–10. c (*p. 549*) Table 23-1

23–11. a (*p. 549*) Table 23-1

23–12. b (*p. 549*) Effects of Regional Analgesia on Instrumental Delivery

23–13. a (*p. 549*) Function of Forceps

23–14. b (*p. 549*) Function of Forceps

23–15. d (*p. 549*) Indications for Forceps

23–16. c (*p. 549*) Indications for Forceps

23–17. a (*p. 549*) Indications for Forceps

23–18. a (*p. 549*) Indications for Forceps

23–19. c (*p. 549*) Elective and Outlet Forceps

23–20. d (*p. 549*) Elective and Outlet Forceps

23–21. b (*p. 550*) Prerequisites for Forceps Application

23–22. a (*p. 550*) Preparation for Forceps Delivery

23–23. b (*p. 551*) Forceps Application

23–24. d (*p. 552*) Traction

23–25. a (*p. 554*) Manual Rotation

23–26. b (*p. 554*) Forceps Delivery of Occiput Posterior

23–27. a (*p. 555*) Forceps Delivery of Occiput Posterior

23–28. b (*p. 555*) Forceps Delivery of Face Presentation

23–29. d (*p. 556*) Maternal Morbidity

23–30. d (*p. 556*) Lacerations and Episiotomy

23–31. d (*p. 556*) Urinary and Rectal Incontinence

23–32. a (*p. 557*) Urinary and Rectal Incontinence

23–33. c (*p. 557*) Febrile Morbidity

23–34. b (*p. 558*) Morbidity from Midforceps Deliveries

23–35. d (*p. 559*) Vacuum Extraction

23–36. a (*p. 559*) Vacuum Extraction

23–37. d (*p. 559*) Vacuum Extraction

23–38. a (*p. 560*) Indications and Prerequisites

23–39. d (*p. 560*) Technique

23–40. c (*p. 560*) Complications

CHAPTER 24

24–1. b (*p. 566*) Introduction

24–2. d (*p. 566*) Etiology

24–3. b (*p. 566*) Complications

24–4. a (*p. 566*) Diagnosis

24–5. b (*p. 566*) Diagnosis

24–6. c (*p. 566*) Diagnosis

24–7. c (*p. 567*) Diagnosis, Abdominal Examination

24–8. a (*p. 567*) Vaginal Examination

24–9. d (*p. 568*) Prognosis

24–10. c (*p. 568*) Vaginal Delivery

24–11. d (*p. 569*) Unfavorable Pelvis

24–12. b (*p. 569*) Hyperextension of the Fetal Head

24–13. d (*p. 571*) Preterm Fetus

24–14. c (*p. 571*) Current Status of Vaginal Breech

24–15. d (*p. 572*) Labor and Spontaneous Delivery

24–16. b (*p. 572*) Partial Breech Extraction

24–17. b (*p. 573*) Fetal Monitoring

24–18. c (*pp. 573-74*) Assisted Frank Breech Delivery

24–19. c (*p. 578*) Mauriceau Maneuver

24–20. a (*p. 578*) Prague Maneuver

24–21. b (*p. 575*) Frank Breech Extraction

24–22. d (*p. 572*) Labor and Spontaneous Delivery

24–23. c (*p. 581*) External Cephalic Version

24–24. d (*p. 582*) Factors Associated w/ Successful Version

24–25. a (*p. 582*) Technique

24–26. a (*p. 582*) Factors Associated w/ Successful Version

24–27. b (*p. 581*) External Cephalic Version

CHAPTER 25

25–1. d (*p. 588*) Historical Background

25–2. c (*pp. 589-90*) Contemporary Status of Cesarean Delivery

25–3. **c** (*p. 590*) Fig 25-2

25–4. **c** (*p. 591*) Dystocia

25–5. **d** (*p. 591*) Fetal Distress

25–6. **c** (*p. 593*) Transverse Incisions

25–7. **d** (*p. 593*) Transverse Incisions

25–8. **a** (*p. 593*) Transverse Incisions

25–9. **d** (*p. 593*) Uterine Incision

25–10. **b** (*p. 595*) Repair of the Uterus

25–11. **c** (*p. 595*) Delivery of the Infant

25–12. **b** (*p. 598*) Abdominal Closure

25–13. **d** (*p. 598*) Technique for Classical Cesarean Incision

25–14. **c** (*p. 592*) Maternal Morbidity and Mortality

25–15. **b** (*p. 599*) Peripartum Hysterectomy

25–16. **a** (*p. 599*) Indications

25–17. **d** (*p. 599*) Indications

25–18. **c** (*p. 603*) Intravenous Fluids

25–19. **b** (*p. 603*) Prevention of Postoperative Infection

CHAPTER 26

26–1. **a** (*p. 609*) Table 26-1

26–2. **c** (*p. 609*) Table 26-1

26–3. **a** (*p. 608*) Magnitude of Risk

26–4. **a** (*p. 609*) Magnitude of Risk

26–5. **d** (*pp. 609, 610*) Costs/Elective Repeat Cesarean Delivery

26–6. **d** (*p. 610*) Table 26-2

26–7. **a** (*p. 610*) Table 26-2

26–8. **d** (*p. 610*) Table 26-3

26–9. **c** (*p. 611*) Type of Prior Uterine Incision

26–10. **b** (*p. 612*) Indication for Prior Cesarean Delivery/Number of Prior Cesarean Incisions

26–11. **c** (*p. 612*) Indication for Prior Cesarean Delivery

26–12. **b** (*p. 612*) Indication for Prior Cesarean Delivery

26–13. **d** (*p. 613*) Cervical Ripening and Labor Stimulation

26–14. **d** (*p. 615*) Diagnosis

26–15. **d** (*p. 615*) Diagnosis

26–16. **d** (*p. 614*) Epidural Analgesia

26–17. **a** (*p. 615*) Uterine Scar Exploration

26–18. **b** (*p. 615*) Classification

26–19. **c** (*p. 615*) Classification

26–20. **c** (*p. 615*) Prognosis

CHAPTER 27

27–1. **a** (*p. 620*) Multiple Placenta with Single Fetus

27–2. **d** (*p. 620*) Succenturiate Lobes

27–3. **b** (*p. 620*) Placental Abnormalities

27–4. **d** (*p. 620*) Ring-Shaped Placenta

27–5. **a** (*p. 620*) Fenestrated Placenta

27–6. **a** (*p. 621*) Extrachorial Placentation

27–7. **a** (*p. 621*) Extrachorial Placentation

27–8. **d** (*p. 621*) Placenta Accreta, Increta, Percreta

27–9. **d** (*p. 621*) Degenerative Placental Lesions

27–10. **c** (*p. 621*) Placental Infarctions

27–11. **a** (*p. 621*) Placental Infarctions

27–12. **c** (*p. 622*) Placental Infarctions

27–13. **d** (*p. 623*) Maternal Floor Infarction

27–14. **c** (*p. 623*) Placental Vessel Thrombosis

27–15. **a** (*p. 623*) Hypertrophic Lesions of Chorionic Villi

27–16. **a** (*p. 624*) Chorioangioma

27–17. **b** (*p. 624*) Chorioangioma

27–18. **b** (*p. 624*) Tumors Metastatic to the Placenta

27–19. **b** (*p. 624*) Meconium Staining

27–20. **b** (*p. 624*) Meconium Staining

27–21. **a** (*p. 624*) Meconium Staining

27–22. **d** (*p. 625*) Meconium Staining

27–23. **b** (*p. 625*) Meconium Staining

27–24. **b** (*p. 625*) Meconium Staining

27–25. **b** (*p. 625*) Chorioamnionitis

27–26. **b** (*p. 626*) Length

27–27. **c** (*p. 626*) Length

27–28. **d** (*p. 626*) Length

27–29. **b** (*p. 626*) Single Umbilical Artery

27–30. **a** (*p. 626*) Cord Coiling

27–31. **a** (*p. 627*) Marginal Insertion

27–32. **a** (*p. 627*) Velamentous Insertion

27–33. **d** (*p. 627*) Vasa Previa

27–34. **c** (*p. 628*) Knots

27–35. **b** (*p. 628*) Knots

27–36. **d** (*p. 628*) Loops

27–37. **d** (*p. 628*) Loops

27–38. **b** (*p. 628*) Torsion and Hematomas

27–39. **d** (*p. 628*) Cysts

27–40. **c** (*p. 628*) Cysts

27–41. **a** (*p. 628*) Pathological Examination

CHAPTER 28

28–1. **a** (*p. 634*) Stimuli to Breathe Air

28–2. **a** (*p. 634*) Stimuli to Breathe Air

28–3. **b** (*p. 634*) Stimuli to Breathe Air

28–4. **d** (*p. 634*) Immediate Care

28–5. **b** (*p. 634*) Newborn Resuscitation

28–6. **c** (*p. 634*) Newborn Resuscitation

28–7. **d** (*p. 635*) Fig 28-2

28–8. **c** (*p. 636*) Ventilation

28–9. **b** (*p. 636*) Ventilation

28–10. **a** (*p. 636*) Ventilation

28–11. **c** (*p. 636*) Endotracheal Intubation

28–12. **b** (*p. 636*) Endotracheal Intubation

28–13. **c** (*p. 637*) Chest Compression

28–14. **d** (*p. 637*) Medications and Volume Expansion

28–15. **a** (*p. 637*) Medications and Volume Expansion

28–16. **b** (*p. 637*) Discontinuation of Resuscitation

28–17. **d** (*p. 637*) Table 28-2

28–18. **b** (*p. 637*) Table 28-2

28–19. **d** (*p. 638*) Apgar Score

28–20. **b** (*p. 638*) Apgar Score

28–21. **c** (*p. 638*) Apgar Score

28–22. **a** (*p. 638*) Table 28-3

28–23. **c** (*p. 638*) Umbilical Cord Blood Acid–Base Studies

28–24. **d** (*p. 639*) Table 28-4

28–25. **b** (*p. 639*) Clinical Diagnosis of Significant Acidemia

28–26. **b** (*p. 640*) Clinical Diagnosis of Significant Acidemia

28–27. **a** (*p. 640*) Clinical Diagnosis of Significant Acidemia

28–28. **d** (*p. 641*) Clinical Diagnosis of Significant Acidemia

28–29. **c** (*p. 641*) Clinical Diagnosis of Significant Acidemia

28–30. **b** (*p. 641*) Clinical Diagnosis of Significant Acidemia

28–31. **a** (*p. 640*) Clinical Diagnosis of Significant Acidemia

28–32. **c** (*p. 641*) Eye Infection Prophylaxis

28–33. **d** (*p. 641*) Eye Infection Prophylaxis

28–34. **a** (*p. 642*) Universal Newborn Screening

28–35. **a** (*p. 641*) Vitamin K

28–36. **d** (*p. 642*) Fig. 28-5

28–37. **b** (*p. 643*) Umbilical Cord

28–38. **c** (*p. 643*) Feeding

28–39. **b** (*p. 643*) Stools and Urine

28–40. **b** (*p. 643*) Circumcision

28–41. **d** (*p. 644*) Table 28-7

28–42. **c** (*p. 644*) Anesthesia for Circumcision

28–43. **a** (*p. 645*) Hospital Discharge

CHAPTER 29

29–1. **c** (*p. 650*) Respiratory Distress Syndrome

29–2. **b** (*p. 650*) Respiratory Distress Syndrome

29–3. **d** (*p. 650*) Clinical Course

29–4. **a** (*p. 650*) Clinical Course

29–5. **a** (*p. 650*) Treatment

29–6. **b** (*p. 651*) Surfactant Treatment

29–7. **d** (*p. 651*) Complications

29–8. **c** (*p. 651*) Amniocentesis for Fetal Lung Maturity

29–9. **b** (*p. 651*) Amniocentesis for Fetal Lung Maturity

29–10. **b** (*p. 652*) Amniocentesis for Fetal Lung Maturity

29–11. **d** (*p. 652*) TOX-FLM

29–12. **b** (*p. 652*) Other Tests

29–13. **d** (*p. 652*) Retinopathy of Prematurity

29–14. **d** (*p. 652*) Intraventricular Hemorrhage

29–15. **c** (*p. 652*) Periventricular Intraventricular Hemorrhage

29–16. **a** (*p. 652*) Periventricular Intraventricular Hemorrhage

29–17. **d** (*p. 653*) Incidence & Severity

29–18. **b** (*p. 653*) Incidence & Severity

29–19. **c** (*p. 653*) Incidence and Severity

29–20. **d** (*p. 653*) Contributing Factors

29–21. **d** (*p. 653*) Prevention and Treatment

29–22. **a** (*p. 653*) Prevention and Treatment

29–23. **c** (*p. 654*) Necrotizing Enterocolitis

29–24. **b** (*p. 654*) Necrotizing Enterocolitis

29–25. c (*p. 654*) Brain Disorders

29–26. c (*p. 654*) Brain Disorders

29–27. d (*p. 654*) Brain Disorders

29–28. d (*p. 654*) Neonatal Encephalopathy

29–29. c (*p. 655*) Neonatal Encephalopathy

29–30. b (*p. 655*) Neonatal Encephalopathy

29–31. b (*p. 655*) Cerebral Palsy

29–32. b (*p. 655*) Incidence and Epid. Corelae

29–33. d (*p. 655*) Incidence and Epid. Corelae

29–34. c (*p. 655*) Incidence and Epid. Corelae

29–35. a (*p. 656*) Apgan Scores

29–36. b (*p. 656*) Umbilical Cord Blood Gas Studies

29–37. c (*p. 657*) Periventricular Leukomalacia

29–38. a (*p. 657*) Periventricular Leukomalacia

29–39. a (*pp. 658-9*) Neuroradiological Imaging

29–40. d (*p. 660*) Neonatal Enceph. at Term

29–41. b (*p. 660*) Mental Retardation

29–42. a (*p. 660*) Neonatal Enceph. at Term

29–43. c (*p. 660*) Infant Outcome in Extreme Premature Birth

29–44. c (*p. 661*) Anemia

29–45. c (*p. 662*) Anemia

29–46. a (*p. 663*) Anemia

29–47. d (*p. 663*) Table 29-6

29–48. b (*p. 663*) Anemia

29–49. b (*p. 664*) Isoimmunization

29–50. c (*p. 664*) ABO Blood Group System

29–51. a (*p. 664*) ABO Blood Group System

29–52. c (*p. 664*) ABO Blood Group System

29–53. c (*p. 664*) ABO Blood Group System

29–54. b (*p. 664*) CDE (Rhesus) Blood Group System

29–55. c (*p. 664*) CDE (Rhesus) Blood Group System

29–56. a (*p. 664*) CDE (Rhesus) Blood Group System

29–57. a (*p. 664*) CDE (Rhesus) Blood Group System

29–58. a (*p. 664*) Other Blood Group Incompatibilities

29–59. b (*p. 665*) Other Blood Group Incompatibilities

29–60. b (*p. 665*) Kell Antigen

29–61. a (*p. 666*) Immune Hydrops

29–62. a (*p. 666*) Immune Hydrops

29–63. b (*p. 667*) Hyperbilirubinemia

29–64. c (*p. 667*) Identification of the Isoimmunized Pregnancy; Predicting Fetal Genotype

29–65. b (*p. 668*) Identification of the Isoimmunized Pregnancy; Predicting Fetal Genotype

29–66. c (*p. 668*) Identification of the Isoimmunized Pregnancy; Predicting Fetal Genotype

29–67. b (*p. 668*) Management of Isoimmunization

29–68. a (*p. 669*) Amnionic Fluid Evaluation

29–69. a (*p. 670*) Fetal Blood Sampling

29–70. d (*p. 670*) Fetal Blood Sampling

29–71. a (*p. 670*) Neonatal Care & Outcome

29–72. b (*p. 671*) Prevention

29–73. b (*p. 671*) Routine Antepartum Administration

29–74. d (*p. 672*) Kernicterus

29–75. d (*p. 672*) Kernicterus

29–76. **c** (*p. 672*) Physiologic Jaundice

29–77. **b** (*p. 672*) Treatment

29–78. **a** (*pp. 672-73*) Etiology

29–79. **d** (*p. 673*) Prognosis

29–80. **d** (*p. 674*) Table 29-8

29–81. **c** (*p. 674*) Maternal Complications

29–82. **c** (*p. 675*) Fetal Cardiac Curhythymia

29–83. **c** (*p. 675*) Respiration Distress Syndrome

29–84. **b** (*p. 675*) Meconium Aspiration Syndrome

29–85. **c** (*p. 675*) Risk Factors

29–86. **d** (*p. 675*) Risk Factors

29–87. **b** (*p. 676*) Prevention

29–88. **d** (*p. 676*) Prophylaxis

29–89. **d** (*p. 677*) Immune Thrombocytopenia

29–90. **c** (*p. 677*) Alloimmune (Isoimmune) Thrombocytopenia

29–91. **d** (*p. 678*) Definition of Fetal Martality

29–92. **d** (*p. 678*) Causes of Death

29–93. **c** (*p. 679*) Placental Causes

29–94. **d** (*p. 679*) Maternal Causes

29–95. **a** (*p. 679*) Laboratory Evaluation

29–96. **d** (*p. 680*) Laboratory Evaluation

29–97. **b** (*p. 680*) Autopsy

29–98. **a** (*p. 681*) Pregnancy After Prior Stillbirth

29–99. **d** (*p. 681*) Pregnancy After Prior Stillbirth

29–100. **d** (*p. 681*) Spontaneous Intracranial Hemorrhage

29–101. **b** (*p. 682*) Fig 29-15

29–102. **c** (*p. 683*) Brachial Plexus Injury

29–103. **c** (*p. 683*) Brachial Plexus Injury

29–104. **d** (*pp. 683-84*) Facial Paralysis

29–105. **a** (*p. 685*) Amnionic Band Syndrome

29–106. **b** (*p. 684*) Muscular Injury

CHAPTER 30

30–1. **c** (*p. 696*) Puerperium

30–2. **a** (*p. 696*) Cervix and Lower Uterine Segment

30–3. **b** (*p. 696*) Involution of the Uterine Corpus

30–4. **d** (*p. 696*) Involution of the Uterine Corpus

30–5. **d** (*p. 696*) Afterpains

30–6. **c** (*p. 696*) Lochia

30–7. **a** (*p. 697*) Subinvolution

30–8. **c** (*p. 697*) Subinvolution

30–9. **b** (*p. 698*) Late Postpartum Hemorrhage

30–10. **b** (*p. 698*) Urinary Tract Charges

30–11. **d** (*p. 698*) Urinary Tract Charges

30–12. **a** (*p. 698*) Urinary Tract Charges

30–13. **c** (*p. 698*) Incontinence

30–14. **a** (*p. 699*) Blood and Fluid Charges

30–15. **b** (*p. 699*) Weight Loss

30–16. **b** (*p. 700*) Colostrum

30–17. **d** (*p. 700*) Milk

30–18. **c** (*p. 700*) Endocrinology of Lactation

30–19. **a** (*p. 700*) Immunological Consequences of Breast Feeding

30–20. **d** (*p. 701*) Lactation Inhibition

30–21. **b** (*p. 702*) Contraception for Breast Feeding Women

30–22. **c** (*p. 702*) Contraindications to Breast
Feeding

30–23. **b** (*p. 702*) Drugs Secreted in Milk

30–24. **a** (*p. 703*) Mastitis

30–25. **a** (*p. 703*) Etiology

30–26. **d** (*p. 703*) Treatment

30–27. **c** (*p. 705*) Early Ambulation

30–28. **b** (*p. 705*) Bladder Function

30–29. **c** (*p. 705*) Subsequent Discomfort

30–30. **b** (*p. 705*) Depression

30–31. **b** (*p. 706*) Obstetrical Neuropathies

30–32. **d** (*p. 706*) Immunizations

30–33. **b** (*p. 707*) Contraception

CHAPTER 31

31–1. **c** (*p. 712*) Pueperal Infection

31–2. **a** (*p. 712*) Puerperal Fever

31–3. **b** (*p. 712*) Differential Diagnosis

31–4. **d** (*p. 712*) Differential Diagnosis

31–5. **a** (*p. 712*) Differential Diagnosis

31–6. **b** (*p. 712*) Differential Diagnosis

31–7. **b** (*p. 712*) Differential Diagnosis

31–8. **d** (*p. 712*) Predisposing Factors

31–9. **c** (*p. 712*) Vaginal Delivery

31–10. **d** (*p. 712*) Cesarean Delivery

31–11. **c** (*p. 713*) Other Risk Factors

31–12. **d** (*p. 713*) Other Risk Factors

31–13. **a** (*p. 713*) Common Pathogens

31–14. **a** (*p. 713*) Table 31-1

31–15. **c** (*p. 713*) Bacteriology

31–16. **b** (*p. 714*) Common Pathogens

31–17. **d** (*p. 714*) Bacterial Cultures/Specific
Antimicrobial Treatment

31–18. **b** (*p. 714*) Clinical Course

31–19. **a** (*p. 714*) Management

31–20. **c** (*p. 714*) Management

31–21. **a** (*p. 714*) Management

31–22. **b** (*p. 714*) Specific Antimicrobial Treatment

31–23. **d** (*p. 715*) Specific Antimicrobial Treatment

31–24. **a** (*p. 715*) Specific Antimicrobial Treatment

31–25. **a** (*p. 715*) Prevention of Infection

31–26. **d** (*p. 716*) Complications of Pelvic
Infections

31–27. **c** (*p. 716*) Wound Infections

31–28. **b** (*p. 716*) Wound Dehiscence

31–29. **c** (*p. 716*) Wound Dehiscence

31–30. **d** (*p. 716*) Necrotizing Fasciitis

31–31. **a** (*p. 716*) Necrotizing Fasciitis

31–32. **b** (*p. 716*) Necrotizing Fasciitis

31–33. **c** (*p. 716*) Peritonitis

31–34. **a** (*p. 717*) Parametrial Phlegmon

31–35. **d** (*p. 717*) Parametrial Phlegmon

31–36. **b** (*p. 718*) Pathogenesis

31–37. **b** (*pp. 718, 719*) Imaging Studies/Clinical
Finding

31–38. **a** (*p. 719*) Clinical Findings

31–39. **c** (*p. 719*) Infections of the Perineum, Vagina,
and Cervix

31–40. **d** (*p. 720*) Pathogenesis and Clinical Course

31–41. **b** (*p. 720*) Pathogenesis and Clinical Course

31–42. **a** (*p. 720*) Treatment

31–43. **c** (*p. 720*) Technique for Early Repair

31–44. **b** (*p. 721*) Necrotizing Fasciitis

31–45. **a** (*p. 721*) Toxic Shock Syndrome

31–46. **a** (*p. 721*) Toxic Shock Syndrome

31–47. **d** (*p. 721*) Toxic Shock Syndrome

31–48. **b** (*p. 721*) Toxic Shock Syndrome

CHAPTER 32

32–1. **d** (*p. 726*) Contraception

32–2. **d** (*p. 726*) Table 32-1

32–3. **a** (*p. 726*) Need for Contraception

32–4. **d** (*p. 726*) Need for Contraception

32–5. **a** (*p. 727*) Fig 32-1

32–6. **c** (*p. 727*) Table 32-2

32–7. **d** (*p. 727*) Table 32-2

32–8. **d** (*pp. 727, 728*) Mechanisms of Action

32–9. **b** (*p. 729*) Pharmacology

32–10. **b** (*p. 729*) Pharmacology

32–11. **c** (*p. 729*) Pharmacology

32–12. **a** (*p. 729*) Pharmacology

32–13. **b** (*p. 729*) Dosage

32–14. **c** (*p. 730*) Drug Interactions

32–15. **c** (*p. 730*) Drug Interactions

32–16. **c** (*p. 726*) Table 32-1

32–17. **a** (*p. 731*) Beneficial Effects

32–18. **d** (*p. 731*) Possible Adverse Effects

32–19. **c** (*p. 732*) Liver Disease

32–20. **c** (*p. 732*) Neoplasia

32–21. **d** (*p. 732*) Neoplasia

32–22. **d** (*pp. 732, 733*) Cardiovascular Effects

32–23. **a** (*p. 733*) Cardiovascular Effects

32–24. **d** (*p. 733*) Cardiovascular Effects

32–25. **a** (*p. 733*) Cardiovascular Effects

32–26. **d** (*p. 733*) Effection Reproduction

32–27. **b** (*p. 733*) Other Effects

32–28. **a** (*p. 734*) Postpartum Use

32–29. **c** (*p. 734*) Table 32-6

32–30. **a** (*p. 735*) Oral Progestins

32–31. **c** (*p. 735*) Benefits

32–32. **d** (*pp. 735, 736*) Disadvantages

32–33. **c** (*p. 736*) Injectable Progestin Contraceptives

32–34. **d** (*p. 736*) Benefits and Disadvantages

32–35. **d** (*p. 736*) Benefits and Disadvantages

32–36. **a** (*p. 736*) Benefits and Disadvantages

32–37. **d** (*p. 736*) Progestin Implants

32–38. **d** (*p. 737*) Advantages & Disadvantages

32–39. **c** (*p. 737*) Intrauterine Devices

32–40. **c** (*p. 737*) Intrauterine Devices

32–41. **a** (*pp. 737, 738*) Levonorgestrel Device (Mirena)

32–42. **b** (*p. 738*) Mechanism of Action

32–43. **b** (*p. 738*) Mechanism of Action

32–44. **b** (*p. 738*) Uterine Perforation and Abortion

32–45. **b** (*p. 738*) Menorrhagia

32–46. **b** (*p. 739*) Infection

32–47. **c** (*p. 739*) Infection

32–48. **c** (*p. 739*) Pregnancy with a Device in Utero

32–49. **c** (*p. 739*) Pregnancy with a Device in Utero

32–50. **b** (*p. 739*) Pregnancy with a Device in Utero

32–51. **d** (*p. 739*) Table 32-8

32–52. **b** (*p. 739*) Table 32-8

32–53. **b** (*p. 741*) Male Condom

32–54. **b** (*p. 741*) Male Condom

32–55. **a** (*p. 742*) Female Condom

32–56. **a** (*p. 742*) Spermicides

32–57. **d** (*p. 742*) Spermicides

32–58. **b** (*p. 743*) Diaphragm & Spermicide

32–59. **d** (*p. 743*) Diaphragm & Spermicide

32–60. **d** (*p. 743*) Contraceptive Sponge

32–61. **d** (*pp. 743, 744*) Periodic (Rhythmic Abstinence)

32–62. **d** (*p. 744*) Contraception in Adolescants

32–63. **a** (*p. 744*) Combination Oral Contraceptions

32–64. **c** (*p. 744*) Contraceptive Choices for Woman, 35

32–65. **c** (*p. 745*) Yuzpe and Estrogen

32–66. **c** (*p. 746*) Progestin Combinations Mechanism of Action

32–67. **a** (*p. 746*) Mifepristone (RU 486) and Epostane

CHAPTER 33

33–1. **d** (*p. 752*) Sterilization

33–2. **c** (*p. 752*) Female Sterilization

33–3. **b** (*p. 752*) Irving Procedure

33–4. **b** (*p. 752*) Pomeroy Procedure

33–5. **d** (*p. 752*) Parkland Procedure

33–6. **a** (*p. 754*) Operative Complications

33–7. **b** (*p. 754*) Operative Complications

33–8. **b** (*p. 754*) Operative Complications

33–9. **d** (*p. 754*) Failure Rates

33–10. **b** (*p. 754*) Long Term Complications

33–11. **d** (*p. 754*) Long Term Complications

33–12. **d** (*p. 755*) Long Term Complications

33–13. **a** (*p. 755*) Long Term Complications

33–14. **b** (*p. 755*) Reversal of Tubal Sterilization

33–15. **c** (*p. 756*) Male Sterilization

33–16. **d** (*p. 756*) Male Sterilization

33–17. **d** (*p. 756*) Male Sterilization

33–18. **b** (*p. 756*) Restoration of Fertility

33–19. **a** (*p. 756*) Long term Effects

33–20. **b** (*p. 756*) Long term Effects

CHAPTER 34

34–1. **b** (*p. 762*) Hypertensive Disorders in Pregnancy

34–2. **b** (*p. 762*) Table 34-1

34–3. **c** (*p. 763*) Diagnosis

34–4. **c** (*p. 763*) Gestational Hypertension

34–5. **c** (*p. 763*) Preeclampsia

34–6. **c** (*p. 763*) Preeclampsia

34–7. **b** (*p. 764*) Severity of Preeclampsia

34–8. **c** (*p. 764*) Table 34-2

34–9. **d** (*p. 764*) Eclampsia

34–10. **c** (*p. 765*) Preeclampsia Superimposed on Chronic Hypertension

34–11. **a** (*p. 765*) Preeclampsia Superimposed on Chronic Hypertension

34–12. **c** (*p. 765*) Preeclampsia Superimposed on Chronic Hypertension

34–13. **c** (*p. 765*) Incidence and Risk Factors

34–14. **a** (*p. 765*) Incidence and Risk Factors

34–15. **b** (*p. 765*) Incidence and Iisk Factors

34–16. **b** (*p. 766*) Etiology

34–17. **a** (*p. 766*) Abnormal Trophoblastic Invasion

34–18. **a** (*p. 769*) Increased Pressor Responses

34–19. **a** (*p. 769*) Increased Pressor Responses

34–20. **a** (*p. 769*) Nitric Oxide

34–21. **b** (*p. 770*) Cardiovascular System

34–22. **a** (*p. 771*) Blood Volume

34–23. **d** (*pp. 772, 773*) Blood and Coagulation

34–24. **a** (*p. 773*) Fragmentation Hemolysis

34–25. **d** (*p. 774*) Volume Hemostasis, Endocrine Changes

34–26. **c** (*p. 774*) Kidney

34–27. **a** (*p. 775*) Anatomical Changes

34–28. **c** (*p. 775*) Anatomical Changes

34–29. **b** (*p. 776*) Brain, Anatomical Pathology

34–30. **a** (*p. 778*) Blindness

34–31. **c** (*p. 778*) Uteroplacental Perfusion

34–32. **d** (*p. 778*) Uteroplacental Perfusion

34–33. **d** (*p. 779*) Roll-Over Test

34–34. **d** (*p. 780*) Prevention

34–35. **a** (*p. 780*) Low Dose Aspirin

34–36. **c** (*p. 764*) Table 34-2

34–37. **a** (*p. 782*) Table 34-5; Antihypertensive Drug Treatment

34–38. **c** (*p. 782*) Table 34-5; Antihypertensive Drug Treatment

34–39. **b** (*p. 787*) Eclampsia

34–40. **c** (*p. 789*) Pharmocology and Toxicology of Magnesium Sulfate

34–41. **b** (*p. 789*) Pharmocology and Toxicology of Magnesium Sulfate

34–42. **c** (*p. 789*) Pharmocology and Toxicology of Magnesium Sulfate

34–43. **c** (*p. 789*) Pharmocology and Toxicity of $MgSO_4$

34–44. **c** (*pp. 789, 790*) Pharmocology and Toxicity of $MgSO_4$

34–45. **c** (*p. 793*) Hydralazine to Control Severe Hypertension

34–46. **b** (*p. 793*) Labetalol

34–47. **a** (*p. 795*) Invasive Hemodynamic Monitoring

34–48. **b** (*p. 797*) Counseling for Future Pregnancies

CHAPTER 35

35–1. **a** (*p. 810*) Obstetrical Hemorrhage

35–2. **c** (*p. 810*) Table 35-1

35–3. **a** (*p. 810*) Antepartum Hemorrhage

35–4. **d** (*p. 813*) Etiology

35–5. **a** (*p. 813*) Etiology; Table 35-3

35–6. **a** (*p. 813*) Etiology

35–7. **a** (*p. 812*) Perinatal Morbidity and Mortality

35–8. **c** (*p. 814*) Etiology, External Trauma

35–9. **d** (*p. 814*) Recurrent Abruption

35–10. **b** (*p. 815*) Clinical Diagnosis; Table 35-4

35–11. **c** (*p. 816*) Consumptive Coagulopathy

35–12. **d** (*p. 816*) Renal Failure

35–13. **c** (*p. 816*) Couvelaire Uterus

35–14. **a** (*p. 817*) Management, Vaginal Delivery

35–15. **a** (*p. 817*) Cesarean Delivery

35–16. **b** (*p. 819*) Placenta Previa, Definition

35–17. **b** (*p. 820*) Incidence

35–18. **d** (*p. 820*) Etiology

35–19. **d** (*pp. 821, 822*) Diagnosis

35–20. **b** (*p. 823*) Management

35–21. **c** (*p. 823*) Delivery

35–22. **d** (*p. 820*) Incidence; Perinatal Morbidity and Mortality

35–23. **c** (*p. 824*) Post Partum Hemorrhage, Definition

35–24. **d** (*p. 825*) Diagnosis

35–25. **c** (*p. 825*) Diagnosis

35–26. **a** (*p. 825*) Sheehan Syndrome

35–27. **c** (*p. 833*) Inversion of the Uterus

35–28. **c** (*p. 826*) Management After Delivery of Placenta

35–29. **c** (*p. 826*) Uterine Atony

35–30. **c** (*p. 827*) Ergot derivatives

35–31. **b** (*p. 827*) Prostaglandins

35–32. **a** (*p. 827*) Prostaglandins

35–33. **a** (*pp. 827, 828*) Bleeding Unresponsive to Oxytocies

35–34. **d** (*p. 828*) Bleeding Unresponsive to Oxytocies

35–35. **d** (*pp. 829-30*) Bleeding Unresponsive to Oxytocies, Uterine Packing

35–36. **c** (*p. 831*) Definitions

35–37. **c** (*p. 831*) Significance

35–38. **c** (*p. 831*) Significance

35–39. **d** (*p. 831*) Etiology

35–40. **a** (*p. 832*) Clinical Course and Diagnosis

35–41. **b** (*p. 833*) Management

35–42. **c** (*p. 834*) Treatment

35–43. **a** (*p. 834*) Treatment

35–44. **d** (*p. 836*) Puerperal Hematomas

35–45. **a** (*p. 836*) Vulvar Hematomas

35–46. **b** (*p. 836*) Vulvar Hematomas

35–47. **d** (*p. 837*) Rupture of the Uterus

35–48. **c** (*p. 838*) Spontaneous Rupture, Table 35-7

35–49. **b** (*p. 839*) Hypovolemic Shock

35–50. **c** (*p. 839*) Hypovolemic Shock

35–51. **d** (*p. 839*) Estimation of Blood Loss

35–52. **b** (*p. 839*) Estimation of Blood Loss

35–53. **c** (*p. 840*) Blood Replacement

35–54. **b** (*p. 840*) Table 35-8, Whole Blood and Blood Components

35–55. **d** (*p. 841*) Table 35-8, Whole Blood and Blood Components

35–56. **a** (*p. 841*) Table 35-8, Whole Blood and Blood Components

35–57. **a** (*p. 841*) Table 35-8, Whole Blood and Blood Components

35–58. **c** (*p. 841*) Whole Blood and Blood Components; Dilational Coagulopathy

35–59. a (*p. 841*) Whole Blood and Blood Components; Type and Screen Us Crossmatch

35–60. b (*p. 841*) Whole Blood and Blood Components; Packed Red Blood Cells

35–61. b (*p. 842*) Whole Blood and Blood Components; Platelets

35–62. c (*p. 842*) Whole Blood and Blood Components; Cryoprecipitate

35–63. c (*p. 842*) Complication of Blood Transfusion

35–64. a (*p. 842*) Complication of Blood Transfusion

35–65. c (*p. 843*) Complication of Blood Transfusion

35–66. d (*pp. 843–44*) Pathological Activation of Coagulation

35–67. d (*p. 845*) Placental Abruption

35–68. d (*p. 844*) Heparin, Epsilon- Aminocaproic Acid

35–69. b (*p. 845*) Fetal Death and Delayed Delivery; Coagulation Changes

35–70. b (*p. 845*) Amnionic Fluid Embolism

35–71. b (*p. 845*) Amnionic Fluid Embolism

35–72. d (*p. 848*) Management

35–73. d (*p. 848*) Prognosis

35–74. a (*p. 848*) Abortion, Coagulation Defects

CHAPTER 36

36–1. b (*p. 856*) Preterm Birth (Chapter Title)

36–2. b (*p. 856*) Preterm Birth (Chapter Title)

36–3. d (*p. 856*) Preterm Birth (Chapter Title)

36–4. c (*p. 856*) Preterm Birth (Chapter Title)

36–5. b (*p. 856*) Preterm Birth (Chapter Title)

36–6. d (*p. 857*) Estimating Survival

36–7. b (*p. 857*) Estimating Survival

36–8. c (*p. 857*) Long-Term Outcomes

36–9. d (*p. 857*) Long-Term Outcomes

36–10. d (*p. 858*) Lower Limit of Survival: Counseling Considerations

36–11. c (*p. 858*) Upper Limit for Adverse Outcomes from Preterm Delivery

36–12. b (*p. 859*) Medical and Obstetrical Complications

36–13. b (*p. 859*) Medical and Obstetrical Complications

36–14. d (*p. 859*) Threatened Abortion

36–15. c (*p. 859*) Lifestyle Factors

36–16. c (*p. 860*) Prior Preterm Birth

36–17. d (*pp. 860–62*) Identification of Women at Risk for Spontaneous Preterm Labor

36–18. b (*p. 862*) Fetal Fibronectin

36–19. a (*p. 863*) Bacterial Vaginosis

36–20. d (*p. 863*) Bacterial Vaginosis

36–21. d (*pp. 863, 864*) Peridontal Disease

36–22. d (*p. 865*) Natural History of Preterm Membrane Rupture

36–23. a (*p. 865*) Natural History of Preterm Membrane Rupture

36–24. c (*pp. 865, 866*) Hospitalization

36–25. b (*p. 866*) Clinical Chorioamnionitis

36–26. d (*p. 866*) Clinical Chorioamnionitis

36–27. a (*p. 867*) Recommended Management of Preterm Membrane Rupture

36–28. d (*p. 867*) Diagnosis

36–29. b (*p. 867*) Management

36–30. b (*pp. 868, 869*) Glucocorticoid Therapy
to Enhance Fetal
Lung Maturity

36–31. d (*p. 869*) Emergency Cerclage

36–32. d (*p. 870*) Beta-Adrenergic Receptor Agonists

36–33. c (*p. 870*) Ritodrine

36–34. b (*p. 870*) Ritodrine

36–35. b (*p. 870*) Table 36-7

36–36. c (*p. 871*) Magnesium Sulfate

36–37. b (*p. 871*) Neonatal Effects of Magnesium

36–38. a (*p. 871*) Prostaglandin Inhibitors

36–39. a (*p. 872*) Calcium-Channel Blockers

36–40. c (*p. 872*) Atosiban

36–41. d (*pp. 872, 873*) Recommended Management
of Preterm Labor

CHAPTER 37

37–1. c (*p. 882*) Postterm Pregnancy
(Chapter Title)

37–2. c (*p. 882*) Postterm Pregnancy
(Chapter Title)

37–3. c (*p. 882*) Incidence

37–4. d (*p. 883*) Perinatal Mortality

37–5. d (*p. 883*) Incidence

37–6. a (*p. 883*) Incidence

37–7. b (*p. 883*) Perinatal Mortality

37–8. a (*p. 884*) Postmaturity Syndrome

37–9. c (*p. 885*) Placental Dysfunction

37–10. d (*p. 885*) Placental Dysfunction

37–11. b (*p. 885*) Fetal Distress and Oligohydramnios

37–12. a (*p. 887*) Management

37–13. d (*p. 890*) Table 37-3

37–14. a (*p. 888*) Unfavorable Cervix

37–15. b (*p. 888*) Unfavorable Cervix

37–16. b (*p. 888*) Induction Versus Fetal Testing

37–17. a (*p. 890*) Intrapartum Management

CHAPTER 38

38–1. a (*p. 894*) Fetal Growth Disorders

38–2. b (*p. 894*) Fetal Growth Disorders

38–3. c (*p. 894*) Fetal Growth Disorders

38–4. d (*p. 894*) Normal Fetal Growth

38–5. b (*p. 894*) Normal Fetal Growth

38–6. d (*p. 894*) Normal Fetal Growth

38–7. c (*p. 894*) Normal Fetal Growth

38–8. a (*p. 895*) Normal Fetal Growth

38–9. b (*p. 895*) Normal Fetal Growth

38–10. c (*p. 895*) Definition

38–11. d (*p. 895*) Definition

38–12. b (*p. 897*) Metabolic Abnormalities

38–13. b (*p. 897*) Metabolic Abnormalities

38–14. b (*p. 897*) Morbidity and Mortality

38–15. c (*p. 898*) Symmetrical Versus Asymmetrical
Growth Restriction

38–16. d (*p. 898*) Symmetrical Versus Asymmetrical
Growth Restriction

38–17. c (*pp. 898, 899*) Risk Factors

38–18. d (*p. 899*) Fetal Infections

38–19. a (*p. 899*) Chromosomal Aneuploides

38–20. b (*p. 899*) Chromosomal Aneuploides

38–21. c (*p. 900*) Placental and Cord Abnormalities

38–22. c (*p. 900*) Antiphospholipid Antibody Syndrome

38–23. b (*p. 901*) Ultrasonic Measurements

38–24. c (*p. 901*) Ultrasonic Measurements

38–25. d (*p. 902*) Ultrasonic Measurements

38–26. d (*p. 902*) Doppler Velocimetry

38–27. c (*p. 905*) Birthweight Distribution

38–28. b (*p. 905*) Risk Factors

38–29. d (*p. 905*) Diagnosis

38–30. b (*p. 906*) Elective Cesarean Section

CHAPTER 39

39–1. b (*p. 912*) Multifetal Gestation

39–2. d (*p. 912*) Multifetal Gestation

39–3. d (*p. 912*) Multifetal Gestation

39–4. c (*p. 913*) Etiology

39–5. d (*p. 913*) Genesis of Monozygotic Twins

39–6. a (*p. 913*) Genesis of Monozygotic Twins

39–7. c (*p. 913*) Genesis of Monozygotic Twins

39–8. c (*p. 914*) Superfetation and Superfecundation

39–9. c (*p. 914*) Frequency of Twins

39–10. b (*p. 915*) Maternal Age and Parity

39–11. a (*p. 915*) Table 39-2

39–12. c (*p. 916*) Infertility Therapy

39–13. b (*p. 916*) Assisted Reproductive Technology

39–14. a (*p. 917*) Sex Ratios with Multiple Fetuses

39–15. d (*p. 917*) Table 39-3

39–16. a (*p. 917*) Ultrasonographic Examination

39–17. b (*pp. 920, 921*) Ultrasonography/Other Diagnostic Aids

39–18. c (*p. 921*) Maternal Adaptation

39–19. c (*p. 921*) Maternal Adaptation

39–20. c (*p. 922*) Birthweight

39–21. d (*p. 922*) Birthweight

39–22. c (*p. 924*) Duration of Gestation

39–23. c (*p. 924*) Duration of Gestation

39–24. a (*p. 924*) Preterm Birth

39–25. b (*p. 925*) Monoamnionic Twins

39–26. b (*pp. 917, 925*) Ultrasonographic Examination/ Monoamnionic Twins

39–27. c (*p. 926*) Monoamnionic Twins

39–28. d (*p. 926*) Conjoined Twins

39–29. d (*p. 928*) Acardiac Twin

39–30. b (*p. 929*) Twin-to-Twin Transfusion Syndrome

39–31. b (*p. 930*) Fetal Brain Damage

39–32. b (*p. 930*) Diagnosis

39–33. c (*p. 932*) Therapy and Outcome

39–34. a (*p. 933*) Diagnosis

39–35. b (*p. 933*) Diagnosis

39–36. d (*pp. 932, 933*) Discordant Twins/ Diagnosis

39–37. **a** (*p. 934*) Death of One Fetus

39–38. **c** (*p. 935*) Diet

39–39. **d** (*p. 936*) Tests of Fetal Well-Being

39–40. **d** (*p. 936*) Prevention of Preterm Delivery

39–41. **c** (*p. 937*) Preterm Labor Prediction

39–42. **a** (*p. 939*) Presentation and Position

39–43. **d** (*p. 940*) Vaginal Delivery

39–44. **a** (*p. 940*) Vaginal Delivery

39–45. **d** (*p. 940*) Vaginal Delivery of the Second Twin

39–46. **d** (*p. 940*) Interval Between First and Second Twins

39–47. **d** (*p. 941*) Triplet or Higher-Order Gestation

39–48. **b** (*p. 942*) Selective Reduction

39–49. **d** (*p. 942*) Selective Termination

CHAPTER 40

40–1. **b** (*p. 950*) Embryogenesis of the Reproductive Tract

40–2. **b** (*p. 950*) Embryogenesis of the Reproductive Tract

40–3. **d** (*p. 950*) Embryogenesis of the Reproductive Tract

40–4. **c** (*p. 950*) Embryogenesis of the Reproductive Tract

40–5. **d** (*p. 950*) Genesis and Classification of Müllerian Abnormalities

40–6. **a** (*p. 950*) Genesis and Classification of Müllerian Abnormalities

40–7. **d** (*p. 950*) Genesis and Classification of Müllerian Abnormalities

40–8. **b** (*p. 950*) Vulvar Abnormalities

40–9. **a** (*p. 951*) Vaginal Abnormalities

40–10. **b** (*p. 952*) Atresia

40–11. **c** (*p. 953*) Diagnosis

40–12. **c** (*p. 953*) Auditory Defects

40–13. **d** (*pp. 953, 954*) Obstetrical Significance

40–14. **d** (*p. 954*) Table 40-2

40–15. **c** (*p. 954*) Unicornuate Uterus

40–16. **a** (*p. 954*) Unicornuate Uterus

40–17. **c** (*p. 955*) Uterine Didelphys (Class III)

40–18. **b** (*p. 956*) Uterine Didelphys (Class III)

40–19. **b** (*p. 956*) Metroplasty

40–20. **b** (*p. 957*) Metroplasty

40–21. **d** (*p. 957*) Diethylstilbestrol-Induced Reproductive Tract Abnormalities

40–22. **c** (*p. 957*) Structural Abnormalities

40–23. **b** (*p. 957*) Reproductive Performance

40–24. **a** (*p. 957*) Preterm Labor

40–25. **d** (*p. 957*) Diethylstilbestrol-Induced Reproductive Tract Abnormalities

40–26. **d** (*p. 958*) Bartholin Gland Lesions

40–27. **d** (*p. 959*) Female Genital Mutilation

40–28. **c** (*pp. 959, 960*) Female Genital Mutilation

40–29. **d** (*p. 960*) Genital Tract Fistulas

40–30. **c** (*p. 960*) Cervical Abnormalities

40–31. **d** (*p. 960*) Retroflexion

40–32. **c** (*p. 961*) Sacculation

40–33. **c** (*p. 961*) Uterine Prolapse

40–34. **a** (*p. 962*) Uterine Leiomyomas

40–35. **c** (*p. 962*) Infertility and Treatment

40–36. **b** (*p. 963*) Effects of Pregnancy on Myomas

40–37. **b** (*p. 963*) Effects of Pregnancy on Myomas

40–38. **c** (*p. 965*) Ovarian Abnormalities

40–39. **a** (*p. 965*) Ovarian Abnormalities

40–40. **c** (*p. 966*) Recommendations

40–41. **c** (*p. 966*) Recommendations

CHAPTER 41

41–1. **d** (*p. 974*) General Considerations and Maternal Evaluation

41–2. **a** (*p. 974*) Table 41-1

41–3. **b** (*p. 975*) Effect of Surgery & Anesthesia on Pregnancy Outcome

41–4. **a** (*p. 975*) Effect of Surgery & Anesthesia on Pregnancy Outcome

41–5. **d** (*p. 975*) Perinatal Outcomes

41–6. **c** (*p. 975*) Table 41-2

41–7. **a** (*p. 975*) Table 41-3

41–8. **d** (*p. 975*) Laparoscopic Surgery During Pregnancy

41–9. **d** (*p. 976*) Maternal and Fetal Effects

41–10. **c** (*p. 977*) Ionizing Radiation

41–11. **c** (*p. 977*) Ionizing Radiation

41–12. **a** (*p. 977*) Animal Studies

41–13. **b** (*p. 979*) Human Data

41–14. **d** (*p. 979*) Human Data

41–15. **a** (*p. 977*) Animal Studies

41–16. **a** (*p. 979*) Radiographs

41–17. **c** (*p. 979*) Radiographs

41–18. **d** (*p. 980*) Computed Tomography

41–19. **a** (*p. 980*) Table 41-7

41–20. **a** (*p. 982*) Nuclear Medicine Studies

41–21. **b** (*p. 982*) Safety

41–22. **b** (*p. 982*) Safety

41–23. **d** (*p. 982*) Magnetic Resonance Imaging

41–24. **b** (*p. 982*) Magnetic Resonance Imaging

41–25. **d** (*p. 982*) Safety

41–26. **d** (*p. 983*) Maternal Indications

41–27. **a** (*p. 984*) Fetal Indications

CHAPTER 42

42–1. **b** (*p. 988*) Obstetrical Intensive Care

42–2. **d** (*p. 989*) Pulmonary Artery Catheter Use

42–3. **b** (*p. 990*) Table 42-3

42–4. **c** (*p. 990*) Acute Pulmonary Edema

42–5. **c** (*p. 991*) Acute Respiratory Distress Syndrome

42–6. **d** (*p. 991*) Definitions

42–7. **b** (*p. 992*) Management

42–8. **a** (*p. 992*) Management

42–9. **d** (*p. 992*) Oxyhemoglobin Dissociation Curve

42–10. **c** (*p. 993*) Fluid Therapy

42–11. **d** (*p. 993*) Fluid Therapy

42–12. **d** (*p. 993*) Other Therapy

42–13. **a** (*p. 994*) Etiopathogenesis

42–14. **d** (*p. 994*) Etiopathogenesis

42–15. **c** (*p. 994*) Etiopathogenesis

42–16. a (*p. 994*) Hemodynamic Changes with Sepsis

42–17. c (*p. 996*) Pressor Agents

42–18. c (*p. 996*) Anti-Inflammatory Agents

42–19. c (*p. 996*) Trauma in Pregnancy

42–20. b (*p. 998*) Table 42-8

42–21. a (*p. 998*) Traumatic Placental Abruption

42–22. a (*p. 999*) Traumatic Placental Abruption

42–23. b (*p. 999*) Penetrating Trauma

42–24. d (*pp. 999–1001*) Management of Trauma

42–25. c (*p. 1001*) Prognosis

42–26. c (*p. 1002*) Cardiopulmonary Resuscitation

CHAPTER 43

43–1. a (*p. 1008*) Obesity

43–2. d (*p. 1008*) Obesity

43–3. c (*p. 1008*) Obesity

43–4. a (*p. 1008*) Definitions

43–5. a (*p. 1008*) Definitions

43–6. a (*p. 1008*) Definitions

43–7. d (*p. 1009*) Metabolic Syndrome

43–8. b (*p. 1009*) Table 43-1

43–9. d (*p. 1009*) Metabolic Syndrome/Prevalence

43–10. d (*p. 1010*) Morbidity and Mortality Associated with Obesity

43–11. a (*p. 1011*) Weight Loss During Pregnancy

43–12. d (*pp. 1011, 1012*) Maternal Morbidity

43–13. a (*pp. 1012, 1013*) Perinatal Morbidity and Mortality

43–14. d (*pp. 1013, 1014*) Pregnancy Following Surgical Procedures for Obesity

CHAPTER 44

44–1. b (*p. 1018*) Cardiovascular Disease

44–2. c (*p. 1018*) Physiological Considerations Associated with Heart Disease in Pregnancy

44–3. b (*p. 1018*) Physiological Considerations Associated with Heart Disease in Pregnancy

44–4. d (*p. 1018*) Physiological Considerations Associated with Heart Disease in Pregnancy

44–5. d (*p. 1018*) Physidogical Considerations Associated with Heart Disease in Pregnancy

44–6. b (*p. 1019*) Table 44-2

44–7. a (*p. 1018*) Table 44-1

44–8. d (*p. 1018*) Diagnostic Studies

44–9. c (*p. 1019*) Electrocardiography

44–10. c (*p. 1019*) Echocardiography

44–11. b (*p. 1019*) Clinical Classification

44–12. a (*p. 1020*) Table 44-3

44–13. a (*p. 1020*) Congenital Heart Disease in Offspring

44–14. d (*p. 1021*) Management of Class I and II Disease

44–15. c (*p. 1021*) Management of Class I and II Disease

44–16. c (*p. 1021*) Labor and Delivery

44–17. a (*p. 1021*) Labor and Delivery

44–18. b (*p. 1022*) Effects on Pregnancy

44–19. **d** (*p. 1022*) Effects on Pregnancy

44–20. **a** (*p. 1023*) Effects on Pregnancy

44–21. **d** (*p. 1023*) Management

44–22. **c** (*p. 1023*) Management

44–23. **a** (*p. 1023*) Management

44–24. **d** (*p. 1024*) Mitral Valvotomy During Pregnancy

44–25. **c** (*p. 1024*) Valvular Heart Disease

44–26. **d** (*p. 1024*) Mitral Stenosis

44–27. **c** (*p. 1024*) Mitral Stenosis

44–28. **b** (*p. 1024*) Mitral Stenosis

44–29. **a** (*p. 1025*) Management

44–30. **a** (*p. 1026*) Aortic Stenosis

44–31. **a** (*p. 1026*) Management in Pregnancy

44–32. **c** (*p. 1027*) Aortic Insufficiency

44–33. **b** (*p. 1027*) Congenital Heart Disease

44–34. **c** (*p. 1027*) Atrial Septal Defects

44–35. **b** (*p. 1027*) Atrial Septal Defects

44–36. **d** (*p. 1027*) Ventricular Septal Defects

44–37. **a** (*p. 1020*) Table 44-4

44–38. **d** (*p. 1027*) Ventricular Septal Defects

44–39. **a** (*p. 1028*) Cyanotic Heart Disease

44–40. **c** (*p. 1028*) Cyanotic Heart Disease

44–41. **b** (*p. 1028*) Labor and Delivery

44–42. **d** (*p. 1028*) Eisenmenger Syndrome

44–43. **d** (*p. 1029*) Pulmonary Hypertension

44–44. **c** (*p. 1029*) Pulmonary Hypertension

44–45. **d** (*p. 1029*) Mitral-Valve Prolapse

44–46. **b** (*p. 1029*) Mitral-Valve Prolapse

44–47. **d** (*p. 1030*) Peripartum Cardiomyopathy

44–48. **b** (*p. 1030*) Idiopathic Cardiomyopathy in Pregnancy

44–49. **d** (*p. 1033*) Table 44-7

44–50. **a** (*p. 1032*) Infective Endocarditis

44–51. **a** (*p. 1032*) Infective Endocarditis

44–52. **a** (*p. 1033*) Obstetrical Procedures

44–53. **d** (*p. 1033*) Arrhythmias

44–54. **d** (*p. 1034*) Arrhythmias

44–55. **a** (*p. 1034*) Arrhythmias

44–56. **d** (*p. 1034*) Diseases of the Aorta

44–57. **b** (*p. 1034*) Diseases of the Aorta

44–58. **c** (*p. 1035*) Effect of Pregnancy (Marfan Syndrome)

44–59. **a** (*p. 1035*) Effects on Pregnancy (Aortic Coarctation)

44–60. **d** (*p. 1036*) Myocardial Infarction During Pregnancy

44–61. **d** (*p. 1036*) Hypertrophic Cardiomyopathy

44–62. **b** (*p. 1037*) Hypertrophic Cardiomyopathy

CHAPTER 45

45–1. **a** (*p. 1045*) Diagnosis

45–2. **b** (*p. 1045*) Treatment in Nonpregnant Adults

45–3. **b** (*p. 1046*) Table 45-2

45–4. **a** (*p. 1045*) Definitions

45–5. **c** (*p. 1044*) Table 45-1

45–6. **d** (*p. 1046*) Preconceptional and Early Pregnancy Evaluation

45–7. b (*p. 1046*) Preconceptional and Early Pregnancy Evaluation

45–8. a (*p. 1047*) Maternal Effects

45–9. b (*p. 1047*) Superimposed Preeclampsia

45–10. b (*p. 1047*) Prevention

45–11. d (*p. 1047*) Fetal and Newborn Effects

45–12. b (*p. 1047*) Fetal Growth Restriction

45–13. d (*p. 1049*) Adrenergic-Blocking Agents

45–14. c (*p. 1049*) Antihypertensive Drugs

45–15. b (*p. 1049*) Angiotensin-Converting Enzyme Inhibitors...

45–16. c (*p. 1051*) Antihypertensive Drug Selection

45–17. d (*p. 1052*) Pregnancy-Aggravated Hypertension...

45–18. c (*p. 1052*) Pregnancy-Aggravated Hypertension...

45–19. c (*p. 1052*) Delivery

45–20. a (*p. 1052*) Postpartum Considerations

CHAPTER 46

46–1. b (*p. 1056*) Pulmonary Disorders

46–2. b (*p. 1056*) Pulmonary Physiology

46–3. a (*p. 1056*) Pulmonary Physiology

46–4. c (*p. 1056*) Pulmonary Physiology

46–5. a (*p. 1056*) Pulmonary Physiology

46–6. d (*p. 1056*) Bacterial Pneumonia, Incidence & Causes

46–7. a (*p. 1056*) Bacterial Pneumonia

46–8. c (*p. 1056*) Incidence & Causes

46–9. d (*p. 1057*) Diagnosis

46–10. b (*p. 1057*) Management

46–11. d (*p. 1057*) Management

46–12. d (*p. 1057*) Management

46–13. b (*p. 1058*) Table 46-2

46–14. a (*p. 1058*) Prevention

46–15. d (*p. 1059*) Prevention

46–16. d (*p. 1059*) Prevention

46–17. b (*p. 1059*) Management

46–18. c (*p. 1059*) Management

46–19. a (*p. 1059*) Varicella Pneumonia

46–20. d (*p. 1059*) Varicella Pneumonia

46–21. d (*p. 1059*) Pregnancy Outcome

46–22. b (*p. 1059*) Prophylaxis

46–23. a (*p. 1059*) Management

46–24. c (*p. 1059*) Prophylaxis

46–25. c (*p. 1060*) Pneumocystis Pneumonia

46–26. a (*p. 1060*) Pneumocystis Pneumonia

46–27. c (*p. 1060*) Fungal Pneumonia

46–28. c (*p. 1060*) Asthma

46–29. d (*p. 1060*) Pathophysiology

46–30. c (*p. 1061*) Effects of Pregnancy on Asthma

46–31. d (*pp. 1061, 1062*) Pregnancy Outcome

46–32. c (*p. 1061*) Table 46-3

46–33. a (*p. 1061*) Table 46-3

46–34. d (*p. 1062*) Clinical Evaluation

46–35. c (*p. 1062*) Clinical Evaluation

46–36. b (*p. 1062*) Management of Chronic Asthma

46–37. b (*p. 1063*) Management of Chronic Asthma

46–38. c (*p. 1064*) Labor and Delivery

46–39. **a** (*p. 1064*) Labor and Delivery

46–40. **a** (*p. 1064*) Tuberculosis

46–41. **c** (*p. 1064*) Tuberculosis

46–42. **d** (*p. 1065*) Treatment

46–43. **c** (*p. 1065*) Treatment

46–44. **a** (*p. 1065*) Treatment

46–45. **d** (*p. 1066*) Sarcoidosis

46–46. **c** (*p. 1066*) Sarcoidosis

46–47. **c** (*p. 1066*) Cystic Fibrosis

46–48. **d** (*p. 1067*) Pathophysiology

46–49. **a** (*p. 1067*) Pathophysiology

46–50. **a** (*p. 1067*) Management

46–51. **d** (*p. 1068*) Treatment

CHAPTER 47

47–1. **c** (*p. 1074*) Table 47-1

47–2. **c** (*p. 1074*) Table 47-1

47–3. **a** (*p. 1074*) Pathophysiology

47–4. **d** (*p. 1074*) Pathophysiology

47–5. **d** (*p. 1075*) Table 47-2

47–6. **a** (*pp. 1075, 1076*) Antithrombin Deficiency

47–7. **b** (*p. 1076*) Protein C Deficiency

47–8. **a** (*p. 1076*) Protein S Deficiency

47–9. **b** (*p. 1076*) Protein S Deficiency

47–10. **c** (*p. 1076*) Activated Protein C Resistance

47–11. **a** (*p. 1076*) Activated Protein C Resistance

47–12. **a** (*p. 1077*) Activated Protein C Resistance

47–13. **a** (*p. 1078*) Hyperhomocysteinemia

47–14. **b** (*p. 1078*) Antiphospholipid Antibodies

47–15. **a** (*p. 1079*) Clinical Presentations

47–16. **c** (*p. 1079*) Venography

47–17. **c** (*p. 1080*) Compression Ultrasonography

47–18. **c** (*p. 1082*) Low Molecular Weight Heparin

47–19. **d** (*p. 1082*) Low Molecular Weight Heparin

47–20. **a** (*p. 1083*) Complication of Anticoagulation

47–21. **b** (*p. 1083*) Heparin Induced Osteoporosis

47–22. **a** (*p. 1084*) Anticoagulation & Delivery

47–23. **b** (*p. 1084*) Superficial Venous Thrombophlebitis

47–24. **b** (*p. 1085*) Ventilation-Perfusion Scintigraphy

47–25. **d** (*p. 1087*) Management

47–26. **b** (*p. 1087*) Thromboembolism Antedating Pregnancy

CHAPTER 48

48–1. **c** (*p. 1094*) Urinary Tract Changes During Pregnancy

48–2. **d** (*p. 1094*) Urinary Tract Changes During Pregnancy

48–3. **d** (*p. 1094*) Assessment of Renal Disease During Pregnancy

48–4. **a** (*p. 1094*) Assessment of Renal Disease During Pregnancy

48–5. **c** (*p. 1094*) Assessment of Renal Disease During Pregnancy

48–6. **a** (*p. 1095*) Orthostatic Proteinuria

48–7. **b** (*p. 1095*) Urinary Tract Infections

48–8. **b** (*p. 1095*) Asymptomatic Bacteriuria

48–9. **b** (*p. 1095*) Significance

48–10. **c** (*p. 1095*) Asymptomatic Bacteriuria

48–11. **b** (*p. 1095*) Significance

48–12. **d** (*p. 1095*) Significance

48–13. **c** (*p. 1096*) Treatment

48–14. **d** (*p. 1096*) Acute Pyelonephritis

48–15. **d** (*p. 1096*) Clinical Findings

48–16. **c** (*p. 1097*) Clinical Findings

48–17. **d** (*p. 1097*) Clinical Findings

48–18. **a** (*p. 1097*) Clinical Findings

48–19. **b** (*p. 1098*) Management

48–20. **d** (*p. 1099*) Management of Non-Responders

48–21. **c** (*p. 1098*) Management of Non-Responders

48–22. **c** (*p. 1099*) Reflux Nephropathy

48–23. **b** (*p. 1099*) Nephrolithiasis

48–24. **a** (*p. 1099*) Stone Disease; Diagnosis

48–25. **b** (*p. 1100*) Glomerulopathies

48–26. **a** (*p. 1100*) Acute Nephrotic Syndrome

48–27. **d** (*pp. 1100, 1101*) Effects of Glomerulonephritis on Pregnancy

48–28. **c** (*p. 1101*) Effects of Glomerulonephritis on Pregnancy

48–29. **c** (*p. 1101*) Effects of Glomerulonephritis on Pregnancy

48–30. **a** (*p. 1101*) Nephrotic Syndrome

48–31. **a** (*p. 1101*) Table 48-4

48–32. **a** (*p. 1102*) Nephrotic Syndrome Complicating Pregnancy

48–33. **b** (*p. 1102*) Nephrotic Syndrome Complicating Pregnancy

48–34. **d** (*p. 1102*) Polycystic Kidney Disease

48–35. **b** (*p. 1102*) Polycystic Kidney Disease

48–36. **d** (*p. 1102*) Polycystic Kidney Disease

48–37. **a** (*p. 1102*) Polycystic Kidney Disease

48–38. **d** (*p. 1102*) Polycystic Kidney Disease & Pregnancy

48–39. **a** (*p. 1102*) Chronic Renal Disease

48–40. **c** (*p. 1103*) Physiological Changes

48–41. **b** (*p. 1103*) Physiological Changes

48–42. **a** (*p. 1104*) Chronic Renal Insufficiency

48–43. **b** (*p. 1104*) Management

48–44. **d** (*p. 1104*) Followup

48–45. **c** (*pp. 1104, 1105*) Pregnancy After Renal Transplant

48–46. **a** (*p. 1104*) Pregnancy After Renal Transplant

48–47. **c** (*p. 1106*) Acute Renal Failure

CHAPTER 49

49–1. **d** (*p. 1112*) Diagnostic Testing

49–2. **b** (*p. 1112*) Laparotomy & Laparoscopy

49–3. **c** (*p. 1112*) Laparotomy & Laparoscopy

49–4. **d** (*p. 1112*) Laparotomy & Laparoscopy

49–5. **b** (*p. 1112*) Nutritional Support

49–6. **d** (*p. 1113*) Nutritional Support

49–7. **c** (*p. 1113*) Hyperemesis Gravidarum

49–8. **d** (*p. 1113*) Hyperemesis Gravidarum

49–9. **d** (*p. 1113*) Complications

49–10. **d** (*p. 1114*) Reflux Esophagitis

49–11. **a** (*p. 1114*) Diaphragmatic Hernia

49–12. d (*p. 1114*) Achalasia

49–13. b (*p. 1115*) Achalasia

49–14. b (*p. 1115*) Peptic Ulcer

49–15. c (*p. 1115*) Peptic Ulcer

49–16. c (*p. 1115*) Upper GI Bleeding

49–17. a (*p. 1116*) Ulcerative Colitis

49–18. c (*p. 1116*) Ulcerative Colitis

49–19. a (*p. 1116*) Table 49-2

49–20. b (*p. 1116*) Ulcerative Colitis

49–21. d (*p. 1116*) Management

49–22. b (*p. 1116*) CROHN Disease

49–23. b (*p. 1117*) Ulcerative Colitis & Pregnancy

49–24. a (*p. 1118*) Ostomy & Pregnancy

49–25. b (*p. 1118*) Intestinal Obstruction

49–26. c (*p. 1119*) Intestinal Obstruction

49–27. c (*p. 1119*) Intestinal Obstruction

49–28. d (*p. 1119*) Appendicitis

49–29. d (*p. 1120*) Effects on Pregnancy

CHAPTER 50

50–1. a (*p. 1126*) Diseases of the Liver

50–2. c (*p. 1126*) Hyperemesis Gravidarum

50–3. d (*p. 1126*) Pathogenesis

50–4. d (*p. 1126*) Pathogenesis

50–5. a (*p. 1126*) Pathogenesis

50–6. b (*p. 1126*) Management

50–7. a (*p. 1127*) Cholestasis & Pregnancy Outcomes

50–8. b (*p. 1127*) Acute Fatty Liver

50–9. b (*p. 1128*) Etiology & Pathogenesis

50–10. d (*p. 1128*) Clinical Findings

50–11. a (*p. 1128*) Clinical Findings

50–12. b (*p. 1129*) Clinical Findings

50–13. b (*p. 1129*) Viral Hepatitis

50–14. b (*p. 1130*) Complications

50–15. b (*p. 1130*) Hepatitis A

50–16. c (*p. 1130*) Table 50-2

50–17. a (*p. 1130*) Immunization

50–18. b (*p. 1130*) Hepatitis B

50–19. d (*p. 1130*) Hepatitis B

50–20. c (*p. 1130*) Hepatitis B

50–21. d (*p. 1130*) Hepatitis B

50–22. d (*p. 1131*) Prevention of Neonatal Infection

50–23. c (*p. 1131*) Hepatitis C

50–24. c (*p. 1131*) Hepatitis C

50–25. c (*p. 1132*) Pregnancy Outcome

50–26. c (*p. 1132*) Treatment

50–27. d (*p. 1132*) Hepatitis E

50–28. a (*p. 1133*) Non-Alcoholic Fatty Liver

50–29. b (*p. 1133*) Cirrhosis

50–30. b (*p. 1133*) Portal Hypertension & Esophageal Varices

50–31. c (*p. 1133*) Portal Hypertension & Esophageal Varices

50–32. a (*p. 1134*) Portal Hypertension & Esophageal Varices

50–33. a (*p. 1134*) Acute Acetaminophen Overdose

50–34. c (*p. 1134*) Liver Transplantation

50–35. **a** (*p. 1135*) Cholelithiasis and Cholecystitis

50–36. **d** (*pp. 1135–36*) Management

50–37. **b** (*p. 1136*) Pancreatitis

50–38. **d** (*p. 1136*) Pancreatitis

50–39. **c** (*p. 1136*) Pancreatitis

50–40. **b** (*p. 1136*) Pancreatitis

CHAPTER 51

51–1. **c** (*p. 1144*) Anemia

51–2. **c** (*p. 1145*) Effects of Anemia on Pregnancy

51–3. **a** (*p. 1145*) Iron-Deficiency Anemia

51–4. **c** (*p. 1145*) Iron-Deficiency Anemia

51–5. **b** (*p. 1145*) Diagnosis

51–6. **b** (*p. 1145*) Iron-Deficiency Anemia

51–7. **b** (*p. 1145*) Diagnosis

51–8. **c** (*p. 1145*) Treatment

51–9. **c** (*p. 1146*) Anemia Associated with Chronic Disease

51–10. **c** (*p. 1146*) Chronic Renal Disease

51–11. **b** (*p. 1146*) Pyelonephritis

51–12. **a** (*p. 1146*) Treatment

51–13. **a** (*p. 1146*) Folic Acid Deficiency

51–14. **d** (*p. 1146*) Treatment

51–15. **d** (*pp. 1146, 1147*) Prevention

51–16. **d** (*p. 1147*) Vitamin B_{12} Deficiency

51–17. **b** (*p. 1147*) Vitamin B_{12} Deficiency

51–18. **c** (*p. 1147*) Autoimmune Hemolytic Anemia

51–19. **d** (*p. 1147*) Autoimmune Hemolytic Anemia

51–20. **a** (*p. 1147*) Autoimmune Hemolytic Anemia

51–21. **c** (*p. 1147*) Drug-Induced Hemolytic Anemia

51–22. **b** (*p. 1147*) Paroxysmal Nocturnal Hemoglobinuria

51–23. **b** (*pp. 1147, 1148*) Paroxysmal Nocturnal Hemoglobinuria

51–24. **d** (*p. 1148*) Paroxysmal Nocturnal Hemoglobinusia

51–25. **b** (*p. 1148*) Hereditary Spherocytosis

51–26. **c** (*p. 1148*) Hereditary Spherocytosis

51–27. **d** (*pp. 1148, 1149*) Hereditary Spherocytosis

51–28. **c** (*p. 1149*) Red Cell Enzyme Def.

51–29. **d** (*p. 1149*) Aplastic Anemia

51–30. **a** (*p. 1150*) Aplastic Anemia & Pregnancy

51–31. **a** (*p. 1150*) Sickle-Cell Hemoglobinopathies

51–32. **c** (*p. 1150*) Inheritance of Sickling Syndrome

51–33. **c** (*p. 1150*) Pregnancy & Sickle Cell Syndrome

51–34. **b** (*p. 1150*) Inheritance of Sickling Syndrome

51–35. **c** (*p. 1151*) Table 51-3

51–36. **d** (*p. 1151*) Management During Pregnancy

51–37. **b** (*p. 1152*) Prophylactic Red Cell Transfusions

51–38. **b** (*p. 1152*) Complications

51–39. **d** (*p. 1153*) Sickle Cell Trait

51–40. **c** (*p. 1153*) Hemoglobin C & C–B Thalassemia

51–41. **d** (*p. 1153*) Hemoglobin C & C–B Thalassemia

51–42. **a** (*p. 1153*) Hemoglobin E

51–43. **c** (*p. 1154*) Alpha-Thalassemia

51–44. **d** (*p. 1154*) Alpha-Thalassemia

51–45. **b** (*p. 1154*) Alpha-Thalassemia

51–46. **a** (*p. 1155*) Beta-Thalassemia

51–47. **c** (*p. 1154*) Alpha-Thalassemia

51–48. **b** (*p. 1155*) Beta-Thalassemia

51–49. **b** (*p. 1155*) Beta-Thalassemia

51–50. **d** (*p. 1155*) Beta-Thalassemia

51–51. **a** (*p. 1156*) Polycythemia

51–52. **b** (*p. 1157*) Inherited Thrombocytopenias

51–53. **a** (*p. 1157*) Immune Thrombocytopenic Purpura

51–54. **b** (*p. 1158*) Fetal and Neonatal Effects

51–55. **d** (*p. 1158*) Fetal and Neonatal Effects

51–56. **b** (*p. 1158*) Detection of Fetal Thrombocytopenia

51–57. **d** (*p. 1158*) Thrombocytosis

51–58. **c** (*p. 1159*) Pregnancy

51–59. **d** (*p. 1159*) Thrombotic Microangiopathies

51–60. **b** (*p. 1159*) Pathogenesis

51–61. **d** (*p. 1159*) Clinical Presentation

51–62. **b** (*p. 1159*) Hematological Abnormalities

51–63. **d** (*p. 1159*) Treatment

51–64. **c** (*p. 1160*) Hemophilia

51–65. **c** (*p. 1160*) Hemophilia

51–66. **c** (*p. 1160*) Hemophilia

51–67. **a** (*p. 1161*) Von Willebrand Disease

51–68. **b** (*p. 1161*) Von Willebrand Disease

51–69. **d** (*p. 1161*) Von Willebrand Disease

51–70. **c** (*p. 1162*) Other Inherited Coagulation Factor Deficiency

51–71. **d** (*p. 1146*) Anemia from Acute Blood Loss

51–72. **c** (*p. 1151*) Table 51-3

51–73. **c** (*pp. 1074, 1162*) Thrombophilias

CHAPTER 52

52–1. **a** (*p. 1170*) Diabetes

52–2. **c** (*p. 1170*) Classification

52–3. **b** (*p. 1170*) Classification

52–4. **b** (*p. 1170*) Classification

52–5. **d** (*p. 1171*) Diagnosis of Overt Diabetes During Pregnancy

52–6. **c** (*p. 1171*) Diagnosis of Overt Diabetes During Pregnancy

52–7. **a** (*p. 1172*) Table 52-3

52–8. **d** (*pp. 1171, 1172*) Table 52-3

52–9. **a** (*p. 1171*) Detection of Gestational Diabetes

52–10. **d** (*p. 1171*) Table 52-4

52–11. **d** (*p. 1172*) Table 52-4

52–12. **d** (*p. 1173*) Gestational Diabetes

52–13. **a** (*p. 1173*) Maternal and Fetal Effects

52–14. **d** (*p. 1173*) Macrosomia

52–15. **d** (*p. 1173*) Macrosomia

52–16. **d** (*p. 1173*) Macrosomia

52–17. **b** (*p. 1174*) Diet

52–18. **d** (*p. 1174*) Plasma Glucose Control

52–19. **c** (*p. 1176*) Postpartum Consequences

52–20. **d** (*p. 1170*) Classification During Pregnancy

52–21. **d** (*p. 1176*) Table 52-6

52–22. **b** (*p. 1177*) Abortion

52–23. **c** (*p. 1177*) Malformations

52–24. d (*pp. 1177, 1178*) Unexplained Fetal Demise

52–25. a (*p. 1180*) Maternal Effects

52–26. b (*p. 1181*) Ketoacidosis

52–27. c (*pp. 1181, 1182*) Infections

52–28. d (*pp. 1177, 1182*) Preconception

52–29. d (*p. 1184*) Contraception

CHAPTER 53

53–1. d (*p. 1190*) Thyroid and Other Endocrine Disorders

53–2. a (*p. 1192*) Table 53-1

53–3. a (*p. 1190*) Thyroid Physiology

53–4. a (*p. 1190*) Thyroid Physiology

53–5. c (*p. 1190*) Thyroid Physiology

53–6. b (*p. 1191*) Autoimmune Thyroid Disease

53–7. c (*p. 1192*) Hyperthyroidism

53–8. c (*pp. 1190, 1192*) Hyperthyroidism

53–9. a (*p. 1192*) Treatment

53–10. b (*p. 1192*) Treatment

53–11. a (*p. 1192*) Treatment

53–12. c (*p. 1192*) Treatment

53–13. b (*p. 1193*) Pregnancy Outcome

53–14. c (*p. 1193*) Table 53-2

53–15. b (*p. 1193*) Thyroid Storm and Heart Failures

53–16. c (*p. 1194*) Fetal and Neonatal Effects

53–17. d (*pp. 1192, 1194*) Subclinical Hyperthyroidism

53–18. b (*p. 1195*) Table 53-3

53–19. a (*p. 1195*) Pregnancy Outcome with Overt Hypothyroidism

53–20. d (*p. 1195*) Subclinical Hypothyroidism and Pregnancy

53–21. d (*p. 1195*) Screening in Pregnancy

53–22. b (*p. 1196*) Iodine Deficiency

53–23. c (*p. 1196*) Congenital Hypothyroidism

53–24. b (*p. 1196*) Congenital Hypothyroidism

53–25. b (*p. 1196*) Postpartum Thyroiditis

53–26. a (*pp. 1196, 1197*) Postpartum Thyroiditis

53–27. d (*p. 1197*) Postpartum Thyroiditis

53–28. b (*p. 1197*) Clinical Manifestations

53–29. d (*p. 1197*) Nodular Thyroid Disease

53–30. b (*p. 1198*) Parathyroid Diseases

53–31. b (*p. 1198*) Parathyroid Diseases

53–32. c (*p. 1198*) Parathyroid Diseases

53–33. d (*p. 1198*) Hyperparathyroidism in Pregnancy

53–34. a (*p. 1199*) Management

53–35. a (*p. 1199*) Hypoparathyroidism

53–36. d (*p. 1199*) Pregnancy-Associated Osteoporosis

53–37. d (*p. 1199*) Adrenal Gland Disorders

53–38. b (*p. 1199*) Pheochromocytoma

53–39. a (*p. 1200*) Pheochromocytoma

53–40. a (*p. 1200*) Management

53–41. a (*p. 1200*) Cushing Syndrome

53–42. d (*p. 1201*) Pregnancy and Cushing Syndrome

53–43. d (*p. 1202*) Adrenal Deficiency

53–44. b (*p. 1202*) Primary Aldosteronism

53–45. **b** (*p. 1202*) Pituitary Diseases

53–46. **d** (*p. 1202*) Prolactinomas

53–47. **d** (*p. 1203*) Prolactinomas and Pregnancy

53–48. **b** (*p. 1203*) Diabetes Insipidus

53–49. **a** (*p. 1203*) Diabetes Insipidus

53–50. **d** (*p. 1203*) Sheehan Syndrome

53–51. **b** (*p. 1203*) Lymphocytic Hypophysitis

CHAPTER 54

54–1. **a** (*p. 1210*) Immunological Aspects

54–2. **a** (*p. 1210*) Immunological Aspects

54–3. **d** (*p. 1211*) Systemic Lupus Erythematosus

54–4. **b** (*p. 1211*) Systemic Lupus Erythematosus

54–5. **c** (*p. 1211*) Systemic Lupus Erythematosus

54–6. **c** (*p. 1211*) Clinical Findings

54–7. **d** (*p. 1211*) Laboratory Findings

54–8. **c** (*p. 1211*) Laboratory Findings

54–9. **b** (*p. 1212*) Diagnosis

54–10. **a** (*p. 1212*) Table 54-2

54–11. **d** (*p. 1212*) Drug-Induced Lupus

54–12. **d** (*p. 1212*) Lupus and Maternal Outcome

54–13. **b** (*p. 1213*) Lupus Nephropathy

54–14. **a** (*p. 1214*) Pharmacological Treatment

54–15. **b** (*p. 1214*) Pharmacological Treatment

54–16. **c** (*p. 1214*) Long-Term Prognosis and Contraception

54–17. **b** (*p. 1215*) Neonatal Lupus

54–18. **a** (*p. 1215*) Congenital Heart Block

54–19. **a** (*p. 1215*) Congenital Heart Block

54–20. **d** (*p. 1215*) Congenital Heart Block

54–21. **c** (*p. 1215*) Congenital Heart Block

54–22. **d** (*p. 1215*) Antiphospholipid Antibodies

54–23. **d** (*p. 1215*) Antiphospholipid Antibodies

54–24. **d** (*p. 1216*) Pathophysiology

54–25. **c** (*p. 1216*) Association of Antiphospholipid Antibodies with Lupus

54–26. **b** (*p. 1216*) Association of Antiphospholipid Antibodies with Lupus

54–27. **b** (*p. 1217*) Antiphospholipid Antibodies in Normal Pregnancy

54–28. **a** (*p. 1217*) Diagnosis of Antiphospholipid Antibody Syndrome

54–29. **c** (*p. 1217*) Diagnosis of Antiphospholipid Antibody Syndrome

54–30. **c** (*p. 1219*) Results of Treatment

54–31. **d** (*p. 1219*) Rheumatoid Arthritis

54–32. **a** (*p. 1219*) Management

54–33. **d** (*p. 1219*) Effects of Pregnancy

54–34. **c** (*p. 1219*) Effects of Pregnancy

54–35. **d** (*p. 1220*) Perinatal Outcome

54–36. **d** (*p. 1221*) Clinical Course

54–37. **a** (*p. 1221*) Clinical Course

54–38. **c** (*p. 1221*) Clinical Course

54–39. **c** (*p. 1221*) Clinical Course

54–40. **d** (*p. 1221*) Clinical Course

54–41. **a** (*p. 1221*) Polyarteritis Nodosa

54–42. **b** (*p. 1222*) Dermatomyositis and Polymyositis

54–43. **c** (*p. 1222*) Marfan Syndrome

54–44. **d** (*p. 1223*) Ehlers-Danlos Syndrome

54–45. **a** (*p. 1223*) Ehlers-Danlos Syndrome

CHAPTER 55

55–1. **d** (*p. 1230*) Diagnosis of Neurological Disease During Pregnancy; Central Nervous System Imaging

55–2. **a** (*p. 1230*) Diagnosis of Neurological Disease During Pregnancy; Central Nervous System Imaging

55–3. **d** (*p. 1230*) Diagnosis of Neurological Disease During Pregnancy; Central Nervous System Imaging

55–4. **c** (*p. 1231*) Migraine Headache

55–5. **b** (*p. 1231*) Migraine Headache

55–6. **b** (*p. 1231*) Effects of Pregnancy

55–7. **c** (*p. 1231*) Management

55–8. **d** (*p. 1231*) Management

55–9. **a** (*p. 1231*) Effects of Pregnancy

55–10. **a** (*p. 1231*) Seizure Disorders

55–11. **d** (*p. 1232*) Pathophysiology

55–12. **b** (*p. 1232*) Epilepsy During Pregnancy

55–13. **b** (*p. 1232*) Epilepsy During Pregnancy

55–14. **a** (*p. 1232*) Epilepsy During Pregnancy

55–15. **b** (*p. 1232*) Management

55–16. **c** (*p. 1233*) Management

55–17. **d** (*p. 1233*) Prenatal Care

55–18. **d** (*p. 1233*) Prenatal Care

55–19. **a** (*p. 1233*) Cerebrovascular Disease

55–20. **b** (*p. 1233*) Cerebrovascular Disease

55–21. **d** (*p. 1234*) Cerebral Artery Thrombosis

55–22. **c** (*p. 1234*) Cerebral Artery Thrombosis

55–23. **a** (*p. 1234*) Cerebral Artery Thrombosis

55–24. **a** (*p. 1234*) Cerebral Embolism

55–25. **d** (*p. 1234*) Cerebral Venous Thrombosis

55–26. **c** (*p. 1235*) Subarachnoid Hemorrhage

55–27. **d** (*p. 1235*) Intracerebral Aneurysm

55–28. **b** (*p. 1235*) Arteriovenous Malformations

55–29. **a** (*p. 1236*) Multiple Sclerosis

55–30. **d** (*p. 1236*) Multiple Sclerosis

55–31. **c** (*p. 1237*) Multiple Sclerosis

55–32. **d** (*p. 1237*) Effects of Pregnancy

55–33. **d** (*p. 1237*) Myasthenia Gravis

55–34. **c** (*p. 1237*) Myasthenia Gravis

55–35. **d** (*p. 1238*) Effects of Pregnancy (Myasthenia)

55–36. **b** (*p. 1238*) Neonatal Effects

55–37. **b** (*p. 1238*) Guillain-Barre Syndrome

55–38. **c** (*p. 1238*) Guillain-Barre Syndrome

55–39. **a** (*p. 1239*) Bell Palsy

55–40. **d** (*p. 1239*) Effects of Pregnancy

55–41. **a** (*p. 1239*) Carpel Tunnel Syndrome

55–42. **d** (*p. 1239*) Spinal Cord Injury

55–43. **d** (*p. 1240*) Spinal Cord Injury

55–44. **d** (*p. 1240*) Spinal Cord Injury

55–45. **a** (*p. 1240*) Benign Intracranial Hypertension

55–46. **b** (*p. 1241*) Effects of Pregnancy

55–47. **a** (*p. 1241*) Effects of Pregnancy

55–48. **c** (*p. 1241*) Chorea Gravidarum

55–49. **d** (*p. 1241*) Adjustment to Pregnancy

55–50. **c** (*pp. 1242, 1243*) Major Depression/Effects of Pregnancy on Mental Illness/Postpartum Depression

55–51. **d** (*p. 1242*) Bipolar Disorder

55–52. **d** (*p. 1242*) Schizophrenia

55–53. **a** (*p. 1243*) Maternity Blues

55–54. **c** (*p. 1243*) Maternity Blues

55–55. **a** (*p. 1243*) Postpartum Depression

55–56. **b** (*p. 1243*) Postpartum Depression

55–57. **c** (*p. 1243*) Postpartum Depression

55–58. **c** (*p. 1243*) Postpartum Depression

55–59. **c** (*p. 1243*) Pregnancy Outcomes/Postpartum Depression

55–60. **d** (*p. 1243*) Postpartum Depression

55–61. **c** (*p. 1245*) Electroconvulsive Therapy (ECT)

CHAPTER 56

56–1. **d** (*p. 1250*) Hyperpigmentation

56–2. **d** (*p. 1250*) Hyperpigmentation

56–3. **c** (*p. 1250*) Hyperpigmentation

56–4. **c** (*p. 1250*) Hyperpigmentation

56–5. **c** (*p. 1250*) Hyperpigmentation

56–6. **c** (*p. 1250*) Hyperpigmentation

56–7. **d** (*p. 1250*) Nevi

56–8. **b** (*p. 1250*) Changes in Hair Growth

56–9. **a** (*p. 1251*) Vascular Changes

56–10. **b** (*p. 1251*) Vascular Changes

56–11. **a** (*p. 1251*) Pruritus Gravidarum

56–12. **b** (*p. 1251*) Pruritus Gravidarum

56–13. **a** (*p. 1251*) Pruritic Urticarial Papules & Plaques of Pregnancy

56–14. **d** (*p. 1251*) Pathophysiology

56–15. **d** (*p. 1251*) PUPPP

56–16. **a** (*p. 1253*) Prurigo of Pregnancy

56–17. **d** (*p. 1253*) Prurigo of Pregnancy

56–18. **b** (*p. 1253*) Herpes Gestationis

56–19. **a** (*p. 1253*) Herpes Gestationis

56–20. **b** (*p. 1253*) Etiopathogenesis

56–21. **c** (*p. 1253*) Etiopathogenesis

56–22. **b** (*p. 1254*) Treatment

56–23. **a** (*p. 1255*) Pruritic Folliculitis

56–24. **b** (*p. 1255*) Pruritic Folliculitis

56–25. **d** (*p. 1255*) Preexisting Skin Disease

CHAPTER 57

57–1. **b** (*p. 1258*) Neoplastic Disease

57–2. **d** (*p. 1258*) Neoplastic Disease

57–3. **c** (*p. 1258*) Surgery

57–4. **d** (*p. 1258*) Surgery

57–5. **c** (*p. 1258*) Radiation Therapy

57–6. **a** (*p. 1258*) Radiation Therapy

57–7. **a** (*p. 1258*) Effect on Pregnancy Outcome

57–8. **b** (*p. 1258*) Effect on Pregnancy Outcome

57–9. **d** (*p. 1259*) Effect on Pregnancy Outcome

57–10. **a** (*p. 1259*) Fertility & Pregnancy After
Cancer Treatment

57–11. **c** (*p. 1259*) Fertility & Pregnancy After
Cancer Treatment

57–12. **a** (*p. 1259*) Breast Carcinoma

57–13. **c** (*p. 1259*) Pregnancy & Breast Cancer

57–14. **c** (*p. 1259*) Pregnancy & Breast Cancer

57–15. **d** (*p. 1259*) Pregnancy & Breast Cancer

57–16. **d** (*p. 1260*) Diagnosis

57–17. **c** (*p. 1260*) Diagnosis

57–18. **b** (*p. 1260*) Diagnosis

57–19. **c** (*p. 1260*) Treatment

57–20. **a** (*p. 1261*) Pregnancy Following Breast
Cancer

57–21. **b** (*p. 1261*) Pregnancy Following Breast
Cancer

57–22. **c** (*p. 1261*) Hodgkin Disease

57–23. **a** (*p. 1261*) Pregnancy & Hodgkin Disease

57–24. **d** (*p. 1261*) Pregnancy & Hodgkin Disease

57–25. **a** (*p. 1261*) Pregnancy & Hodgkin Disease

57–26. **c** (*p. 1262*) Long-Term Prognosis

57–27. **b** (*p. 1262*) Long-Term Prognosis

57–28. **c** (*p. 1262*) Non-Hodgkin Lymphomas

57–29. **c** (*p. 1262*) Leukemias

57–30. **d** (*p. 1262*) Pregnancy & Leukemia

57–31. **a** (*pp. 1262, 1263*) Perinatal Outcome

57–32. **d** (*p. 1263*) Malignant Melanoma

57–33. **a** (*p. 1263*) Pregnancy & Melanoma

57–34. **b** (*p. 1263*) Pregnancy & Melanoma

57–35. **d** (*pp. 1264, 1265*) Intraepithelial Neoplasia

57–36. **a** (*p. 1265*) Intraepithelial Neoplasia

57–37. **a** (*p. 1265*) Intraepithelial Neoplasia

57–38. **d** (*p. 1265*) Intraepithelial Neoplasia

57–39. **c** (*p. 1265*) Invasive Cervical Cancer

57–40. **a** (*p. 1265*) Invasive Cervical Cancer

57–41. **a** (*p. 1267*) Prognosis

57–42. **d** (*p. 1268*) Colorectal Cancer

57–43. **d** (*p. 1268*) Renal Tumors

57–44. **a** (*p. 1264*) Table 57-3

CHAPTER 58

58–1. **a** (*p. 1276*) Fetal and Newborn Immunology

58–2. **c** (*p. 1276*) Fetal and Newborn Immunology

58–3. **d** (*p. 1276*) Varicella-Zoster

58–4. **a** (*p. 1276*) Prevention

58–5. **c** (*p. 1277*) Prevention

58–6. **b** (*p. 1277*) Fetal Effects

58–7. **b** (*p. 1277*) Fetal Effects

58–8. **c** (*p. 1277*) Fetal Effects

58–9. **a** (*p. 1277*) Prevention

58–10. **d** (*p. 1278*) Treatment

58–11. **a** (*p. 1278*) Fetal Effects (Influenza)

58–12. **a** (*p. 1278*) Mumps

58–13. **b** (*p. 1278*) Fetal Effects (Mumps)

58–14. **b** (*p. 1279*) Measles

58–15. **c** (*p. 1279*) Respiratory Viruses

58–16. **a** (*p. 1279*) Hantavirus

58–17. **d** (*p. 1279*) Coxsackie Virus

58–18. b (*p. 1279*) Parvovirus

58–19. c (*p. 1280*) Parvovirus

58–20. c (*p. 1280*) Fetal Effects

58–21. d (*p. 1280*) Prevention (Parvovirus)

58–22. b (*p. 1281*) Diagnosis

58–23. a (*p. 1282*) Congenital Rubella Syndrome

58–24. a (*p. 1282*) Congenital Rubella Syndrome

58–25. d (*p. 1282*) Maternal Infection

58–26. d (*p. 1283*) Congenital Infection

58–27. a (*p. 1283*) Prenatal Diagnosis

58–28. c (*p. 1283*) Treatment

58–29. b (*p. 1283*) Prevention

58–30. d (*p. 1284*) Group A Streptococcus

58–31. c (*p. 1284*) Group B Streptococcus

58–32. c (*p. 1285*) Group B Streptococcus

58–33. b (*p. 1285*) Neonatal Sepsis

58–34. b (*p. 1285*) Neonatal Sepsis

58–35. d (*p. 1285*) Recommended Prevention Strategies

58–36. b (*p. 1286*) Recommended Prevention Strategies

58–37. b (*p. 1287*) Listeriosis

58–38. c (*p. 1288*) Listeriosis

58–39. a (*p. 1288*) Listeriosis

58–40. d (*p. 1288*) Treatment

58–41. b (*p. 1288*) Salmonellosis

58–42. c (*p. 1288*) Salmonellosis

58–43. d (*p. 1288*) Shigellosis

58–44. c (*p. 1289*) Lyme Disease

58–45. a (*p. 1289*) Treatment

58–46. c (*p. 1289*) Lyme Disease

58–47. a (*p. 1289*) Prevention

58–48. d (*p. 1289*) Toxoplasmosis

58–49. c (*p. 1290*) Toxoplasmosis

58–50. d (*p. 1290*) Toxoplasmosis

58–51. d (*p. 1290*) Treatment

58–52. c (*p. 1291*) Prevention

58–53. b (*p. 1291*) Effects on Pregnancy

58–54. b (*p. 1291*) Prophylaxis

58–55. c (*p. 1292*) West Nile Virus

58–56. a (*p. 1292*) West Nile Virus

58–57. d (*p. 1292*) Severe Acute Respiratory Syndrome

58–58. b (*p. 1292*) Severe Acute Respiratory Syndrome

58–59. a (*p. 1293*) Methicillin-Resistant Staph Aureus

58–60. b (*p. 1293*) Smallpox

58–61. c (*p. 1294*) Anthrax

CHAPTER 59

59–1. c (*p. 1302*) Syphilis

59–2. d (*p. 1302*) Syphilis

59–3. d (*p. 1302*) Syphilis

59–4. d (*p. 1302*) Fetal and Neonatal Infections

59–5. d (*p. 1302*) Pathology

59–6. a (*p. 1303*) Serological Diagnosis

59–7. a (*p. 1303*) Serological Diagnosis

59–8. c (*p. 1303*) Fetal Diagnosis

59–9. b (*p. 1303*) Fetal Diagnosis

59–10. d (*p. 1304*) Treatment

59–11. d (*p. 1304*) Treatment

59–12. c (*p. 1304*) Table 59-1

59–13. d (*p. 1304*) Treatment

59–14. b (*p. 1304*) Treatment

59–15. c (*p. 1304*) Treatment

59–16. d (*p. 1304*) Lumbar Puncture

59–17. a (*p. 1305*) Treatment of Congenital Syphilis

59–18. d (*p. 1305*) Gonorrhea

59–19. a (*p. 1305*) Gonorrhea

59–20. a (*p. 1305*) Treatment

59–21. d (*p. 1305*) Treatment

59–22. a (*p. 1305*) Disseminated Gonococcal Infections

59–23. c (*p. 1306*) Chlamydial Infections

59–24. d (*p. 1306*) Maternal Infections

59–25. a (*p. 1306*) Symptomatic Infection

59–26. b (*p. 1306*) Neonatal Infections

59–27. c (*p. 1306*) Neonatal Infections

59–28. b (*p. 1306*) Pneumonitis

59–29. c (*p. 1307*) Treatment

59–30. d (*p. 1307*) Treatment

59–31. a (*p. 1307*) Lymphogranuloma Venereum

59–32. a (*p. 1307*) Virology

59–33. d (*p. 1308*) Antibodies

59–34. a (*p. 1308*) Primary Infection

59–35. c (*p. 1308*) Primary Infection

59–36. a (*p. 1309*) Diagnosis

59–37. b (*p. 1309*) Viral Shedding at Delivery

59–38. c (*p. 1309*) Fetal and Neonatal Disease

59–39. d (*p. 1310*) Fetal and Neonatal Disease

59–40. a (*p. 1310*) Fetal and Neonatal Disease

59–41. b (*p. 1310*) Fetal and Neonatal Disease

59–42. b (*p. 1310*) Fetal and Neonatal Disease

59–43. b (*p. 1311*) HIV Infection

59–44. d (*p. 1311*) Etiology

59–45. c (*p. 1311*) Etiology

59–46. c (*p. 1311*) Clinical Manifestations

59–47. c (*p. 1312*) Clinical Manifestations

59–48. b (*p. 1312*) Serological Testing

59–49. b (*p. 1312*) Serological Testing

59–50. d (*p. 1312*) Screening

59–51. d (*p. 1317*) Prevention of Vertical Transmission

59–52. b (*p. 1312*) Maternal and Fetal-Neonatal Infection

59–53. d (*p. 1312*) Maternal and Fetal-Neonatal Infection

59–54. a (*p. 1316*) Management During Pregnancy

59–55. a (*p. 1316*) Prevention of Vertical Transmission

59–56. b (*p. 1317*) Prevention of Vertical Transmission

59–57. a (*p. 1317*) Breast Feeding

59–58. b (*p. 1317*) Human Papillomavirus

59–59. c (*p. 1318*) Treatment

59–60. a (*p. 1318*) Neonatal Infection

59–61. b (*p. 1319*) Chancroid

59–62. c (*p. 1319*) Chancroid

59–63. c (*p. 1319*) Trichomoniasis

59–64. d (*p. 1319*) Treatment

Index

The numbers following each entry indicate chapter and question numbers.